Sounds, Structures and Senses

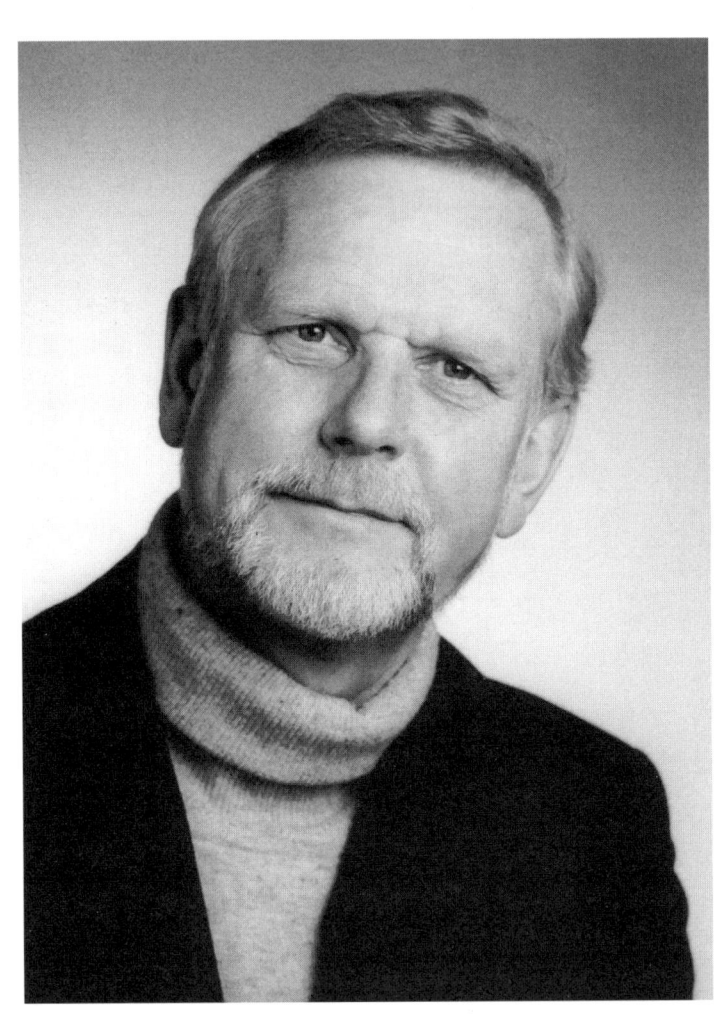

Sounds, Structures and Senses

Essays Presented to Niels Davidsen-Nielsen
on the Occasion of his Sixtieth Birthday

Edited by Carl Bache and Alex Klinge

Odense University Press

This book has been published with the generous financial support
of the Copenhagen Business School

© The Authors and Odense University Press 1997
Printed in Denmark by Special-Trykkeriet Viborg a-s
Cover by Designco
ISBN 87-7838-307-2

Odense University Press
Campusvej 55
DK-5230 Odense M

Tel. +45 66 15 79 99
Fax. +45 66 15 81 26
E-mail: Press@forlag.ou.dk
www-location: http://www.ou.dk/press

Contents

Carl Bache: Another Look at the Order of Premodifying Adjectives in English 9

John M. Dienhart: A Linguistic Analysis of Archibald MacLeish's *Ars Poetica* 29

Per Durst-Andersen: The English Progessive 55

Dorrit Faber and Finn Sørensen: Remarks on *if*, *when* and *where* 71

Peter Harder: Futurity in English: A Case for Messy Structure 79

Michael Herslund: Predication and the Nominal Clause 95

Bente Lihn Jensen: On the Use of Mood and Modal Verbs in Italian and Danish 109

Per Anker Jensen: On the Semantics of Agentive *af* in Danish 127

Stig Johansson and Berit Løken: Some Norwegian Discourse Particles and their English Correspondences 149

Alex Klinge: Modality and Morphology: The Case of *-able* 171

Fritz Larsen: The Danish and English Sound Systems: Complications of a Contrastive Analysis 189

Hans F. Nielsen: The Appeal of Otto Jespersen's *Growth and Structure of the English Language* 205

Bent Preisler: Tendencies in the Syntax of the Verb in American and British English 215

Torben Thrane: Understanding Semantics 235

Torben Vestergaard: 'Free Adjuncts' in English 251

Carl Vikner and Sten Vikner: The Aspectual Complexity of the Simple Past
   in English. A Comparison with French and Danish 267

List of contributors with their affiliation... 285

Foreword

A tradition has developed in the academic world by which birthdays and anniversaries of scholars of eminence prompt former students and fellow scholars to join together in celebrating a mentor and colleague. The celebration takes the form of a dedicated publication which affords contributors the opportunity to reflect on, respond to and honour a significant scholarly achievement. Such are also the circumstances which have brought together the linguists who contribute to this Festschrift for Professor Niels Davidsen-Nielsen on the occasion of his sixtieth birthday.

However, the motivation underlying the present Festschrift goes beyond the bounds of tradition. The scope of the contributions bears testimony to the depth and diversity of academic affiliations and friendships Niels Davidsen-Nielsen has established throughout his career. His immediate points of academic contact have been as a lecturer at the University of Copenhagen, as an external lecturer at the University of Odense and, since 1985, as a professor in the English Department of the Copenhagen Business School. His research interests have resulted in numerous guest lectures in Denmark and abroad and have taken him on sabbaticals overseas, and in recent years to Lancaster and Cambridge. Thematically his work and interests have spanned phonology, phonetics and several aspects of contrastive grammar, where the categories of the verb phrase have been the focus of his attention. In the process of capturing intricate aspects of grammar, he has contributed to a better understanding not only of English but also of Danish, most significantly in the domain of modality and the modal auxiliaries, and in connection with discourse particles. His preoccupation in the past few years has been with co-authoring a comprehensive grammar of English addressing the needs of both research colleagues and advanced students.

Niels Davidsen-Nielsen is a highly effective communicator in both his oral and his written presentations. To the benefit of students and colleagues alike, readability and accessibility are hallmarks of his publications. Within the past twenty years generations of Danish and Norwegian students of English have found their way into English phonetics via his textbook *Engelsk udtale i hovedtræk*, currently available in a revised translation of the second edition as *An Outline of English Pronunciation* (see the contribution by Fritz Larsen below for further remarks). Indeed his concern for the communicability of complex linguistic issues has ensured that he remains an always popular lecturer who takes a genuine interest in the trials and tribulations of his students.

All who have collaborated with Niels Davidsen-Nielsen in matters of research or teaching will have appreciated the high degree of conscientiousness which he brings to his work. Coupled with his dedication and wit, this always makes it a delight to work with him. We are confident that as editors we speak on behalf of contributors, colleagues and students when we say that we look forward to many more years of cooperation and inspiration.

Carl Bache & Alex Klinge

Another Look at the Order of Premodifying Adjectives in English

Carl Bache

1. Introduction

In this paper[1] I offer a description of the order of premodifying adjectives in English. This topic has already received a great deal of attention in Bache 1978. But, while some of my suggestions there certainly seem to have influenced later descriptions of adjective order (cf. e.g. Quirk et al. 1985, Vestergaard 1993), the essentially *functional* approach that I developed on the basis of Teyssier 1968 has been largely ignored. In what follows, I want to explore the functional element of adjective order and integrate it in what I shall refer to as 'the functional domain' of noun groups. At the same time, the paper gives an overview of positions which are more independent of functional considerations.

2. Preliminaries

Let me begin by clarifying some of the terminological conventions and theoretical assumptions on which the description is based. First of all, it is important to note that I operate with a rigid form/function distinction in the syntactic analysis of sentences. Thus, for example, the adjective *fine* in *a fine achievement* is not only an adjective (form) but also a dependent (function) in relation to the head noun *achievement* (head = function, noun = form); for introductions to the full system, see Bache et al. 1993, Bache 1996, Bache & Davidsen-Nielsen *in press*, chapter 3. The terms 'nominal' and 'adjectival' are general *form* terms covering both groups (noun groups, adjective groups) and single words with head potential in groups (nouns, adjectives).

For the description of major form types it is convenient to operate not just with their syntactic function in relation to other constituents but also with their *functional domain*. The functional domain of a constituent type is its communicative function at its most general. The reason for calling it a 'functional domain' (rather than simply a '(main) function') is that this term has associations of something spacious

---

[1] The data and analyses presented here appear in a short Danish version in Bache 1997 and are integrated in a more comprehensive presentation of noun groups and adjective groups in Bache & Davidsen-Nielsen *in press*, especially chapters 10 and 12. I would like to thank John Dienhart, Niels Davidsen-Nielsen, Peter Harder, Leo Hoye, Alex Klinge, Fritz Larsen, Jens Nørgård-Sørensen and Christian Heyde Petersen for useful comments on earlier drafts and presentations.

and thus invites a description of internal structure and complexity: a functional domain is typically very composite, involving many different, interacting lower-level functions. As we shall see, an important subfunction in the functional domain of nominals is *modification*. This subfunction is typically but not exclusively realized by premodifying adjectives. It is in fact appropriate to say that modification itself is a functional domain of premodifying adjectives – a domain with its own subfunctions. The aim of the present paper is to show that the functional domain of modification is structured subfunctionally in a way that often determines the order of premodifying adjectives (and thus has clear syntactic repercussions). I shall also argue that the proposed internal structure of modification is non-random in the larger functional context of nominals, as described in Bache & Davidsen-Nielsen *in press*.

3. The functional domain of nominals

The functional domain of nominals can be defined in traditional terms as the expression of meaning as 'entities' (concrete or abstract, personal or nonpersonal, etc.). Nominals enable us to code what we want to talk about as entities with the degree of specificity required for our communicative purposes: speakers encode meaning in nominals in the shape of entities and listeners decode such constituents accordingly. Nominals are used for a variety of more specific communicative functions, such as to *refer* to entities:

(1)   *The restaurant* was crowded.

(2)   *The bastards* won't get away with it.

or to *mention* 'type of entity':

(3)   I told her I wanted *an apple*.

(4)   *Teachers who work overtime* must be very idealistic.

or to *describe* an already established referent:

(5)   Most of the diners were *Japanese tourists*.

(6)   Rose is a *very good student*.

or to *specify* the 'situation' expressed by the verb in examples of syntactic and semantic fusion between predicator and object (cf. Bache & Davidsen-Nielsen *in press*, section 7.3.4. [I]):

(7)   The meeting *took place* yesterday. (*took place* = 'happened')

(8)   We *caught sight of* her. (*caught sight of* = 'saw', 'sighted')

For the expression of entities, nominals rely on cognitively loaded lexical material (such as the head noun) as well as interactive elements (such as determiners), both contributing to a set of contrasts, some of which are context-dependent, others more context-independent. To describe the resulting delimitation (or 'singling out') of (types) of entities, I use the term 'contrast-formation': nominals provide a set of *contrasts*, lexical as well as morphological and syntactic, with which to discriminate between entities. Roughly, contrast-formation seems to work as follows. By using the definite article in a nominal like *the small yellow key*, the speaker signals that there will be enough information in the nominal for the listener to construe the referent as unique in the context. There is thus an abstract but highly context-dependent contrast between unique and non-unique. This interactively derived contrast is combined with three lexical contrasts, the first two of which are provided by the adjectives *small* and *yellow*. The meanings denoted by these ('smallness' and 'yellowness') must be considered in relation to the third and more context-independent contrast, the one provided by the head noun *key*. The particular combination of various contrasts evoked by *the small yellow key* enables the listener to delimit the entity intended by the speaker.

There is often more contrast-formation in nominals than we actually need in order to identify the intended referent in a particular context. For example, in a construction like:

(9)   Have you met *my beautiful wife* yet?

we cannot say that the adjective *beautiful* is criterial for establishing who the referent of the construction *my beautiful wife* is, unless of course the speaker has more than one wife and only one of them is beautiful. Instead it simply offers a description of the referent. Though this description clearly involves a (subjective) contrast (beautiful versus non-beautiful entities), this contrast is, strictly speaking, redundant from the point of view of establishing the referent: an expression like *my wife* will usually do the job with sufficient precision. In general, whether or not contrast-formation is redundant (from the point of view of establishing the referent of a construction) may depend entirely on the context of the utterance. Consider:

(10)   *The unhappy mother* left at once.

If the context is such that there is only one mother present, the adjective *unhappy* is 'merely' intended as a description of that mother: it could be left out without making the noun group referentially unclear. If the context is such that there are several mothers present but only one of them is unhappy, *unhappy* provides information without which the listener cannot establish which mother left: without the adjective the noun group becomes referentially unclear (by implying that there is only one mother in the context) and is thus likely to confuse the listener if he or she knows that there is more than one mother in the context. For the listener, the communicative status of the contrast provided by *unhappy* as either descriptive elaboration or identificatory clue must be worked out in context.

We may accordingly distinguish between *restrictive* and *non-restrictive* contrast-formation. This distinction is a fundamental, but also very general, subfunction of the functional domain of noun groups. The chart below provides a first approximation to our description of the relationship between functional domain (shaded cells) and internal syntactic structure (white cells) ('pre-H' stands for pre-head dependents, 'H' for the nominal head, 'post-H' for post-head dependents):

expression of meaning as entities		
contrast-formation: restrictive/non-restrictive		
pre-H	H	post-H

As yet, the constituents of the noun group are not individually and separately related to specific subfunctions. However, such relationships can, and will shortly, be established. Note also that in a construction like *the small, yellow key* I consider the noun rather than the definite article to be the head of the construction. One important reason why the definite article is sometimes viewed as the head is that it anchors the construction in communicative interaction and thus in a sense governs the construction within the context of specific communicative interaction (cf. e.g. Heltoft 1996). However, if I am right in assuming that the functional domain of nominals at its most general is indeed 'expression of entities', the specific function of an expression in communication presupposes the cognitive element underpinning the lexical choice of a noun, if only as a potential to be realized. Using Harder's terminology (cf. Harder 1995: 276ff), I choose the noun as head for its *operand* status in the nominal rather than the article, which has *operator* status. An operation – an instance of communication – certainly always requires an *operator* but it just as clearly presupposes an *operand*: what the operator does may vary from one instance of communication to another but the operand is a constant, a meaning potential to be operated on.

One factor contributing to pre-head complexity is the distinction between two communicative subfunctions of the functional domain of nominals: *determination* and *modification*. These two subfunctions, as realized by pre-head dependents, can be thought of in terms of *zones* in the noun group arranged more specifically in the following canonical order:

determination	modification	H	post-H dependents

Determination is realized by articles, pronouns and genitive constructions, while modification is chiefly realized by adjectives, as in the following examples:

determination	modification	H	post-H dependents
the	little	girl	with the shy smile
an	old	friend	from London
this	very dull	visit	to her parents
no	additional	staffing,	academic or secretarial,
any	delicious	dessert	that you can think of
my	best	student,	who left school early,
what a	hearty, cheerful	talk	we had the other day
the	sudden	death	of my father
my neighbour's	thick fibrous	clothes	from Woolworth's

In all these examples, the head noun is both determined and modified by pre-head dependents. Determination is, strictly speaking, a cover term for a number of more specific operator meanings, such as *definiteness* (as expressed by the definite article *the*, the possessive pronoun *my*, the demonstrative pronoun *this* and the genitive noun group *my neighbour's*) and *indefiniteness* (as expressed by the indefinite article *an* and the indefinite pronoun *any*). As we shall see, modification is also a cover term for a number of more specific meanings.

The communicative task performed by the head of a noun group is to provide a close lexical match for the entity that the speaker has in mind. The head normally represents the entity as a member of a *category* of things, persons, etc., or as a type. For example, the function of the head noun *girl* in *the little girl with the shy smile* is to categorize the person expressed *as a girl* (rather than as a woman, a boy or a man, etc.). The nucleus in the functional domain of nominals is thus *categorization*:

determination	modification	categorization	post-H dependents

Since the main focus in this paper is on pre-H dependents, I simply note in passing that post-head dependents are used for a variety of communicative functions, e.g. modification (as in *the little girl with the shy smile*) and complementation (as in *the visit to her parents*). We shall therefore simply operate with one post-head *multifunctional* zone. Note also that the important subfunction of *quantification* potentially affects all parts of a noun group and combines with elements realizing other subfunctions (cf. *these books / a short meeting / numerous girlfriends / whiskey in large quantities*).

The following chart summarizes our discussion so far of the functional domain of nominals:

expression of meaning as entities				
contrast-formation: restrictive/non-restrictive				
quantification				
determination	modification	categorization	(multi-functional)

As this chart shows, nominals are used to express entities. The primary, but also most general means of serving this functional domain is contrast-formation (restrictive/non-restrictive). The functional domain is fragmented into contributing subfunctions, some of which are closely associated with certain syntactic zones within the structure of the noun group. Communicative interaction often requires an interplay of contrast-formation, determination, modification, categorization, complementation and quantification.

4. The functional domain of adjectivals

Adjectivals are typically used to express properties in relation to entities (for more detailed discussion, see e.g. Ferris 1993). This functional domain is realized on different syntactic levels, depending on the speaker's communicative intention. As subject and object complements, they denote an ATTRIBUTE or a RESULT, e.g. *The children were unhappy / She got pretty mad at me / Tyson knocked Bruno unconscious* (cf. Bache & Davidsen-Nielsen *in press*, section 7.3.4). In such cases the assignment of a property to an entity is the primary communicative purpose of the sentence. As dependents, adjectivals serve a secondary communicative role, as in e.g. *The happy children returned to the kindergarten*, which primarily reports on the situation of 'returning', with *happy* merely describing one of the two participants of this situation. But the function of such adjectivals is basically the same: to assign a property. In this paper I am going to look more closely at the functional domain of adjectivals serving as premodifying dependents.

Premodifying adjectivals can be defined broadly as constituents appearing between central determiner position and head noun, e.g.:

(1)   the *same* approach   the *interesting* novel
      these *two* problems   a *sleeping* child
      numerous solutions   his *black* hat
      the *first* chapter   her *French* husband
      my *only* consolation   an *historical* account
      your *own* house   a *medical* dictionary
      her *major* spending empire   the *human* nervous system
      a *specific* theory   a *fugitive* heiress
      a *beautiful* garden   *solar* energy
      a *very happy* child   the woman's *silver* ring
      a *well-known* colour movie   the *paratrooper* battalions
      that *small* green-house   etc.

The price we pay for operating with such a broad class is its heterogeneity. One way of dealing with this heterogeneity is to describe the class in prototype terms as consisting of *central* and *peripheral* members (cf. e.g. Crystal 1967, Coates 1971, Huddleston 1984, 1988, Greenbaum & Quirk 1990). Central adjectives, unlike peripheral adjectives, allow modification by degree adverbs (like VERY and EXTREMELY), comparison and predicative use; compare:

(2)   HAPPY: a happy child   a very happy child
                                              a happier child
                                              the child was happy

(3)   SOLAR: this solar energy   *this very solar energy
                                              *this more solar energy
                                              *this energy was solar

Semantically, central adjectives *describe* the entity expressed by the head noun and are therefore called *descriptive adjectives*. In the list in (1) above, *beautiful, small, well-known* and *interesting* are clear examples of descriptive adjectives.

There are two main types of peripheral adjective: *classifying* adjectives and *specifying* adjectives. Classifying adjectives *subcategorize* the head they modify. For example, a *medical dictionary* is a special kind of dictionary and *solar energy* is a special kind of energy. Classifying adjectives narrow down the potential referents of the head and thus help establish precisely what sort of entity is involved in the expression. In the list in (1), *French, historical* and *human* are other clear examples of classifying adjectives.

Specifying adjectives help *single out* or *quantify* the referent of the construction in relation to some context. For example, in *the same approach* and *my former colleague*, the specifying adjectives *same* and *former* have determiner-like properties. In the list in (1), *first*, *only*, *numerous*, *two* and *own* are other clear examples of specifying adjectives.

It is important to note that the division of adjectives into descriptive, classifying and specifying adjectives is function-based: an adjective cannot be identified unambiguously as one or the other in isolation. In each case the relationship between the adjective and the head noun in a particular noun group must be carefully examined and interpreted. Rather than speaking of three subclasses of adjectives, it is therefore more appropriate to operate with three *subfunctions* of modification which adjectives may assume in relation to a noun: specification, description or classification. This approach, which circumvents the 'circularity' problem in connection with traditional order classes (for discussion, see Annear 1964, Martin 1968, Oller & Sales 1969 and Bache 1978), is supported by such data as:

CIVIL:	*civil reply*	(description)
	civil rights	(classification)
BLACK:	*black cloud*	(description)
	black coffee	(classification)
PRIMARY:	*my primary concern*	(specification)
	this primary election	(classification)
WILD:	*a wild party*	(description)
	Australian wild birds	(classification)
DANISH:	*Danish cheese*	(classification)
	a very Danish approach	(description)
SECRET	*a secret plan*	(description)
	the Polish secret service	(classification)
WOODEN:	*wooden bed*	(classification)
	wooden methods	(description)
ONLY:	*an only child*	(classification)
	the only child	(specification)
etc.		

In these constructions, one and the same adjective functions in two of the three different ways depending on how it relates to the head noun.

The three subfunctions of modification: specification, description and classification, are arranged in different syntactic zones. In other words, they impose a certain positional order on attributive pre-head adjectives: when two or more such premodifying adjectives appear together in a noun group, specifying adjectives precede descriptive adjectives, which in turn precede classifying adjectives, as shown in the table below. To emphasize the positional characteristics of the three subfunctions, we refer to specification as Mod. I (= 'modificational zone I'), description as Mod. II and classification as Mod. III. Each of these zones may accommodate zero, one or more than one adjective.

Determination	Modification			Categorization
	Specification (Mod. I)	Description (Mod. II)	Classification (Mod. III)	
the	usual	sound	English	stock
her	own	handsome	naval	officer
the	same	beautiful	French	actress
the	next	interesting	congressional	procedure
	certain	serious	organic	diseases
the	last	mighty	German	attack
the	earliest	important	Aboriginal	carvings
	many	eager	medical	students
this	particular	informal	linguistic	rule
	other	horrid	psychological	tricks

In strings of premodifying adjectives belonging to different Mod. zones, it appears that those adjectives which are closest in function to determination, viz. specifying adjectives, are placed closest to the determiner and those adjectives which are closest in function to categorization, viz. classifying adjectives, are placed closest to the head of the noun group. This means that there is no strict separation between determination, modification and categorization but rather a continuum of functional values from determination to categorization: from the left determination fades into modification via specification and from the right categorization fades into modification via classification. In the middle we have modification at its purest: description. The term 'central adjective' (which was replaced by 'descriptive adjective' above) thus acquires new functional and syntactic significance: a central adjective appears in central position in the modificational zone and is functionally pure (i.e. left untainted by determination and categorization).

We thus claim that adjective order is first and foremost a question of the functional characteristics of adjectives in relation to the head noun. It follows that the same adjective may appear in different positions depending on its subfunction. That this is indeed the case is shown in the following data:

(4a)	Scottish *popular* ballads	(III + III)
(4b)	*popular* Scottish ballads	(II + III)
(5a)	the *first* brilliant chapter	(I + II)
(5b)	the brilliant *first* chapter	(II + III)
(6a)	the antique *occasional* table	(III + III)
(6b)	the *occasional* antique table	(I + III)
(7a)	this *good* international turn	(II + III)
(7b)	this international *good* turn	(III + III)
(8a)	English *dirty* books	(III + III)
(5b)	*dirty* English books	(II + III)

In each of these constructions, the italicized adjective changes its modificational subfunction in relation to the noun (e.g. *popular*, which subclassifies *ballads* with respect to genre in (4a) and simply describes it in (4b) – I leave it to the reader to work out the interpretations of the other examples).

5. Inherent Mod. I, Mod. II and Mod. III adjectives

Despite the fact that we have characterized specifying, descriptive and classifying adjectives in functional terms rather than as subclasses of adjectives seen in isolation, it is convenient to regard adjectives as *inherent* Mod. I, Mod. II or Mod. III adjectives, according to their typical usage. Thus, for example, GOOD, DIRTY and BRILLIANT are inherent Mod. II adjectives, ENGLISH, INTERNATIONAL and MEDICAL are inherent Mod. III adjectives, and SAME, FIRST and OTHER are inherent Mod. I adjectives. The point of treating adjectives as inherent members of Mod. zones is to be able to offer a description of some of the mechanisms in English for affecting the subfunction of an adjective.

One effective way of changing an inherent Mod. II or Mod. III adjective to a Mod. I adjective is to give it contrastive stress (indicated by capitals):

(1)   I'm taking about the BIG girl not the SMALL one.

As the specifying force of the adjectives is made clear by prosodic means, it is possible to keep the normal positional order of the unstressed, classifying adjective rather than the one associated with the derived, specifying function:

(2a)   I'm talking about the good yellow chair. (II + III)

(2b)   I'm talking about the good YELLOW chair. (II + I)

But in some cases, the order is made to conform with the derived function (cf. Martin 1968: 37ff):

(2c)   I'm talking about the YELLOW good chair. (I + II)

Another way of changing inherent Mod. II adjectives, which are typically gradable (cf. section 4 above), to Mod. I adjectives is to subject them to comparison:

(3)   The *smarter* kids quickly learned how to avoid grounding.

This too may affect the positional order, compare:

(4)   The other great achievement was to beat Celtic. (I + II)
(5)   The *greatest* other achievement was to beat Celtic. (I + I)

Inherent Mod. I and Mod. II adjectives are sometimes changed to Mod. III adjectives by being placed immediately before the head noun, i.e. after any other adjective:

(6)   the intersting *first* chapter
      (cf. the first intersting chapter)

(7)   this international good turn
      (cf. this good international turn)

Even one of the inherent determiners, the genitive, sometimes occupies this position (the so-called *classifying genitive*) and thus becomes a Mod. III adjective:

(8)   artificial silk *women's* underwear
(9)   a standard tourist's guide
(10) some black *Indian's* hair

Inherent Mod. III adjectives are occasionally changed to Mod. II adjectives by means of adverbs of degree superimposing gradability on the originally classifying meaning of the adjective:

(11) That was a *very English* remark.
(12) He gave a *fairly political* lecture.

Using these techniques of varying the modificational subfunction of adjectives, including positional order, we can offer examples in which the same adjective functions in three different ways:

(13a) the *BLACK* new car   (*I* + II)
(13b) a small, thin, *very black* figure   (II + II + *II*)
(13c) strong, sweet *black* coffee   (II + II + *III*)
(14a) the *more popular* Scottish ballads   (*I* + III)
(14b) *popular* Scottish ballads   (*II* + III)
(14c) Scottish *popular* ballads   (III + *III*)

Many adjectives are of course functionally more restricted than BLACK and POPULAR.

6. Structure in and across Mod. zones

There is often more than one adjective in the same Mod. zone:

(1a)	the first few primaries	(I + I)
(1b)	the greatest subsequent numbers	(I + I)
(1c)	the only other solution	(I + I)
(2a)	a new, strange way	(II + II)
(2b)	the sweet warm stale air	(II + II + II)
(2c)	a healthy and virtuous girl	(II + II)
(3a)	one Republican congressional leader	(III + III)
(3b)	classical Greek drama	(III + III)
(3c)	tactical nuclear weapons	(III + III)

If one wants to ascertain that the analysis of strings of non-central adjectives (such as (1a) to (1c) and (3a) to (3c)) is correct, one can always try inserting an inherent Mod. II adjective (such as e.g. INTERESTING or INFLUENTIAL): if the original adjectives are to the left of the inherent Mod. II adjective in its most appropriate position, they are Mod. I adjectives (as in *the first few interesting primaries*); if the original adjectives are to the right of the inherent Mod. II adjective, they are Mod. III adjectives (as in *one influential Republican congressional leader*); and if the inherent Mod. II adjective squeezes in between the original adjectives, we have a Mod. I and a Mod. III adjective (as in e.g. *the only interesting Greek drama*).

Adjectives in Mod. I, in Mod. III and in combinations of Mod. I, Mod. II and Mod. III are *hypotactically* related, while adjectives in Mod. II are paratactically related. In Mod. II, many adjectives are separated by comma and/or conjunction (cf. (2a) and (2c) above). If they are not, it is always possible to separate them by such means without changing the meaning of the construction:

(4) the sweet warm stale air
   = the sweet, warm, stale air
   = the sweet, warm and stale air

Furthermore, in many strings of Mod. II adjectives, the order can be reversed with little or no semantic change:

(5) its dark soft eyes
   = its soft dark eyes

(6) a new, strange way
   = a strange, new way

(7) equally mindless and vicious types
   = equally vicious and mindless types

By contrast, within Mod. I or Mod. III, adjectives are not separated by comma and/or conjunction except to express *alternative specification* (in Mod. I) or *alternative classification* (in Mod. III):

(8) the third and smallest class
≠ the third smallest class

(9) white, Protestant women
≠ white Protestant women

In *the third and smallest class*, the class referred to could be specified precisely enough by *third* alone or by *smallest* alone. The construction thus provides alternative specification of the third class but, in addition, we get the information that the third class is also the smallest class. By contrast, in the unbroken sequence *the third smallest class*, there is complex, progressive specification. In the broken sequence *white, Protestant women*, the head noun *women* is subclassified separately and individually by *white* and *Protestant*. The two ways of classifying *women* are viewed as parallel, *Protestant* being an alternative to *white*. The implication is 'if white, then Protestant'. By contrast, in the unbroken sequence *white Protestant women*, there is complex, regressive classification: *Protestant* classifies *women*, and *white* subclassifies *Protestant women*.

Separation of adjectives is carried one step further in cases where parenthetical adjectival insertions elaborate or rephrase a preceding adjective:

(10) a less central, or peripheral, position

(11) purely abstract, but in some sense objective, entities

(12) a further, and much more complex, question

Adjectives from different Mod. zones are not normally separated:

(13) an interesting economic strategy   (II + III)

(14) the same beautiful girl   (I + II)

(15) the first medical dictionary   (I + III)

When separation does occur, it is usually semantically significant, as in the following examples:

(16a) a second context-sensitive rule   (I + III)

(16b) a second, context-sensitive rule

(17a) the helpful local dealers   (II + III)

(17b) the helpful, local dealers

Here (16b) and (17b) with the broken sequences differ in meaning from (16a) and (17a) with the unbroken sequences. (16a), unlike (16b), implies the existence of a 'first context-sensitive rule'. In (17a) *helpful* restrictively or non-restrictively describes *local dealers*, while in (17b) the description provided by *helpful* and the classification provided by *local* are viewed as separate, parallel properties of *dealers*, with the implication that there is some notional relationship between them.

7. Zone-internal order

In this section we shall comment on the internal order in each Mod. zone:

A) Mod. I: In this zone we can distinguish four major groups of adjectivals which prove reasonably order sensitive:

(i) precise and fuzzy ordinal numbers, like FIRST, SECOND, SEVENTH, NEXT, FINAL, etc.

(ii) precise and fuzzy cardinal numbers, like TWO, FOUR, FEW, MANY, COUNTLESS, NUMEROUS, etc.

(iii) compared forms like *older, smaller, better-known, finest, most beautiful*, etc.

(iv) others, like ONLY, OWN, SAME, OTHER, SUBSEQUENT, FORMER, MAJOR, SIMILAR, DIFFERENT, MAIN, CHIEF, GENERAL, SPECIFIC, PRIMARY, CERTAIN, etc.

A string of two or more Mod. I adjectives provides increasing specification. There is a *tendency* for the adjectives in the four groups to appear in the order in which they have just been presented, i.e. 'ordinals *before* cardinals *before* compared forms *before* others':

(1)   the first five primaries
(2)   the two major categories
(3)   six smaller children
(4)   the greatest subsequent importance

It is important to note, however, that some Mod. I adjectives may contract more closely with the definite article for the expression of definite specific reference, in which case they precede other Mod. I adjectives, irrespective of their membership of the four groups presented above:

(5)   the same particular phenomena
(6)   the other six more positive roles
      (cf. *the six other more positive roles*)
(7)   the only two utterances
      (cf. *the two only utterances*)
(8)   the most beautiful two young ladies
      (cf. *the two most beautiful young ladies*)

Not surprisingly, therefore, positional order is occasionally dependent on the presence or absence of the definite article, compare:

(9a)   three other Nixon associates
(9b)   *other three Nixon associates
(9c)   the other three Nixon associates

B) Mod. II: In this paratactic, descriptive zone there are few hard and fast rules for adjective order. Often, as we have seen (cf. section 6), the order seems random and can be reversed with little or no change of meaning (e.g. *a harsh thin light* versus *a thin harsh light*). There are, however, certain *tendencies* or *preferences*:

(i) short adjectives tend to precede long adjectives (therefore underived adjectives typically precede derived adjectives):

(10)   a deep quiet sleep
(11)   a charming, hard-working child
(12)   a loud booming voice
(13)   a slight disdainful smile

(ii) deverbal adjectives tend to precede denominal adjectives:

(14)   undulating hilly slopes
(15)   predictable wishful distortions
(16)   quivering dusky maidens
(17)   prolonged painful squeal

(iii) adjectives denoting size, length and height tend to precede other Mod. II adjectives:

(18)   that big, tough guy
(19)   large, warm eyes
(20)   a tall, thin creature
(21)   long blank periods

(iv) adjectives denoting size, length and height tend to appear in just that order:

(22)   big, long things
(23)   big, high cheek bones
(24)   long, low sheds
(25)   Long Tall Sally (the title of a Beatles song)

(v) emotionally loaded adjectives like BEAUTIFUL, WONDERFUL, LOVELY, HORRIBLE, DREADFUL, NASTY, etc. tend to precede other Mod. II adjectives, even those denoting size, height and length:

(26) the beautiful creamy paper
(27) lovely soft hands
(28) a horrible ghoulish enjoyment
(29) a nasty cold wind
(30) a fine big fellow
(31) a terrible small room

Note in this connection that emotionally loaded adjectives occasionally enter a close relation to the following adjective and assume an almost adverb-like status:

(32) a great big dog
 (= 'a very big dog')
(33) a tiny little tumour
 (= 'a very little tumour')
(34) an awful long trip
 (= 'a very long trip')

It is important, finally, to emphasize the fact that adjective order in Mod. II is extremely variable and cannot be captured by any strict rules.

C) Mod. III: In this zone hypotaxis prevails, each adjective (sub)classifying the following adjective(s) and the head noun. Like the order in Mod. I, the order in Mod. III is relatively fixed. When variation does occur, it affects the way in which the head noun is (sub)classified, cf. e.g.:

(35a) classical Greek drama
(35b) Greek classical drama
(36a) the paramilitary Protestant organizations
(36b) the Protestant paramilitary organizations
(37a) some therapeutic non-hypnotic technique
(37b) some non-hypnotic therapeutic technique

But usually the order is fixed and can be described in terms of certain well-defined groups of adjectives:

(i) deverbal adjectives, like LEADING, SLEEPING, INTERNALIZED, RECOGNIZED, SUSCEPTIBLE, HYPNOTIZABLE, etc.

(ii) adjectives denoting colour, like GREEN, RED, YELLOW, BLACK, etc.

(iii) adjectives denoting nationality, like ENGLISH, FRENCH, CHINESE, etc.

(iv) (other) denominal adjectives, like INDUSTRIAL, PRESIDENTIAL, NUCLEAR, WOOLLEN, MEDICAL, CULTURAL, POLITICAL, AUTOMATIC, FISCAL, etc.

(v) nominals serving as premodifiers, like METAL, SILK, FOREIGN POLICY, TOURIST, AIRLINE, etc.

The linear order is 'deverbal *before* colour *before* nationality *before* denominal *before* nominal':

(38) handwritten green pages
(39) a retired Indian Judge
(40) internalized linguistic representation
(41) Mao's supposed deathbed benediction
(42) white American men and women
(43) her pink woollen Dior
(44) a yellow silk handkerchief
(45) the American political system
(46) the increasing Russian military strength
(47) the Democratic foreign policy establishment
(48) an electronic metal detector

Mod. III adjectives which denote 'locality' or 'time' often precede (other) denominal or nominal modifiers but follow deverbal adjectives and adjectives denoting colour and nationality:

(49) *local* economic independence
(50) the *national* political scene
(51) the giant *Memphis* grain-export firm
(52) *daily* physical evaluation form
(53) the *annual* aquatic contest
(54) the *long-term* California Governor
(55) a mostly white *Atlanta* district
(56) a growing American *national* concern
(57) patched-up *nineteenth-century* houses

Non-inherent Mod. III adjectives (i.e. inherent Mod. I or II adjectives) always immediatly precede the nominal head, forming a compound-like relationship with it:

(58) South-African *wild* birds
(59) Australian *fast* bowler Jeff Thomson
(60) the various French *secret* services
(61) unreconstructed *cold* warriors
(62) this international *good* turn

(63) key *primary* states

(64) the five-times-wed *former* actress

The same place is occupied by one of the inherent determiners when serving as a modifier, the classifying genitive (cf. Bache & Davidsen-Nielsen *in press*, section 10.3.8 [A]):

(65) a muggy London *summer's* day

(66) a standard *tourist's* guide

(67) black *Indian's* hair

(68) artificial silk *women's* underwear

Finally it should be noted that LITTLE, OLD and YOUNG, which are best interpreted as inherent Mod. II adjectives, often occur immediately before the head noun with no intervening Mod. III adjectives and seem to enter a kind of compound-like relation with the head (e.g. *little girl, old man, young people*). But in strings of adjectives from both Mod. zones, they usually follow (other) Mod. II adjectives and precede Mod. III adjectives:

(69) a very attractive little American girl

(70) a handsome young Italian doctor

(71) funny old driven snow

8. Conclusion

In this paper I have assessed the extent to which the order of premodifying adjectives is functionally determined. The overriding principle seems to be that adjectives are ordered according to their relationship with the head noun: specifying adjectives precede descriptive adjectives, which in turn precede classifying adjectives. These three different kinds of adjective are not 'order classes' in the traditional sense but 'function classes' associated with certain hypotactically related modificational zones between determination (as realized by e.g. dependent articles) and categorization (as realized by the head noun) in the functional domain of nominals. These zones are referred to as Mod. I (specification), Mod. II (description) and Mod. III (classification). The order in which these zones appear is seen as non-random: specification is the kind of modification that is most like determination and therefore immediately follows it; and classification is the kind of modification that is most like categorization and therefore immediately precedes it. The specific function of an adjective cannot be determined in isolation but only in relation to the head noun it modifies. Many adjectives may thus have different functions (i.e. may appear in different Mod. zones) in different examples. Nevertheless it is convenient to operate with inherent membership, as this allows us to describe certain mechanisms for varying the function of an adjective: change of relative position, prosodic prominence, comparison, modification. In constructions with two or more adjectives in Mod. I or in Mod. III, it appears that the adjectives are hypotactically related and that the order is functionally determined, though in a somewhat weaker sense: in Mod. I we get progressive specification and in Mod. III we get regressive classification. Though variation does occur within this framework, the order of adjectives is here relatively fixed. In Mod. II, in which adjectives are paratactically related, the order is relative free. Though it is certainly possible to describe Mod. II in terms of certain order preferences or tendencies, there seems to be little or no correlation with function, even in a weak sense. It thus appears that hypotaxis and modificational function generally go hand in hand.

References

Annear, S. S. (1964). The Ordering of Pre-Nominal Modifiers in English. *Project on Linguistic Analysis Report* No. 8, Ohio State University Research Foundation, 95-120.

Bache, C. (1978). *The Order of Premodifying Adjectives in Present-Day English*. Odense: Odense University Press.

Bache, C. (1996). Presentation of a pedagogical sentence analysis system. *Hermes* 17, 11-35.

Bache, C. (1997). Adjektivers funktionelt betingede rækkefølge i engelsk. In L. Falster Jakobsen & G. Skytte (eds) *Ny Forskning i Grammatik* 4, Odense: Odense University Press.

Bache, C., M. Davenport, J. Dienhart & F. Larsen (1993). *An Introduction to English Sentence Analysis, 2nd edition revised*. Copenhagen: Munksgaard.

Bache, C. & N. Davidsen-Nielsen (in press). *Mastering English: An Advanced Grammar for Non-native and Native Speakers*. Berlin & New York: Mouton de Gruyter.

Coates, J. (1971). Denominal Adjectives: A Study in Syntactic Relationships between Modifier and Head. *Lingua* 27, 160-169.

Crystal, D. (1967). English. *Lingua* 17, 24-56.

Ferris, C. (1993). *The Meaning of Syntax: A Study in the Adjectives of English*. London & New York: Longman.

Greenbaum, S. & R. Quirk (1990). *A Student's Grammar of the English Language*. London: Longman.

Harder, P. (1996). *Functional Semantics: A Theory of Meaning, Structure and Tense in English*. Berlin & New York: Mouton de Gruyter.

Heltoft, L. (1996). Det danske nominals udtryks- og indholdssyntaks – et dependensanalytisk forsøg. In M. Herslund (ed) *Ny Forskning i Grammatik* 3. Odense: Odense University Press, 7-34.

Huddleston, R. (1984). *Introduction to the Grammar of English*. Cambridge: Cambridge University Press.

Huddleston, R. (1990). *English Grammar: an Outline*. Cambridge: Cambridge University Press.

Martin, J. E. (1968). *A Study of the Determinants of Preferred Adjective Order in English*. Unpublished doctoral dissertation, Urbana, Illinois: University of Illinois.

Oller, J. W., B. D. Sales & R. V. Harrington (1969). A Basic Circularity in Traditional and Current Linguistic Theory. *Lingua* 22, 317-328.

Quirk, R., S. Greenbaum, G. Leech & J. Svartvik (1985). *A Comprehensive Grammar of the English Language*. London: Longman.

Teyssier, J. (1968). Notes on the Syntax of the Adjective in Modern English. *Lingua* 20, 225-249.

Vestergaard, T. (1993). *Engelsk Grammatik*. 2nd impression, Schønberg.

A Linguistic Analysis of Archibald MacLeish's *Ars Poetica*

John M. Dienhart

1. Introduction

Archibald MacLeish (1892-1982) was born in Illinois. He graduated from Yale (1915) and from Harvard law school (1919), and then practiced law in Boston for several years. In 1923 he quit his law practice and, desiring to try to make his living from writing poetry, he moved to Paris with his wife and two children. There he stayed until 1928, when he returned to the United States. He became a very prolific writer of poetry, but his multi-faceted talent took him into many other fields as well. In addition to publishing numerous poems, plays and essays, he was, at various times in his career, head of the Library of Congress (1939-1944), Assistant Secretary of State under Roosevelt (1944-1945), instrumental in the founding of UNESCO, and Professor of Rhetoric and Oratory at Harvard (1949-1962).[1] MacLeish's willingness and ability to combine his love of poetry with public service has been frequently commented upon:

> During the war years he had the qualities that the time of crisis demanded; he set aside his first love, poetry, to serve his country and risked irreparable damage to his chosen work and its development; however, he returned to poetry and proved that public service and lyric expression are not incompatible. (Falk 1965: 169)

In 1926, MacLeish published a collection of poems entitled *Streets in the Moon*. In this volume is a poem which has been referred to as "MacLeish's ultimate expression of the art-for-art's-sake tenet" (Falk 1965: 41). The poem is *Ars Poetica*. It is this poem which I wish to examine in this paper.

The poem consists of 12 couplets, but there is some disagreement about whether or not these couplets should be linked together in any fashion. In the most recent publication of the poem which I have come across (Lynn 1994: 24f), there is no attempt to group the couplets into any higher units. The poem simply appears to have 12 very short stanzas, each stanza consisting of one couplet. The same form is found in Bergman and Epstein (1983: 386f). Perkins et al. (1985: 1196f) put a bit of extra space after every fourth couplet. This is closer to MacLeish's intention, but not quite satisfactory, since the reader is likely to overlook this slight difference in spacing. In the anthologies which MacLeish himself was responsible for, an asterisk is used to separate the couplets into three loosely linked eight-line stanzas (see, for

---

[1] For a biography of MacLeish, see Falk (1965).

example, MacLeish 1952: 40f and 1972: 106f, not to mention the original publication, MacLeish 1926: 37f). It seems reasonable, therefore, to adopt this form here, and to view the poem as consisting of three stanzas.[2]

Ars Poetica

A poem should be palpable and mute
As a globed fruit,

Dumb
As old medallions to the thumb,

5   Silent as the sleeve-worn stone
Of casement ledges where the moss has grown –

A poem should be wordless
As the flight of birds.

*

A poem should be motionless in time
10   As the moon climbs,

Leaving, as the moon releases
Twig by twig the night-entangled trees,

Leaving, as the moon behind the winter leaves,
Memory by memory the mind –

15   A poem should be motionless in time
As the moon climbs.

*

A poem should be equal to:
Not true.

For all the history of grief
20   An empty doorway and a maple leaf.

For love
The leaning grasses and two lights above the sea –

A poem should not mean
But be.

---

[2] In the body of the paper, however, I occasionally present selections from the poem without displaying the blank lines between the couplets. This is simply a space-saving convention. It does not violate the form of the poem, since that has already been supplied.

2. The nature of the analysis

I have, on earlier occasions (Dienhart 1989, 1994), commented on some of the reservations I have regarding much published commentary which purports to analyze a given poem. Traditional analyses often deal primarily, if not solely, with the interpretation of various kinds of imagery in the poem. Or they are concerned chiefly with trying to relate the given poem to works by other poets. Or they characterize the poem in such vague generalities that no real information is communicated to the reader.

Now I am not, in principle, opposed to any analytical approach which helps us appreciate a poem more fully. I am merely asserting that, in my view, the first steps of any analysis should always involve a careful examination of the poem itself – the form and nature of the language, the shape of the lines, the character of the rhyme and meter.

My general reservations have not been lessened by the various commentaries I have encountered regarding "Ars Poetica". In some cases the remarks are so startlingly unhelpful that one wonders why they were written at all. Consider the following characterization by someone who is capable of much better:

> "Ars Poetica" is more than an extension of poetic language; beneath its successful experiments in timing, interior rhyme and suspension, it says a number of pointed and profound things which have nothing to do with timeliness and changing tastes. The tone of these verses may be as new as this generation; the spirit which moves beneath them is as old as the sung phrase and the unspoken word. (Untermeyer 1962: 451)

This may be charming prose, but it says little about MacLeish's poem. Rather more to the point is the following observation by Grover Smith (1975: 30f):

> One of the most often cited anthology pieces from *Streets in the Moon* is the paradoxical and enigmatic "Ars Poetica." ... The central paradox of "Ars Poetica" is that it makes sense only when the reader accepts its sense as a function of form ... The real subject of "Ars Poetica" is itself, by a sort of narcissism of the written word as "pure poetry"; this poem exhibits aestheticism circling round, as it were, and returning like the equator upon the round earth.

Smith clearly has a valid point here: "Ars Poetica" provides an intellectual paradox. By stating at the end of the poem that *A poem should not mean / But be*, MacLeish appears to be discouraging any investigation into the "meaning" of this (or any) poem. But at the same time, it is obvious that we cannot appreciate the sense of this dictum, unless we understand the meaning of the couplet. Having pointed out the paradox, Smith should then go on to try to resolve it – by investigating the form of the poem itself. This he does not do. Instead he adopts that very fashionable gambit of linking MacLeish's poem to the work of other poets:

> "Ars Poetica," somewhat Yeatsian like various other short poems in the volume, looks also Keatsian: the whole poem speaks with a voice which, like that of the Grecian urn when it equates beauty and truth, belongs to a realm of ideality and is relevant only to that. (Smith 1975: 31)

Valid as these comparisons may be, they do not in themselves constitute an analysis of the poem, even when carried out in some detail, as another commentator, Victor Staudt (1957) has done.

Staudt begins his short commentary on "Ars Poetica" by addressing MacLeish's paradox from the point of view of a literature teacher confronted by a wily and recalcitrant student:

> In the past decade or so, there is probably not a teacher of literature in America who has not had the quotation "A poem should not mean / But be" thrown at him. There is, of course, something about the analysis of poems which the student finds inimical to his own anarchical interests; accordingly he seizes whatever ammunition is at hand in an attempt to dispose of the tiresome business. The implication of the lines themselves he takes to be a condemnation of any attempt to "explain" or to "seek meaning" in a poem. (Staudt 1957: 28)

To start with, this is a very patronizing characterization of the student. Why should we assume that "of course" the student will rebel when it comes to the "tiresome business" of analyzing poetry?

I suggest that the answer might lie in the way the analysis is performed. I think we should sympathize with any student who finds vague generalities unilluminating. We should also be aware that not all students, or readers in general, are equipped with sufficient background knowledge to find Yeatsian and Keatsian echoes in "Ars Poetica".

Staudt continues his condescending remarks by observing that "the sensitive reader becomes aware of a startling number of allusions to or echoes of Keats", after which he gives us a list of "a few of the more obvious" ones (Staudt 1957: 28).

Leaving tone aside, analyzing a poem in this way – by searching for related literary objects outside the poem itself – is a fairly common practice. Again, let me stress that I am not claiming that connections among poetic objects do not exist, nor am I advocating that they not be sought out. Obviously, the richer one's poetic background, the richer one's interpretation of any given poem. And, as we shall see at a later point in this paper, the reference to Keats is useful and informative. My point, simply, is this: an analysis of a poem should begin not by seeking outside connections, but by examining relationships internal to the poem itself.

More particularly, it should begin, as I said above, by focusing on the form of the poem – the shape and organization of the lines, the orthography, the lexical choices, the phonological and syntactic patterns. Once these internal patterns have been uncovered and described, the analyst may, if he so wishes, go on to seek out connections between the poem under analysis and other elements in the literary universe.

There is, of course, nothing new or startling in this view. But I feel it needs to be stressed at the outset, since it seems to be in clear and constant danger of being forgotten or ignored. Needless to say, I believe further that this focus on the form of the poem is precisely what MacLeish is urging us to undertake – not only in the case of "Ars Poetica", but in the case of all poems.

3. Form and meaning

MacLeish is clearly advocating that the reader "listen" to the form of the poem instead of (or as well as) trying to decipher the meaning of each word, phrase, and sentence. Put more briefly: the poem is the poem.

MacLeish is, of course, not alone in making such a claim. In one sense or another, all poets and readers accept this dictum in varying degrees. If a poem involved only the meaning of the words in it, then there would be no reason to write a poem. Simple prose would do. Prose would, in fact, be more effective, since the writer would be freed from the formal prosodic constraints which a poem imposes.

Unlike other major forms of art, such as painting, sculpture, and music, the medium of poetry, which is language, has a voice of its own, and this voice is in constant competition with the other voice, which is the poem itself. A painter's tools are the canvas and his paints. He does not have to fear that a given color, or combination of colors, will begin to speak to the observer in any linguistic sense. But a poet, whose basic tools are words, has to combat the unruly voices of the words themselves. Auden has expressed this point very nicely:

> It is both the glory and the shame of poetry that its medium is not its private property, that a poet cannot invent his words and that words are products, not of nature, but of a human society which uses them for a thousand different purposes. (Auden 1962: 23)

As Saussure long ago made clear, a word is a sign, and a sign has both form and meaning. MacLeish is urging us, as other poets have urged us, not to let the message of the form be overpowered by the message of the meaning. Look and listen to the forms themselves, and observe the poet at work as he chooses his materials from the paintbox of language.

In a magnificent lecture on the nature of poetry, Housman (1933: 37) posed the following questions to his Cambridge audience:

> Poetry is not the thing said but a way of saying it. Can it then be isolated and studied by itself? [F]or the combination of language with its intellectual content, its meaning, is as close a union as can well be imagined. Is there such a thing as pure unmingled poetry, poetry independent of meaning?

Housman's unqualified answer is yes: "Meaning is of the intellect, poetry is not" (Housman 1933: 38). As an illustration, Housman refers the reader to the poetry of William Blake:

> For me the most poetical of all poets is Blake. I find his lyrical note as beautiful as Shakespeare's and more beautiful than anyone else's; and I call him more poetical than Shakespeare, even though Shakespeare has so much more poetry, because poetry in him preponderates more than in Shakespeare over everything else, and instead of being confounded in a great river can be drunk pure from a slender channel of its own. Shakespeare is rich in thought, and his meaning has power of itself to move us, even if the poetry were not there: Blake's meaning is often unimportant or virtually non-existent, so that we can listen with all our hearing to his celestial tune. (Housman 1933: 40)

With this kind of support and advice from poets as diverse as Housman, Auden and MacLeish, let us now turn our attention to the object of our analysis, the poem "Ars Poetica".

4. Stanza one: unsilent silence

The first stanza of the poem is marked lexically by four near synonyms: *mute*, *dumb*, *silent*, and *wordless*. The use of this set of terms takes us directly into that seeming paradox which we touched on above: a poem is not to be comprehended solely by focusing on the meaning of the words which appear in the poem. These meanings have to be silenced, so that we can hear the poem itself speak, through its form.

These four words of silence clearly constitute the major structural pillars of the first stanza. Each of the four words forms part of a two-line couplet. This links the couplets semantically. The couplets are also related structurally by the repetition of a syntactic *as*-construction. This *as*-construction establishes, within each couplet, a concrete simile for a poem itself. Furthermore, three of the four words of silence participate in end rhymes, thus establishing phonological links between words of silence and other words in the similes. All these relationships are shown in the following reproduction of the first stanza (words of silence are capitalized, similes are italicized, and relevant end-rhymes are underlined):

> A poem should be palpable and MUTE
> *As a globed fruit.*
>
> DUMB
> *As old medallions to the thumb,*
>
> 5   SILENT *as the sleeve-worn stone*
> *Of casement ledges where the moss has grown –*
>
> A poem should be WORDLESS
> *as the flight of birds.*

Observe how the similes wax and wane in length. The longest simile follows the word, *silent*, which is the only one of the four silent words which does not participate in an end-rhyme. Instead we sense its presence by means of the alliteration on its initial /s/. The alliteration is found throughout the couplet (the number of instances would increase if we also include the voiced counterpart of /s/, namely /z/, in *as*, *ledges*, and *has*):

5   SILENT as the sleeve-worn stone
    Of casement ledges where the moss has grown –

By allowing these words of silence to participate in such phonological patterns as full rhyme and alliteration, MacLeish actually highlights their presence, thus contradicting their very content. This adds to the paradox in this stanza, since we have silence speaking out. This seeming contradiction reinforces the poet's claim: it is the form of the poem that does the speaking.

Consider, too, the metrical nature of the first stanza. Since the lines are not isometric,[3] there is no fixed metrical pattern in the lines themselves. But it is nonetheless clear that the poet has adopted a general pattern of starting each line with an unstressed syllable. In fact, this is a characteristic not only of the first stanza, but of the poem as a whole. Consequently, lines that start with a stressed syllable are singled out. Note that in stanza one, only lines 3 and 5 begin with a stressed syllable. And once again it is a word of silence (*dumb* in line 3, *silent* in line 5) which breaks the pattern. Metrically, too, then, these silent words speak out.

There are other formal devices in this stanza which relate to the concept of silence. Look at the first three lines of the poem. They can be seen to decrease drastically in length, until we reach the third line, which consists of the single word, *dumb*. Here the poet is making superb use of the result of his decision to adopt the principle of non-isometric lines. By permitting himself the liberty of allowing the number of syllables in each line to vary, he can use line length as a meaningful device in the form of the poem. Line three is the shortest line in the poem. It consists of one word, which itself consists of only one syllable. And this word is *dumb*. So the line itself is practically silent.

Now, consider the options MacLeish has at this point. He has decided to create a one-word line using one of the four words of silence. He has four synonyms to choose from: *mute*, *dumb*, *silent*, and *wordless*. The latter two can be dismissed, because they are too long. Two-syllable words are not as silent as one-syllable words. So the choice is between *mute* and *dumb*. MacLeish has chosen *dumb*, and

---

[3]Lines in a poem are isometric if they are of the same metrical length – for example, if they are all iambic pentameter (five iambic feet = a metrical line of 10 syllables).

his choice is an inspired one. Consider the phonological makeup of *dumb*. It consists of three phonemes: /dʌm/.[4] The final phoneme is a bilabial nasal, which means that it is articulated by closing the two lips. The word, and therefore the line, thus ends with the mouth shut. This is a fine physical reinforcement of the mental concept of silence. But the iconic relationship does not end here. Consider, too, the orthography. The word *dumb* ends in a silent letter, the letter *b*. So the word itself, and thus, again, the line, ends in silence.

Note how this silent *b* continues to play a role throughout the poem. We find it next in the rhyme word for *dumb*, namely *thumb* (l. 4). And it appears twice in the second stanza, in the word *climbs* (ll. 10, 16). Furthermore, in a tiny miracle of form, the silent *b*, becomes unsilent at the very end of the poem. The last word, the last syllable of the poem itself, is the sound /bi/. The poet has linked the orthographically silent *b* of the silent word *dumb* with the semantically silent copula verb *be*, and given them a resounding significance as the final syllable of the poem – before it, too, falls into silence.

5. Stanza two: motionless motion

Just as the first stanza focuses on absence of sound, the second stanza focuses on absence of motion. Or, better, on very slow motion. The primary image in this stanza is the moon – as seen, at various times, behind the branches of trees. The stanza opens with *A poem should be motionless in time / As the moon climbs* (ll. 9-10). There is, of course, the potential ambiguity of *As*, which could mean either "while" (cp. *As I was leaving the house, the phone rang*) or "like". Though both interpretations are possible, the second reading is particularly appropriate, since it sets up a direct parallel with the opening two lines of the first stanza: *A poem should be palpable and mute / As a globed fruit*. This establishes one of the many formal links between the two stanzas.

Note that once again we have a seeming contradiction: a poem should be motionless in the way that the moon climbs in the sky. There is a tension between the adjective *motionless* and the verb *climbs*. The resolution of the conflict can be found in considering how the moon rises. It is difficult to actually see the moon in motion, no matter how steadfast one's gaze. Instead, we are aware of the motion by noting the position of the moon at different times. This is the image which MacLeish supplies in the lines, *the moon releases / Twig by twig the night-entangled trees* (ll. 11-12). In just this nearly motionless way, a poem leaves *Memory by memory the mind* (l. 14). Consider, in this connection, the convoluted syntax of lines 11-14:

---

[4]The phonemic symbols used in this paper conform to those found in Bauer, Dienhart, Hartvigson, and Jakobsen (1980). The consonant symbols are self-evident. The vowel symbols which are used are: /i/ as in *beat*, /u/ as in *boot*, /ʌ/ as in *butt*, /aI/ as in *bite*.

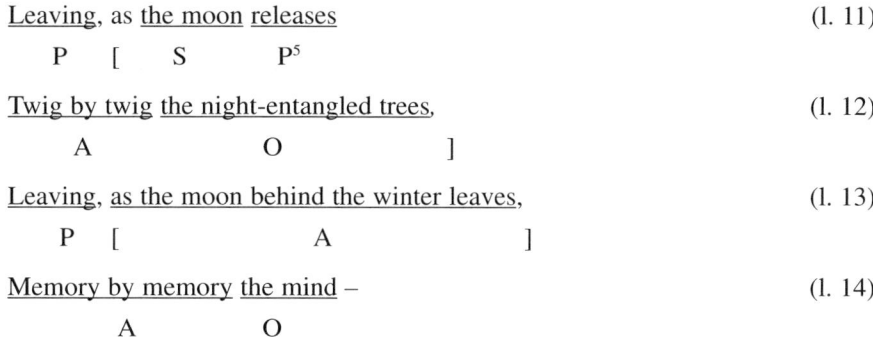

The matrix clause here is *Leaving ... memory by memory the mind*. Normal word order would have given us: *Leaving the mind, memory by memory*. Thus, instead of the standard POA, we are given the unusual structure, PAO, in which the adverbial separates the object from its verb. The same pattern is found in the subordinate clause: *as the moon releases / Twig by twig the night-entangled trees* (instead of the more normal word order: *The moon leaves the night-entangled trees, twig by twig*). This syntactic parallelism strengthens the link MacLeish is creating between a poem on the one hand, and the moon on the other.

Furthermore, the subordinate *as*-clause itself functions as an adverbial (A) interposed between the predicator *Leaving* (l. 11), and its object, *the mind* (l. 14). The resulting discontinuity is so great that the predicator *Leaving* is repeated in line 13. The result is that when the reader encounters the first instance of *Leaving* (l. 11), he has to make a mental journey through 22 words before encountering the direct object (*the mind*) that belongs with this verb. This is complicated syntax indeed.

But the complication does not stop here. The syntax contains even more complexity than the double PAO structures and the long-distance object. Consider next the string of words, *Leaving, as the moon*, which appears in line 11 and again in line 13. The reader naturally assumes that the two strings will be processable in the same way. This is not the case, however. The poet has set a syntactic trap for us. In the first instance (*Leaving, as the moon releases / Twig by twig the night-entangled trees*), we eventually work out that the moon is subject of a subordinate clause, and *as* functions as a subordinate conjunction. In the second case, however (*Leaving, as the moon behind the winter leaves / Memory by memory the mind*), both *the moon* and *as* take on different functions. No matter how hard we may try, we cannot make sense of a reading where the moon continues to be the subject: "the

---

[5]The symbols and terminology used in my discussion of syntax in this paper are those employed in the "Odense model", as described in Bache, Davenport, Dienhart, and Larsen (1993). In this system, capital letters represent syntactic functions: S = Subject, P = Predicator, O = Object, A = Adverbial. The square brackets ([...]) in the analyses here of lines 11-13 delimit the two *as*-constructions; in this way, it can be seen that the first is a subordinate clause (with the structure SPAO), whereas the second – despite its superficial syntactic similarity to the preceding *as*-clause – is a simple manner adverbial (A) in the form of a nominal group (with *moon* as the head of the group).

moon (which is behind the winter) leaves". The trap has been set first by the double use of the non-finite verbal form, *leaving* (ll. 11 and 13), and then by the use of the word *leaves* (l. 13). It is natural to interpret *leaves* as another instance of the verb *to leave*, this time in its finite form (third person singular, present tense). A finite verb requires a subject, so the mind backs up, tries *winter* (*the winter leaves*), fails to make this work, backs up again, tries *the moon* (*the moon*, behind the winter, *leaves*), and again gets a nonsensical reading. At this point it probably dawns on the reader that *leaves* is not a verb here at all, but rather a plural form of the noun *leaf*. This at last makes sense: the moon is behind the winter leaves. So in this case, *the moon* functions as head of a nominal group (rather than subject of a subordinate clause), and *as* functions as a preposition (rather than a subordinate conjunction). This is an ingenious touch of linguistic artistry.

It is reasonable, now, to ask why the poet has created all these linguistic difficulties for the reader. The answer is that the convoluted syntax in lines 11-14 mirrors *the night-entangled trees* (l. 12) through which the moon passes. By working its way through this tangled syntax, the mind of the reader is forced to enact the movement of the moon.

The poet employs other devices to reinforce this image of the moon moving through the branches. Note, for example, how many times the word *moon* appears in this stanza. We find it in lines 10, 11, 13, and 16. The effect of this repetition can be made visible as follows:

>   A poem should be motionless in time
> 10   As the **MOON** climbs,
>
>   Leaving, as the **MOON** releases
>   Twig by twig the night-entangled trees,
>
>   Leaving, as the **MOON** behind the winter leaves,
>   Memory by memory the mind –
>
> 15   A poem should be motionless in time
>   As the **MOON** climbs.

The moon is literally climbing through the stanza. At the risk of attributing too much ingenuity to the poet, I would like to suggest that the moon actually appears in two additional lines in this stanza, namely lines 9 and 15, in the word motionless:

>   A poem should be **MOtiON**less in time

In this case, however, the word *moon* is made discontinuous by the presence of *ti*. But that, of course, is the way the moon would appear behind twigs – discontinuous, or fragmented. Note, too, that the letters *t* and *i* which are causing the discontinuity in *motionless* both appear in the word *twig*.

If we grant this interpretation, then the moon can be seen in every line of stanza two except lines 12 and 14. So why stop now? It is not hard to find an even more tenuous and fragmented moon in line 14:

>MeMOry by memOry the miNd –

And if this is acceptable, why not find a fraction of the moon in the one remaining line in the stanza where no moon has yet appeared:

>Twig by twig the night-entaNgled trees, (l. 12)

Here, only a tiny portion of the moon is visible, but then this is the line where the thicket of twigs may be most dense, since it is the line containing the word *entangled*. Of course, there are three possible choices for the relevant *n* (one in *night*, two in *entangled*). I have simply selected the one that seems to me most deeply entangled in the word *entangled* itself. The actual choice is not important. What may be significant is that the moon is nearly invisible in this particular line, there being not a single occurrence of the other letters in *moon*, namely *m* and *o*.[6] If we now highlight all these proposed images of the moon in this stanza, we have the following picture:

>A poem should be **MOtiON**less in time
10   As the **MOON** climbs,

>Leaving, as the **MOON** releases
>Twig by twig the night-enta**N**gled trees,

>Leaving, as the **MOON** behind the winter leaves,
>Me**MO**ry by mem**O**ry the mi**N**d –

15   A poem should be **MOtiON**less in time
>As the **MOON** climbs.

Seen in this light, the moon is clearly climbing through the individual words, the convoluted syntax, and the stanza itself. This is an ingenious use of linguistic forms, and gives us another clear example of how a poem can "be". No prose discussion of this image can capture the image itself. We can only point out the technique employed by the poet, and then turn to the poem to witness its application.

Consider next, the parallels between stanzas one and two. We have the four couplets in each stanza. Both stanzas are framed (that is, start and end) with a couplet which opens with the words *A poem should be*. Furthermore, stanza two, like stanza one, contains four similes, all introduced by *as*:

---

[6]If the reader thinks that it is quite natural for a line of poetry to be without the two letters, *m* and *o*, he might examine other lines of poetry, starting with this poem. Of the other 23 lines in this poem, only one is without *m* and *o*, namely the very last line, *But be*.

A poem should be motionless in time
10 **As the moon** climbs,

Leaving, **as the moon** releases
Twig by twig the night-entangled trees,

Leaving, **as the moon** behind the winter leaves,
Memory by memory the mind –

15 A poem should be motionless in time
As the moon climbs.

At the same time, however, there is an important difference. The similes in this stanza all relate to the moon. Contrast this with the similes in the first stanza:

As a globed fruit (l. 2)

As old medallions to the thumb (l. 4)

... as the sleeve-worn stone (l. 5)

As the flight of birds (l. 8)

In the first stanza, the similes involve comparisons with different objects, and all these objects are stationary – that is, *as* is followed solely by a nominal group. In the second stanza, on the other hand, the similes involve a single object (the moon) and that object is involved in a process – (that is, *as* is followed by constituents in a clause, with the moon functioning as subject):

As the moon climbs (l. 10)

... as the moon releases (l. 11)

As the moon climbs (l. 16)

The single exception, as was noted above, is the expression in the middle of the stanza:

... as the moon behind the winter leaves (l. 13)

where the *as*-construction hovers between the two types (group and clause) until the reader deciphers the complex code in favor of the pattern in stanza one.

We have thus seen that stanza two contains a number of parallel states involving repeated patterns. The simplest pattern is the repetition of the word *moon* itself. A larger pattern involves the phrase *as the moon* (ll. 10, 11, 13, 16). Even longer strings are repeated, however. We have already noted the repetition of *Leaving, as the moon* (ll. 11, 13). But most remarkable of all is the fact that the first two lines of the stanza are repeated in full at the end of the stanza:

      A poem should be motionless in time
10   **As the moon climbs,**

      Leaving, as the moon releases
      Twig by twig the night-entangled trees,

      Leaving, as the moon behind the winter leaves,
      Memory by memory the mind –

15   **A poem should be motionless in time**
      As the moon climbs.

These repetitions have the effect of capturing the seemingly contradictory notion of motionless motion. An object (the moon, a word, a group of words) is encountered unchanged but in different locations. We do not see the movement but we see the effect of the move: the object appears in a new position. And after all this "movement", the moon is still in the same place it started in.

Metrically and phonologically, too, a sense of movement in non-movement is provided. As we noted in the first stanza, the predominant stress pattern for line openings is to start with an unstressed syllable. This pattern is continued in the first two lines and the last two lines of the second stanza as well. But in the middle of the stanza (ll. 11-14) the pattern is broken. Each of these four lines, which contain the tangled syntax, starts with a stressed syllable: *Leav*ing (l. 11), *Twi*g (l. 12), *Leav*ing (l. 13), and *Me*mory (l. 14). Thus we see the meter becoming more complex, just as the syntax becomes complex. Note, too, how nicely these four openings establish the simile: the moon leaves the twigs, the poem leaves the memory.

Consider next the word *climbs* (ll. 10, 16). This verb is involved in a whole array of lexical and phonological networks in this poem. First of all, it counterpoints the word *motionless* (ll. 9, 15). In the same way that stanza one contains an aural paradox (unsilent silence), stanza two contains a visual one (motionless motion). There is tension between the word *motionless* and the word *climbs* – between state and process.

But *climbs* has a much wider array of associations. Note that it contains within it the word *limbs*, which links up semantically with *twig* (l. 12), *trees* (l. 12), and *leaves* (l. 13). Furthermore, it contains a silent *b*, thus linking it to *dumb* (and *thumb*) in the first stanza. Motion and silence are thus orthographically linked.

In addition, the vocalic nucleus of *climbs* is the diphthong, /aɪ/, which echoes the first syllable of *silent*, another word of silence in stanza one. In its own stanza, stanza two, this diphthong assonates with its rhyming partner, *time* (ll. 9, 15), as well as with *mind* (l. 14).

An examination of the nature of the diphthong itself reveals that it is a "climbing" one, moving from the open vowel position of [a] toward the half-close vowel position of [ɪ]. Try pronouncing the diphthong /aɪ/ in isolation, and you will feel the lower jaw rise, or climb, as the diphthong is enunciated. The climbing continues as you articulate the following /m/, resulting in a complete closure of the lips.

If we look at the nature of the end rhymes in stanza two, we see that the rhyming technique is different from that used in the first stanza. Instead of pairs of full rhymes, we find assonance (and some consonance). Five of the lines end in words containing the diphthong /aɪ/, while three end in words with /i/:

/aɪ/	*time, climbs*	(ll. 9, 10)
/i/	*rel<u>ea</u>ses, trees, leaves*	(ll. 11, 12, 13)
/aɪ/	*mind, time, climbs*	(ll. 14, 15, 16)

Note how the /aɪ/-lines envelop the /i/ lines. Phonologically, the middle lines have "climbed" even higher than the opening lines of stanza two, as indicated by the following diagram, which displays the vowel movement of /aɪ/ and the very high position of /i/:

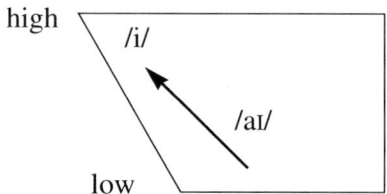

Having examined some of the linguistic devices employed by MacLeish in stanzas one and two, let us now turn our attention to the final stanza, where the poet continually breaks with the parallels set up in the first two stanzas.

6. Stanza three: pattern breaks

We have seen that stanza one focuses on a series of similes in which nominal groups are introduced by *as*. We have also seen that stanza two follows a similar pattern, though here *as* introduces primarily clausal similes rather than nominal ones. In stanza three, however, the similes disappear altogether. Compare the openings of the three stanzas:

Stanza 1:	A poem should be palpable and mute	(l. 1)
	As a globed fruit.	(l. 2)
Stanza 2:	A poem should be motionless in time	(l. 9)
	As the moon climbs,	(l. 10)
Stanza 3:	A poem should be equal to:	(l. 17)
	Not true.	(l. 18)

In the third stanza, the simile pattern (manifested by *as*-constructions) is broken. Recall that the *as*-constructions were found not only in the opening couplets of stanzas one and two, but in every single couplet in these stanzas. By breaking with this pattern in stanza three, the poet establishes his new theme: a poem is not like anything else. A poem is a poem. Hence similes will not suffice.

Let us examine more carefully the opening couplet in this third and last stanza. It is not easy to decipher. In the first line of the couplet (l. 17), I sense a contrast between *be equal to* and the implied *be like* of stanzas 1 and 2, even though the second element of the equation appears to be missing: equal to what? The next line – *Not true* – is even more difficult to decode. Two interpretations recommend themselves.

On one reading, this line contradicts the preceding one: it is not true that "A poem should be equal to". On this reading, one could account for the missing second element in the equation by assuming that the poet has interrupted himself in mid-sentence. The reason the second element is missing is that the poet has decided that the line was heading in the wrong direction, and hence is declared to be "not true" – that is, false. The implication in this reading is that one should not only avoid saying that a poem is *like* something else, one should also avoid saying that a poem is *equal* to something else.

There is (at least) one more reading, however. On this reading, line 18 does not contradict line 17, but rather continues it: "A poem should be equal to" *and* "Not true". That is, a poem is neither true nor false. A poem simply is. This, then, would anticipate the closing statement: *A poem should not mean / But be*. If a poem has no propositional meaning, then clearly it can not be subject to a test of truth or falsity.

It is possible to entertain both of the above readings simultaneously, in that both lead to the claim that a poem is not like anything but itself. In fact, since MacLeish insists that *A poem should not mean* (l. 23), it would seem to follow, as was pointed out earlier, that the very exercise we are here carrying out – namely attempting to decode the message of this couplet (ll. 17-18) – is itself a denial of that statement. So a third possibility is that the poet has planted here a string of words that do not "mean", but just "are".

This line of thought gains some support from an examination of the rest of the stanza. Whereas the syntax is quite regular in stanza one, and tangled but decipherable in stanza two, in stanza three it seems to be "ungrammatical". We have already seen that the first couplet, though it ends in a full stop, forms a very curious sentence. The next two lines (ll. 19-20), though also followed by a full stop, do not form a complete sentence at all:[7]

---

[7]Note how the punctuation in the third stanza breaks with the pattern set up in stanzas one and two. In the first place, there is a difference in the series of punctuation marks at the end of each of the four couplets. In stanzas one and two the series is , , – . In stanza three the series is . . – . The result is that the subject of the first couplet in stanzas one and two participates in the syntactic structure of the second and third couplets in each stanza. In stanza three, on the other hand, the first couplet is effectively cut off from the next two. This contributes to the sense of fragmentation which is found in the third stanza. In the second place, the first couplet itself is fragmented in the third stanza by the introduction of the colon at the end of line 17 (*A poem should be equal to:*).

> For all the history of grief
>
> An empty doorway and a maple leaf.

The same is true of the next two lines (ll. 21-22):

> For love
>
> The leaning grasses and two lights above the sea –

It is not really clear, however, whether this is meant to be the end of a "sentence", since line 22 ends in a dash, not a full stop. However, the syntactic parallels which lines 21 and 22 show with lines 19 and 20 suggest a major break at the end of line 22.

Being incomplete sentences, with no apparent subject or predicator, these two couplets (ll. 19-20, 21-22) are quite difficult to interpret. Perkins (1987: 51), I believe, finds the right key. In his view, MacLeish is making use of "the method of the elliptical image", whereby a phrase such as *an empty doorway* or *a maple leaf* can be used "to express 'all the history' of an experience that ends in grief". Lynn (1994: 27) makes a similar point in a more mathematical fashion. In Lynn's view, each of these couplets has the form "for X, (substitute) Y". That is, for an abstraction such as grief, a poet should substitute something concrete – such as an empty doorway, or a maple leaf. Similarly for love. This interpretation not only makes syntactic sense of these difficult couplets, it also ties in nicely with MacLeish's use of concrete similes in the earlier stanzas to suggest the nature of a poem.[8]

In the final couplet of the poem (ll. 23-24) the poet returns to the form of a complete sentence. In fact, this couplet is the only complete sentence in all of stanza three, and even it is a bit odd, since the verb *mean* is here used intransitively (rather than transitively, which is its normal use) and the copula verb, *be*, which normally takes some sort of complement, does not do so here:

> A poem should not mean
> But be.

The linguistic devices MacLeish makes use of in this stanza all contribute to the poet's efforts to wrest the words of the poem from the daily functions they perform in general communication. Recall Auden's lament: "It is both the glory and the shame of poetry that its medium is not its private property". MacLeish is making these words into his own private property. By using old words in new ways he loosens our grip on the meanings of the words, forcing us to attend increasingly to the forms.

Let us, therefore, look more closely at the forms of the words in this final stanza,

---

[8]This is clearly related to T. S. Eliot's notion of "objective correlative", as described in Eliot's essay, "Hamlet and His Problems", published in 1919. MacLeish was no doubt well acquainted with the concept when he wrote "Ars Poetica".

and explore some of the linguistic networks that these words and their fragmented images enter into with other parts of the poem.

Consider first the images themselves: the history of grief, an empty doorway, a maple leaf, the leaning grasses, two lights above the sea. Though apparently incomplete and disconnected at first sight, upon closer examination they can each be seen to bear a relationship to images in the preceding stanzas.

Thus, *the history of grief* (l. 19) connects with *old medallions* (l. 4), in that both images involve the passing of time. *An empty doorway* (l. 20) links up with the *sleeve-worn stone of casement ledges where the moss has grown* (ll. 5-6). A casement is defined as "a window that opens like a door" (*Longman Dictionary of Contemporary English* 1978: 158), so both images refer to openings in a house. Furthermore, both of these openings appear to be deserted or to have fallen into disuse (the door is empty, the casement ledges overgrown with moss). Recall, too, the verb *leaving*, which plays such an important role in stanza two. With its associations of departure, this word, too, ties in with *empty*.

A *maple leaf* (l. 20) echoes the twigs and leaves of stanza two (as well as the verb, *leaving*, thus also connecting with the image of emptiness). The *two lights above the sea* (l. 22) is a difficult image to interpret, but the moon is a prime candidate for one of the lights,[9] thereby linking this image to the climbing moon of stanza two (a link which also reaches into stanza one through the word *globed* in line 2). Note, too, that the diphthong of *lights* echoes the vowel which plays such an important role in *climbs*, linking this word to the already existing network which includes, in addition to *climbs*, also *time* and *mind*.

Phonologically, too, the last stanza establishes formal links with the first two. Consider the rhyme scheme of the last stanza. On one level, we find three pairs of rhymes, and two lines with no matching rhyme: aa bb cd ed. The full rhymes, with the corresponding vowel nuclei, are:

/u/ *to, true*   (ll. 17, 18)
/i/ *grief, leaf*   (ll. 19, 20)
/i/ *sea, be*   (ll. 22, 24)

The unrhymed words are:

---

[9]The other light may also be the moon. Thus MacLeish speaks of an important event in his life (more on this below) when one night he looked up into the "icy, absolutely clear sky" and saw "the new moon with the old moon in its arms" (Drabeck and Ellis 1986: 20). The second light could, of course, also be the sun, since the sun and the moon can often be seen in the sky at the same time. The sun/moon theme shows up, for example, in one of MacLeish's conversations with the moon in an autobiographical sketch:
 Why do you always turn your face away? I asked the moon. Why do you keep your face turned toward the sun no matter where the sun may lead you? Why do you blind yourself with sunlight? (MacLeish 1978: 75)

/ʌ/   love   (l. 21)
/i/   mean   (l. 23)

On another level, however, line 23 ties in, through assonance, with lines 19, 20, 22, and 24 – since these lines all end in words whose stressed syllable contains the vowel /i/. From this point of view, the rhyme scheme is aa bb cb bb, and the relevant vowel sequence is a = /u/, b = /i/, c = /ʌ/.

We are now prepared to illuminate the multiple phonological links which stanza three has with the preceding two stanzas. In the first place, stanza three combines, in one stanza, the rhyming techniques found in stanzas one and two: like stanza one, stanza three makes use of full rhyme, but like stanza two, it also makes use of assonance.

Additional concrete phonological links are established by the assonating vowels themselves. The vowel /u/ in the first pair of rhymes in stanza three echoes the vowel in the opening pair of rhymes in stanza one (*mute, fruit*), while the vowel in the two other rhyming pairs (/i/) echoes the vowel in the middle three lines of stanza two (*releases, trees, leaves*).

Consider, finally, the lonely vowel /ʌ/ of *love* in stanza three (l. 21) – the only line-ending which does not find a rhyming mate at the end of any other line in the stanza. This is phonological symbolism. It tinges the notion of love with a sense of forlornness, which ties in with *grief* and the *empty doorway* (and contrasts with the image of <u>two</u> *lights above the sea*, in the same couplet). Love is not all alone, however, for the vowel does find a distant echo – in stanza one, where it links up with *dumb* (and *thumb*). In fact, the phonological parallels between *love* and *dumb* are quite extensive: not only do they share the same vowel sound, but the opening and closing consonants in both words are articulatorily similar. /l/ and /d/ are both alveolar, while /v/ and /m/ are both labial:

alveolar	shared vowel	labial
/l/	/ʌ/	/v/
/d/	/ʌ/	/m/

The last pattern I would like to examine is the one found within the couplets framing the three stanzas. Each stanza starts and ends with a couplet whose grammatical subject is the same in every case: *A poem* (ll. 1 and 7; 9 and 15; 17 and 23). Note that this parallel extends to the next word, the modal verb *should*, as well. The result is full identity of the first three words in each of these lines: *A poem should*. Each stanza is thus framed by an opening and a closing set of words tying in directly with the semantics of the title itself: "Ars Poetica", the art of poetry.

But something interesting happens when we consider the fourth word in each of the relevant lines (ll. 1 and 7; 9 and 15; 17 and 23). With the exception of line 23, the fourth word is *be*: *A poem should be*. But this pattern is broken in the final couplet of the poem. A contrast is thereby set up as the word *be* gives way to the word *not* in line 23 (*A poem should not*). Observe that the "missing" *be* is not lost altogether, but is postponed for three syllables, to become the last word, and thereby perhaps the most significant word, of the poem itself: *A poem should not mean / But be*.

7. Conclusion

We have now examined some of the linguistic and prosodic features of "Ars Poetica". I hope I have shown that the patterns are there to be found, and that finding them can help illuminate the structure of the poem and thereby amplify the voice by which the poem speaks to us.

As I remarked at the beginning of this essay, many commentators are prone to try to link a given poem to the work of other poets and to events in the life of the poet himself. As I said, I am not opposed to this type of exercise, provided that the search for such external ties does not take the place of an examination of the internal relations within the poem itself.

I referred earlier to two sources (Staudt 1957 and Smith 1975) who find "Keatsian" traits in MacLeish's "Ars Poetica". Smith does not specify what the Keatsian features are, except to say that MacLeish's poem "speaks with a voice ... like that of the Grecian urn" (Smith 1975: 31). Staudt (1957: 28f), however, claims to have found a number of concrete parallels to words and images in Keats's works. Some of these are quite convincing, others less so. For example, he feels that MacLeish's *globed fruit* echoes Keats's *globed peonies* in "Ode on Melancholy". In Keats's "Ode to a Nightingale" Staudt finds a counterpart to *sleeve-worn casements* in the phrase *charmed magic casements*, while *leaning grasses*, we are told, echoes *the alien corn*. In "Ode on a Grecian Urn", Staudt sees in *an empty doorway* an allusion to *emptied of this folk, this pious morn*, while *maple leaf* echoes *what leaf-fringed legend*. He also refers the reader to Keats's "On Seeing the Elgin Marbles" and "Bright Star! Would I were Steadfast as Thou Art" for (very!) loose connections to, respectively, *old medallions*, and *two lights above the sea*.

Let us consider these suggestions in more detail. Lexically, the observed parallels consist of a) two cases of lexical identity (*globed* and *casements*), b) two uses of the same lexical items, but in different forms (*empty* vs. *emptied*, and *maple leaf* vs. *leaf-fringed*), c) a kind of botanical parallel (*leaning grasses* vs. *alien corn*), and finally d) loose thematic links: *old medallions* remind Staudt of the Elgin marbles in the British Museum, and *two lights above the sea* brings to Staudt's mind Keats's final sonnet about a "bright star" (presumably, the moon). These latter associations are, in my view, too vague and general to be given serious consideration. Were we to grant these connections, we could be forced to seek out connections between "Ars Poetica" and every other poem mentioning old man-made objects and heavenly bodies.

Let us therefore restrict our attention to those cases where Staudt sees lexical parallels between "Ars Poetica" and works by Keats. First of all, it should be stressed that the English lexicon, the paint-box of the poet, offers every poet roughly the same words to choose from. Naturally, duplications are inevitable. Thus no one would dream of pointing out that MacLeish has used words such as *and*, *be*, *for*, *of*, *to*, *the*, etc. and that all of these words also appear in Keats's "Ode on a Grecian Urn". These function words are basic elements in English phrases and clauses. But even words with more content, such as *trees*, *leaves*, *moon*, *fruit*, *poem*, and *time*, can hardly be said to be the property of any one poet. Thus I find some of Staudt's lexical comparisons questionable – at least when considered in isolation. This is particularly true of those involving *leaf* and *empty*, not to mention the *leaning corn* vs. *alien grass*. More thought-provoking, however, are the two instances of less common words: *globed* and *casements*. Here, I agree, there may be a faint Keatsian echo, albeit from two different poems.

But Staudt is not finished. He finds in MacLeish's focus on silence and motionlessness an echo of Keats's line, "Thou foster-child of silence and slow time" (Staudt 1957: 29). Here I believe that Staudt is on very firm ground – the connection is well spotted. Keats's line comes from the opening stanza of his "Ode on a Grecian Urn":

> Thou still unravish'd bride of quietness,
>> Thou foster-child of Silence and slow Time,
>
> Sylvan historian, who canst thus express
>> A flowery tale more sweetly than our rhyme:

This is Keats, speaking to a Grecian urn, where time and motion are frozen forever. It is indeed difficult for any reader who is aware of these lines not to link MacLeish and Keats – not to link "Ars Poetica" and "Ode on a Grecian Urn". And having done this, I believe we can take the comparison even further than Staudt does. Keats, in these opening lines, claims that the urn, which is silent and motionless in time, speaks "more sweetly than our rhyme". MacLeish, on the other hand, gives this silent voice to the poem, to poetry itself. Thus his is a mild refutation of the Keatsian claim – a poem's voice *can* compete with that of the urn. In a sense the poem is "equal to" the urn. I believe that the numerous concrete images supplied by MacLeish in "Ars Poetica" can be seen as a kind of poetic counterpart to the concrete scenes depicted on the Grecian urn, and described so poignantly by Keats.

Now, once this connection between the two poems has been established, semantic parallels are strengthened that were at best tenuous before. We now can hear echoes in "Ars Poetica" of such lines in "Ode on a Grecian Urn" as:[10]

---

[10] My citations from "Ode on a Grecian Urn" are taken from *The Complete Poetical Works and Letters of John Keats*, edited by Horace Scudder (1899: 135).

What leaf-fringed legend haunts about thy shape	(l. 5)
Oh happy, happy boughs! that cannot shed	(l. 21)
Your leaves, nor ever bid the Spring adieu;	(l. 22)
What little town by river or sea shore,	(l. 35)
Or mountain-built with peaceful citadel,	(l. 36)
Is emptied of this folk, this pious morn?	(l. 37)
And, little town, thy streets for evermore	(l. 38)
Will silent be; and not a soul to tell	(l. 39)
Why thou art desolate, can e'er return.	(l. 40)
O Attic shape! Fair attitude! with brede	(l. 41)
Of marble men and maidens overwrought,	(l. 42)
With forest branches and the trodden weed;	(l. 43)
'Beauty is truth, truth beauty,' – that is all	(l. 49)
Ye know on earth, and all ye need to know.	(l. 50)

Here the references to leaves and trees and branches, to marble men and maidens, to an empty, desolate town, to truth – all in the same poem about "silence and slow time" – these reverberate heavily through the lines of "Ars Poetica". Even the phrase *trodden weed* seems to find its echo now in MacLeish's *leaning grasses* (far better, in my view, than *the alien corn*, which Staudt takes from a different poem). So Staudt is right: "Ars Poetica" does contain echoes of Keats's "Ode on a Grecian Urn". He is also right about additional echoes from "Ode to a Nightingale". Consider the following excerpts:

Away! away! for I will fly to thee,	(l. 31)
Not charioted by Bacchus and his pards,	
But on the viewless wings of Poesy,	
Though the dull brain perplexes and retards:	
Already with thee! tender is the night,	
And haply the Queen-Moon is on her throne,	
Cluster'd around by all her starry Fays;	
But here there is no light,	
Save what from heaven is with the breezes blown	
Through verdurou glooms and winding mossy ways.	(l. 40)

>   Perhaps the self-same song that found a path   (l. 65)
>   Through the sad heart of Ruth, when, sick for home,
>   She stood in tears amid the alien corn;
>   The same that oft-times hath
>   Charm'd magic casements, opening on the foam
>   Of perilous seas, in faery lands forlorn.   (l. 70)

Here we find a bird, the moon, night, seas, moss and casements. Taken as a whole, these associations lend credence to Staudt's insistence (1957: 29) on the "cumulative value of all these Keatsian reverberations". But I do not side with Staudt in his further claim that these reverberations force us "to insist that whatever conclusions we draw about 'Ars Poetica' should be drawn within the Keats canon and should conform to his position in relation to the nature of poetry" (Staudt 1957: 29). What they establish, in my mind, is simply that we have to do here with an additional set of relations: namely extrinsic connections between one text and other texts. These add a further dimension to the voice of the poem, an extension of the intrinsic relations which we have uncovered within the poem itself. As is well known, a poem speaks to us on many levels. The richer the reader's background, the richer the voice of any given poem. MacLeish's poem stands on its own feet, though it trods the ground that other poets have trod and echoes the voices of those who have gone before. In a nice reversal of who relates to whom, Cleanth Brooks (1975: 151) has suggested that "[t]here is much in the poetry of Keats which suggests that he would have approved of Archibald MacLeish's dictum, 'A poem must not mean / But be'".

Let me conclude with an investigation of one last connection, this one to Archibald MacLeish's own personal history.

We have seen that the moon plays an important role in this poem. It is therefore appropriate to point out that the moon seems to have had a special significance for MacLeish. In fact, the moon appears to have been intimately linked with what MacLeish no doubt viewed as the most significant moment in his life. As I mentioned at the beginning of this paper, MacLeish decided at the age of thirty-one to change his career. He abruptly quit the practice of law, a profession which, by his own account, he was quite good at,[11] packed up his family and headed for Paris to devote his full time to the study and the writing of poetry. MacLeish tells the story in an address which he delivered to the Cosmos Club in Washington, D.C. when he

---

[11] During the last decade of his life, MacLeish allowed himself to be interviewed in an extensive series of tape recordings. Here he spoke frankly, informatively, and eloquently about his life and his views on many topics. The interviews were conducted by Bernard Drabeck and Helen Ellis, who published a verbatim transcription of the tapes in 1986, in a book entitled *Archibald MacLeish – Reflections*. Pages 20-21 contain a description of his years as a young lawyer. What made leaving the profession particularly difficult, MacLeish tells us, was the fact that he was turning out to be "a pretty good lawyer" (Drabeck and Ellis 1986: 20).

was past the age of sixty. The address had the apt title, "Conversation with the Moon".[12] Let us listen to his own account of the fateful evening when that decision was made:

> I know when it happened – a cold, clear, winter evening in February of 1923 when I was five years out of the Great War and four years out of Harvard Law School and trying to support myself and my wife and my two small children by practicing law in a Boston office and teaching a course in Legal Procedure in a night school – trying to find time to write on Saturday afternoons and Sunday mornings when there was a Saturday or a Sunday ...
>
> To go home to Coolidge Hill in Cambridge from the law office on State Street in Boston you walked to Park Street Under, took the subway to Harvard Square and any transportation you could get the rest of the way – usually your own legs. It took half an hour more or less, and you made it with your mind on something else – usually, for me, the witness I'd have on the stand next morning.
>
> That night the ritual changed. When I came out from the narrow downtown streets to the open Common I saw to westward in the icy sky a new moon waiting – seeming in that hastening wind to wait. And when I smelled the familiar subway smell, that warm, moist, fetid, daily exhalation, I knew why. It was for me the moon was waiting. I turned back up the subway stair, crossed Tremont Street between the inching cars and headed west across the Common ... I climbed the Common hill. The moon was waiting still among the bare, black branches ... Charles Street. The Public Garden. Sidewalks empty in the winter wind. The great black elms on Commonwealth before me. I saw the silver silence through the elm trees. (MacLeish 1978: 72ff)

When he got home after that long walk, his wife was distraught. Where had he been? He told her. And he told her of the decision that was pressing in on him – the decision to quit his law practice and his teaching job, and focus on his writing. They talked all night. By morning they were agreed. MacLeish went to his law office that morning and resigned. That summer they moved to Paris, where his wife went back to the singing she had discontinued when they married, and MacLeish started writing poetry in earnest, and providing himself with the literary education he felt he had never received. They did not return to the United States until 1928, two years after the publication of *Streets in the Moon*, containing "Ars Poetica". There can be no doubt that in this poem we can hear the echo of that fateful evening in 1923. So strong was the experience, that the details of that evening remained vivid in the mind of the poet for the rest of his life: "there is always a moon left even when you're old if you will only look for it", says MacLeish. "Conversations with the moon go on and on. Sometimes sixty years or longer" (MacLeish 1978: 80, 81).

---

[12] This address was later published under the title "Autobiographical Information" in MacLeish's *Riders on the Earth – Essays and Recollections* (1978: 69-81). This is my source.

References

Auden, W. H. (1962). *The Dyer's Hand and Other Essays*. London: Faber and Faber.

Bache, C., M. Davenport, J. Dienhart & F. Larsen (1993). *An Introduction to English Sentence Analysis*, second edition (first edition, 1991). Copenhagen: Munksgaard.

Bauer, L., J. Dienhart, H. Hartvigson & L. Kvistgaard Jakobsen (1980). *American English Pronunciation*. Copenhagen: Gyldendal.

Bergman, D. & D. Epstein (eds) (1983). *The Heath Guide to Poetry*. Lexington, Massachusetts: D. C. Heath & Company.

Brooks, C. (1975). *The Well Wrought Urn – Studies in the Structure of Poetry*. New York: Harcourt, Brace & World (first published 1947).

Donoghue, D. (ed). (1975). *Seven American Poets – From MacLeish to Nemerov, An Introduction*. Minneapolis: University of Minnesota Press (first published 1963).

Dienhart, J. (1989). "Form and Function in Ted Hughes's Poem 'The Jaguar'". *English Studies* 70/3, 248-252.

Dienhart, J. (1994). "Phonological Ingenuity in 'Five Songs' by W. H. Auden". In F. G. Andersen and L. O. Sauerberg (eds) *Traditions and Innovations – Papers Presented to Andreas Haarder* (*PEO Special Issue*) Odense University, 63-102.

Drabeck, B. & H. Ellis (eds) (1986). *Archibald MacLeish – Reflections*. Amherst: University of Massachusetts Press.

Falk, S. (1965). *Archibald MacLeish*. New York: Twayne Publishers, Inc.

Housman, A. E. (1933). *The Name and Nature of Poetry* (The Leslie Stephen Lecture, delivered at Cambridge on May 9, 1933). Cambridge: Cambridge University Press.

Longman Dictionary of Contemporary English. (1978). London: Longman Group Limited.

Lynn, S. (1994). *Texts and Contexts – Writing about Literature with Critical Theory*. New York: Harper Collins College Publishers.

MacLeish, A. (1926). *Streets in the Moon*. Boston: Houghton Mifflin Company.

MacLeish, A. (1952). *Collected Poems – 1917-1952*. Boston: Houghton Mifflin Company.

MacLeish, A. (1972). *The Human Season – Selected Poems 1926-1972*. Boston: Houghton Mifflin Company.

MacLeish, A. (1978). *Riders on the Earth – Essays and Recollections*. Boston: Houghton Mifflin Company.

Perkins, D. (1987). *A History of Modern Poetry: Modernism and After.* Cambridge, Massachusetts: The Belknap Press of Harvard University Press, 47-52.

Perkins, G., S. Bradley, R. Beatty & E. Long (eds) (1985). *The American Tradition in Literature*, sixth edition (first edition 1956). New York: Random House.

Scudder, H. (ed) (1899). *The Complete Poetical Works and Letters of John Keats*. Cambridge: Houghton Mifflin Company.

Smith, G. (1975). "Archibald MacLeish". In Donoghue (ed) *Seven American Poets – From MacLeish to Nemerov, An Introduction*, Minneapolis: University of Minnesota Press, 16-54.

Staudt, V. (1957). "'Ars Poetica' and the Teacher". *College English* 19, 28-29.

Untermeyer, L. (ed) (1962). *Modern American Poetry*. New York: Harcourt, Brace & World, Inc.

The English Progressive

Per Durst-Andersen

1. Introductory remarks

The present topic has been selected for several reasons. First, it forms part of English verbal semantics, which is an area to which Niels Davidsen-Nielsen has made major contributions (e.g. Davidsen-Nielsen 1990). Secondly, the progressive vs. non-progressive distinction in English has been treated along the same lines as the perfective vs. imperfective distinction in Russian, which I think is wrong. Thirdly, the distinction between lexical semantics and aspectual semantics is not always as clear in English linguistics as I feel it should be. In the following I shall attempt to present some of the main results of an analysis of the English progressive which is meant to overcome most of the difficulties of previous theories.

2. Two types of aspectual systems

If we compare the acquisition of tense forms by Danish children and the acquisition of similar forms by English children, we observe a striking difference (cf. Durst-Andersen 1984). What seems amazing at first sight is that Danish children very early acquire the distinction between the present perfect (e.g. *har spildt* 'has spilt') and the imperfect (e.g. *spildte* 'spilt') and that from the very beginning these two forms are used side by side, whereas English children initially have no distinction between the corresponding two English past forms, thus letting the simple past (≈ imperfect) act as a substitute for the present perfect. Instead they have two present tense forms: a progressive and a non-progressive form (see e.g. Bloom et al. 1980, Fletcher 1985, Gathercole 1986, C. Johnson 1985, Rispoli & Bloom 1985).

The Danish child's initial grammar can be said to be identical to the Russian child's (cf. Gvozdev 1949): it has one present tense form (which is used by the Danish child as the imperfective present in Russian) and two past tense forms, viz. the present perfect which is used as the perfective preterite in Russian as well as the imperfect which is used as the imperfective preterite in Russian (cf. Durst-Andersen 1984). As we see, the initial Russian and Danish child-grammar involves two oppositions: one of tense, and another of aspect, which is restricted to past tense forms. The given system can be regarded as being a representative of a prototype system (This appears very clearly from the great number of languages examined by Dahl (1985) on the basis of identical questionnairies). If we return to the acquisition of past tense forms in English, we may say that an early acquisition of the present perfect must be blocked by the aspectual system developed by the English child within the present tense. Thus since the initial English child-grammar has the aspectual distinction within the present tense and no such distinction in the past tense, it seems as if this system represents another prototype which should be distinguished from the above-mentioned one.

Both prototype systems consist of three forms which enter into two oppositions – one of aspect and another of tense. They differ however in the way the three forms are distributed in the structure. The initial Danish child-grammar has the aspectual distinction anchored in the past tense, whereas the English aspectual distinction is rooted in the present tense. This is tantamount to saying that the aspectual distinction in English is acquired before the past vs. non-past distinction. Since this is the case and since the aspectual distinction made by the Danish child occurs simultaneously with the past vs. non-past distinction, it makes sense to claim what has been generally accepted since Slobin 1977, namely that aspectual notions have greater accessibility to children than temporal distinctions. It seems, however, that the progressive vs. non-progressive distinction in English is more accessible than the perfective vs. non-perfective distinction or that the grammar behind the semantic distinction in English is more natural and obvious for children. This is furthermore supported by the fact that the English child does not overgeneralize the use of ING-forms – at least not to an extent that is striking for child linguists (see Mapstone and Harris 1985). One might of course say that an overgeneralization is almost impossible in English, since – as Dahl (1985: 94) and Comrie (1976: 32) point out – in comparison with other languages having the same kind of aspect the English progressive is an 'overgeneralization' of uses found in other languages. The point, however, is – and here Mapstone and Harris (1985) agree – that English children never extend ING-forms to state verbs which have no possibility of taking this form or seldomly do, e.g. *believe, belong, contain, hate, know, like, need, possess, relate, want*, etc. (cf. Kuczaj 1978).

The conclusion to be drawn is that a grammar of the progressive aspect should be able to explain that the progressive vs. non-progressive distinction is even more obvious and even more easily acquired than the perfective vs. non-perfective distinction, and moreover, be capable of explaining why and how children manage to avoid expanding ING-forms to verbs which do not accept this form, and, finally, be able to explain how it is possible for English children to generalize the initial grammar of ING-forms to an extent that it seems almost impossible to find a simple theory that can describe and explain all uses of this form in a consistent way. In the following sections I shall come up with some solutions to these problems, but before that I want to dwell a little bit on the main tradition in English linguistics.

3. On the traditional approach

It turns out that the majority of linguists who have been concerned with the progressive vs. non-progressive distinction in English from a more general perspective consider the progressive aspect as having something to do with the temporal distinction or contour of an event (Hockett 1957: 237), with the internal temporal constituency of a situation (Comrie 1976), with reference to one of the temporally distinct phases in the evolution of an event through time (M. Johnson 1981: 152), or with the relation of an event or state to a particular reference point located before, after, around (i.e. the progressive aspect) or simply at a particular point in time (J. M. Anderson 1973: 39). This view which implies that aspect is treated as a kind of relative or secondary tense concerned with the internal time structure of a situation makes it possible to view the progressive and imperfective aspects as being tokens of the same type – a type which is called 'imperfectivity' by Comrie (1976), Brinton (1987) and Freed (1979), or 'durativity' by Friedrich (1974) and Verkuyl (1972).

By taking the progressive aspect in English and the imperfective aspect in Russian as being different manifestations of a universal semantic primitive, one ignores not only linguistic evidence from first language acquisition (cf. section 2), but also certain signs from languages having these two aspects. Thus it is not a coincidence that the progressive aspect is the marked member of the opposition in English, whereas the perfective aspect is the marked member of the opposition in Russian. What is marked will – as I see it – always be a symptom of the ontogenesis of the category itself: the marked member will indicate the mental basis of the origin of the linguistic category itself. If we pursue this way of thinking, we may conclude that the origin of the progressive vs. non-progressive distinction must be totally different from the origin of the perfective vs. non-perfective distinction. This follows from the fact that the progressive aspect is marked in English, whereas the perfective aspect is marked in Russian. These two systems are simply grounded on a different mental basis. One cannot simply lump together the progressive and imperfective aspects under the same heading, because the progressive aspect is a positive manifestation of what is mentally obvious and natural for a child to arrive at as a hypothesis about a situation in the *present* world, whereas the imperfective aspect is a negative definition of the perfective aspect, which in itself is a positive manifestation of what is mentally obvious and natural for a child to make as a hypothesis about a situation in the *past* world. That the progressive and imperfective aspect have common uses should not astonish us, since both grammatical categories divide the same discourse universe into two parts – in that way they cannot but share some part of it. It should, however, be noted that the basic meaning of the present progressive (cf. *He is always smoking*) and the basic meaning of the simple present tense form (cf. *He always smokes*) are in fact covered by the present tense of the imperfective aspect in Russian (cf. *On vsegda kurit*) and could never be used in the perfective aspect. In other words, the Russian imperfective aspect seems to jump over the aspectual distinction made by the English language. This observation is crucial.

Against this background it is predictable that theories about the progressive vs.

non-progressive distinction in English which borrow feature oppositions proposed for the Russian language and just invert the marking relations have nothing substantial to add to our understanding of the progressive aspect from a theoretical point of view, despite the fact that they may give us some new insight. This is, for instance, true of Bache (1986 and 1995) and Smith (1983 and 1991) who both use the feature '[totality]' which is well-known from the literature on Russian aspect. They both assign [-totality] to the progressive form and [+totality] to the simple form. I here ignore the fact that in Bache 1986 [+totality] is understood as external situational forms, and [-totality] as internal situational forms and that Bache also uses other feature oppositions in order to account for non-standard uses of the progressive aspect. It is argued that the feature [-totality] assigned to the progressive aspect, the marked member of the opposition, implies an internal perspective from which the endpoints of an event is ignored. If one did not know that Smith and Bache were talking about the progressive aspect in English, one could have believed that they were talking about the Russian imperfective aspect, because this is exactly the standard definition of the Russian imperfective aspect.

Although, admittedly, it is tempting to see all languages as being different varieties of the same invariant, or manifestations of two different choices of prominence, it is nevertheless a distortion of both English aspect and Russian aspect to put them under the same heading (see Dahl 1985: 92f for some general arguments against this identification). There is, however, another important reason for rejecting the totality-theory proposed by Smith and Bache – which is comparable with the incompleteness-theory proposed by Jespersen (1924 and 1931) and continued and further developed by Reichenbach (1947), John M. Anderson (1973), and Brinton (1988) and which is found in the majority of works on English aspect. Despite the fact that the theory is intuitively appealing to linguists, because [-totality] seems to imply all what can be attributed to the progressive form, i.e. incompleteness and duration in general as well as in the specific sense that event time extends over reference time (cf. Reichenbach 1947 and Saurer 1984), it fails simply because the theory can in no way account for the fact that the progressive aspect is acquired as the first verbal category by English children: the negatively defined feature should suggest that the positively marked member of the opposition, i.e. the simple aspect, was acquired before the progressive and was more obvious and natural for a child.

English aspectologists make a distinction which is important to our understanding of the ontogenesis of the progressive aspect. They sharply differentiate *standard uses* and *non-standard uses*. They assign non-standard uses of ING-forms to state verbs and standard uses to all other verbs which are subsumed, respectively, under events by Smith (1983) and under dynamic situations by Lyons (1977). The singling out of state verbs seems to be very important. As pointed out, for instance by Brown (1973: 363ff) and Fletcher (1985: 120ff) early English child language shows no ING-forms in connection with state verbs. This seems plausible enough, since verbs like *believe, belong, contain, hate, know, like, possess, relate* and *want* either do not take ING-forms or – if they take – create highly special effects, i.e. are felt to be highly marked by English speakers. I need to point out that in some varieties of English some of the verbs mentioned here cannot occur with the ING-form – British English is an exception in this regard, cf. Mapstone and Harris 1985. There are, however, some state verbs which very easily and without being felt to be 'marked' occur with ING-forms. This concerns, for instance, *lie, sleep, stand, sit*, etc.

The first child-grammar of ING-forms should thus exclude state verbs, but at the same time be capable of explaining why some verbs can occur and other cannot occur with ING-forms. Although Brown (1973: 374) explains this by dividing state verbs into voluntary (e.g. *sit* and *stand*) and involuntary state verbs (e.g. *know* and *need*) – which seems to be a natural distinction for a child to make – I do not think that this conceptual distinction is the real one – it is rather a concomitant effect of the real distinction which I shall try to explicate below.

Before doing so I want to mention some works on the English progressive which, unfortunately, have lead an unnoticed life – perhaps, because these works, in fact, do not propose a complete theory. Hatcher (1951) distinguishes verbs denoting overt activity which most frequently occur in the expanded form, and verbs denoting covert activity which most frequently occur in the simple form. Andersen et al. (1978) assign a special kind of description to the ING-form in the present tense which implies that the situation referred to by the verb with an ING-form is characterized in 'an immediately recognizable manner'. The theory proposed by Andersen et al. (1978) is more or less identical to the theories found in Woisetschlaeger 1985 [1976] and Goldsmith & Woisetschlaeger 1982 as well as in Conrad & Schousboe 1989.

4. The ontogenesis of the progressive vs. non-progressive distinction in English

I assume that the first verb class distinction to be made by the English child is the activity vs. state distinction. This distinction is drawn by means of receiving and recognizing two different kinds of pictures, viz. *stable* and *unstable pictures*. Since unstable pictures play a more prominent and salient role for the child (Weisstein & Wong 1986), I propose to substitute the activity vs. non-activity distinction for the traditional stativity vs. non-stativity distinction, which does not predict that activities are more important to the child – quite on the contrary. The unstable pictures will be prominent because besides a stable element they have an extra element in comparison with stable pictures which are stable throughout. This corresponds to the fact that an activity in reality is always produced against the background of a certain state. In other words, both a state and an activity involve a figure-ground relationship, but besides that an activity also involves what I call a *primary figure*, i.e. the perceptual counterpart of the notion of topic.

It is my hypothesis that the distinction between stable and unstable pictures, which matches the distinction between states and activities, forms the very basis of the child's acquisition of the progressive vs. non-progressive distinction. When an English child is confronted with an utterance involving an ING-form of verbs such as *playing*, *crying*, *walking*, *doing*, *cooking*, *drinking*, *smiling*, *laughing*, *climbing*, *stepping*, *touching* or *ironing* it will either be the case – depending on who is performing the activity referred to by the verb – that at the moment of speech the child is receiving an unstable picture (e.g. *Mommy/Daddy is drinking*) or that the child is being looked at by the speaker when it is performing an activity (e.g. *Stevie is walking*). At the same time, an English child observes that when Mommy or Daddy are producing utterances involving a simple form in the present tense (e.g. *want*, *need*, *know*, *hear*, *like*, etc.) it either receives a stable picture in which only part of the situation referred to is present (e.g. *Stevie like(s) that cake*) or it simply does not receive any picture which could have something to do with the situation referred to (e.g. *Stevie want(s) to eat?*).

The child will only construct a grammar of two forms if its *here-and-now analysis* gives different answers when applied to utterances which involve the two 'conflicting' forms – in this case the ING-form and the NON-ING-form (cf. Durst-Andersen 1984). I suggest that the child's grammar of ING-forms is constructed on the basis of receiving an unstable picture simultaneously with auditorily receiving an utterance which involves an ING-form. When confronted with an ING-form the child will ask the following question: What is the case exactly at the moment of speech? The child will receive the following answer: It is the case that I am receiving an unstable picture of the situation referred to by the verb (It is an activity verb). When the same analysis is applied to NON-ING-forms, he will receive the opposite answer: it is not the case that I am receiving a picture of the situation referred to by the verb (It is a state verb). In this way, the ING-form is coupled to activity verbs and NON-ING-forms to state verbs. But what is more important, the ING-form becomes associated with pictures being received by the child and NON-ING-forms with non-pictures. This association is not only important for our understanding of the mental basis of the generalization of ING-forms, but also for our understanding of the English language as a representative of image-based languages.

5. The ideal vs. real grammar of the English progressive

The perceptually based acquisition of ING-forms explains in a natural manner why children use ING-forms in connection with activity verbs and why the progressive vs. non-progressive distinction is learnt very early and very easily – and before the perfective vs. non-perfective distinction which is conceptually based. The theory, however, has other advantages. It explains why certain state verbs cannot occur with ING-forms and why certain state verbs can or simply must occur with ING-forms given the appropriate conditions for using this form. Thus it is predictable that state verbs which refer to situations that cannot be visualized are not capable of taking the ING-form, i.e. *know, believe, possess, own, need, relate*, etc. (But when the situation becomes visualizable it becomes possible for one to use the verbs just mentioned, cf. *She is knowing more and more*). State verbs which refer to situations that normally are visualizable take the ING-form without any difficulty, cf. *She is sitting over there!* In other words, *She is sitting over there* is uttered when the speaker has a picture of the situation he is referring to at the moment of speech. As we see, this is a generalization of the initial child-grammar because the picture being received by the speaker is stable.

From the grammar just proposed it is furthermore predictable that when ING-forms are used in the so-called non-standard uses they will either have a *visualization effect* (cf. 1) or an *activity-creating effect* (cf. 2) on the hearer.

(1) ... when you turn the corner, the statue of Nelson is standing right in the middle of Trafalgar Square.

In (1) the ING-form conveys to the hearer that when he turns the corner, he will *see* the statue of Nelson, i.e. the speaker has placed himself in the hearer's place and is on his way to the statue together with the hearer. This is not implicated by the simple form (cf. *When you turn the corner, the statue of Nelson stands in the middle of Trafalgar Square*) which is a pure instruction.

(2) You are being foolish now.

The utterance conventionally implicates that the person behaves like a fool and that this appears from the picture the speaker is receiving. In that way one might say that the progressive aspect presents the situation denoted by the verb as being a quality of a picture, and not a quality of a person which is taken care of by the simple form (cf. *You are foolish*). Note here that the notions of agency and control assigned by Smith to an utterance like (2), viz. *He is being polite* (cf. Smith 1983: 487) has nothing to do with the ING-form itself, but with the quality of politeness which in all normal worlds is a kind of behaviour controlled and consciously evoked by a person. The ING-form only presents the possessor of the given quality as one who produces politeness. This suggests that the voluntary vs. involuntary distinction among state verbs has no real existence in English, although it can in fact explain the majority of data representing non-standard uses of the progressive aspect.

After having based the ontogenesis as well as the phylogenesis of the progressive aspect on the sense of vision and having linked it to unstable pictures corresponding to activity situations in reality, it seems plausible for a child to expand the distinction to other senses as well. As a matter of fact, there is evidence for such an extension:

(3) The meat is smelling good.

It appears that (3) can be seen as a description of an olfactory picture which is being received by the speaker at the very moment of speech – here the meat is looked upon as a producer or an activator of that olfactory picture, i.e. it is an active source. One might say that the utterance is an index of the speaker's olfactory picture which in itself is an icon of a situation. Moreover, the fact that the speaker is receiving a picture makes him an active experiencer. All these qualities are totally absent in the simple form of the same verb:

(4)   The meat smells good.

This utterance is not a description of an olfactory picture, but a characterization of the meat – the meat is assigned a certain property by the speaker on the basis of a subjective olfactory experience.

It seems as if states based on experience in general may be treated as if they were sense impressions:

(5)   Jennifer is hating her uncle.

This utterance not only conveys that Jennifer is producing hate, but also that her emotional experience of her uncle or her feelings towards him are permanently present on her emotional screen – to an extent that her hate is visible to others. The same appears from the following example (from Smith 1983: 491):

(6)   I have been wanting to talk to you for a long time.

Here the speaker presents himself as having been an active experiencer of a certain wish which can be complied with now. It is as if his wish had been present for a long time on his 'screen of desires' whereby all other desires are felt literally to be backgrounded.

As we see from (6), there is no visualization effect on the hearer, because *want* cannot be visualized. This effect, however, seems to be replaced by an internal *screen-making effect* accompanied by an activity-creating effect. This replacement might be restricted to utterances which involve the first person:

(7)   I am feeling cold.
(8)   Are you feeling cold?

(7) need not imply that the hearer or hearers receive an unstable picture where the speaker is trembling out of cold. This seems, however, to be the case, when for instance one asks the question presented as (8) (see Andersen et al. 1978 for a further discussion).

Up to now I have confined myself to a description of the meaning conveyed by ING-forms in connection with state and activity verbs in the present tense – on which the progressive vs. non-progressive distinction is grounded. But already at this stage it should be obvious that a grammar of the progressive aspect cannot be straightforward due to the extension of this form to all verbs. In other words, if we just assign the grammar a feature opposition, the grammar will be an idealized grammar – a grammar which only explains ideal data, not real data. In that respect, all previous grammars of the progressive aspect are more or less idealized grammars which are only felt intuitively adequate if the right data occur to the reader. For instance, I find it extremely difficult to see that the data presented so far should convey duration (see e.g. Miller and Johnson-Laird 1976: 438 and Lyons 1977: 687) or that the progressive aspect presents an interior perspective from which the endpoints of the event (in Smiths's terms) is ignored (Smith 1983). If we take the feature [-totality] assigned to the progressive aspect by Smith and Bache, it seems to me that the feature involved could also be [+totality], since the progressive aspect views the situation indirectly referred to as a picture of the total situation. Contrary to this, I find it more easy to understand why Barwise and Perry (1983: 35 and 288f) find that the progressive is deictic in that it refers to a specific point in time. Although ING-forms are not tense forms – as suggested by them – it is true that they are felt to be deictic. This is, however, not an inherent property of the form itself, but a concomitant effect of the fact that the ING-form presents the situation denoted by the verb as being a quality or a property of a picture – and since a picture is always confined to a specific situation in reality, and to a specific point in time, it automatically gets a deictic connotation. Note that when you look at a picture you frame reality and the situation pictured (corresponding to *writing* in (9)) seems to continue, seems to extend over a real event (corresponding to *entered* in (9)) which enters into the frame created by the picture itself (cf. Jespersen's frame-theory):

(9)   He was writing a letter, when I entered the room.

In (9), which represents a piece of ideal data for previous grammars, it makes sense to say that the ING-form refers to an incompleted action, presents an action as an ongoing process, or that event time extends over reference time (cf. Reichenbach 1947 and Soga 1983: 6f). This suggests that previous grammars should be able to explain the meaning of progressive aspect in connection with action verbs which – in opposition to state verbs – are a natural extension of the progressive aspect, since action verbs contain a natural reference to activities and therefore create unstable pictures (for further discussion, see Durst-Andersen 1992). But, unfortunatley, it is not possible to assign the meaning of an ongoing process to all action verbs without distorting data. Admittedly, it is true of many utterances involving ING-forms:

(10a)   He is reading a book.
(10b)   She is explaining her hypothesis.

Here the progressive aspect can be said to present the action as an ongoing process by assigning the truth-value "T" to the activity description and "F" to the state description (which completes the description). However, this does not apply to the following utterances:

(11a)   He is starting his lecture now.
(11b)   I am leaving tomorrow.

64 *Per Durst-Andersen*

Here the ING-form conveys the meaning of a planned action – i.e. it is either intended by the person himself (it is agent-desired) or by the world (it is world-desired). Nor does it apply to utterances such as the following:

(12a)   She is convincing him now.

(12b)   He is dying.

Here the ING-form conveys the meaning of an approaching event. Although there is a certain correlation between these three meanings and my distinction between three subclasses of action verbs, i.e. implementation verbs, punctual verbs, and attainment verbs (cf. Durst-Andersen 1992: 153ff), the hypothesis of identity between a specific meaning of the ING-form and a specific subclass of verbs seems to fall to ground when it appears that one and the same verb can have all three meanings:

(13a)   Mr. Jones is taking her home (*planned action*).

(13b)   Mr. Jones is taking the oath (*ongoing process*).

(13c)   Mr. Jones is taking the prize (*approaching event*).

This suggests that what matters in English is not the single verb – as it is in Russian where the meaning of aspect is predictable from the verb itself – but the whole verb phrase (a finding which is implicit in Vendler (1967), but explicit and distorted in Saurer (1984). Another and better way of putting it is that the meaning of the ING-form is dependent on that situation in reality that the utterance is a symbolic representation of. If ING-forms are based on unstable pictures, it is predictable that *start* and *leave* cannot be used to convey the meaning of an ongoing process, because they have no separate activity at all – they are punctual verbs where the very activity marks the change itself. 'Starting and leaving situations' may, however, be visualized. If one does that the picture becomes all those visual stimuli being received prior to the actual change and which leave you with an impression of a person who is about to do something. This appears quite clearly from the following question:

(14)   Are you leaving?

This question is asked by the speaker because the hearer is doing something which leaves the impression that he is about to leave. What the hearer is doing is received by the speaker as a visual picture which is unstable. By linking the physical preconditions for leaving and starting and all other punctual actions, it seems natural to extend them to the phychological preconditions for performing an action, viz. an action which is planned and scheduled. Note here the screen-making effect again.

The same applies to verbs like *convincing* and *dying*. In order to visualize an understanding of these actions on the basis of what is happening in reality, one has to be very near the change of state. In other words, the visual stimuli should leave you the impression that the person is about to change his opinion or is about to leave the world. If the ING-form were based on a conceptional understanding of the world, the meaning of the ING-form in connection with these two attainment verbs would have been that of an ongoing process, i.e. a certain person was trying to make another person change his opinion. The fact that the meaning of the ING-form in (12) is that of an approaching event thus supports the claim that the progressive aspect is based on unstable pictures and frames the whole situation in a single total picture.

6. On the propositional and discourse semantics of the two aspectual forms

If we want a non-idealizing grammar of the progressive and non-progressive aspect, we have to say that ING-forms and NON-ING-forms of the same verb denote the same situation, but present it in different ways.

To sit and *to be sitting* both name a state where somebody is located in a particular way at a certain place. But they differ in the way they present this state. The simple form presents the state referred to as a property of a person, whereas the progressive form presents the state referred to as a property of a picture. This means that *He sits there* is a characterization of a certain person – you characterize him by ascribing him a certain quality. In the example *He is sitting there* you describe the situation being received as a picture.

To smoke and *to be smoking* both name an activity where somebody produces a certain kind of activity based on a certain state where somebody has something in his mouth. But whereas *He smokes* presents this activity as being a property of that person, *He is smoking* presents the activity referred to as a property of a picture. The simple form thus characterizes this person by ascribing him a certain quality – he is qualified as a person, who produces smoking activity, be it sometimes, often or always. This use has been called *dispositional use* and has been said to be equivalent to *He is a smoker*. This is, however, not true, since this utterance is a categorization of that person – i.e. he is included in a set which consists of all members sharing the property of producing smoking-activity. In the case of the progressive utterance, we are neither talking about characterization nor categorization. When using the progressive form the speaker describes the situation being received as a total picture. Note that the visualization effect also occurs if the utterance is separated from the here-and-now by adding *always*:

(15)   He is always smoking.

This utterance can be paraphrased as follows:

(15´)   'Whenever I see him, he is producing smoking-activity'.

To kill and *to be killing* name the same complex situation, viz. that somebody is producing an activity which implies a state, where somebody is not on world-location anymore. *He kills people* presents the action referred to as being a property of that person whereby the speaker characterizes the person by ascribing him a certain quality: he is qualified as a person, who produces killing. This use can be compared with the so-called experiential use of the present perfect:

(16)   He has been in the army.

Here one refers to a past state, but presents it as being a present property of that person. This qualification has been true, since he was in the army, and is therefore also true at the very moment of speech. *He is killing people*, however, presents the action referred to as a property of a total picture being received or which can be received under the appropriate conditions. This utterance is thus a description of a situation which has a visual copy.

What has been called the habitual use of the simple form, in fact, has nothing to do with the form itself (for a historical overview of different treatments of the habitual meaning assigned to English verbal forms, see Brinton 1987). The 'habitual reading' of utterances involving the simple present tense forms is a side-effect of the characterization-function of this form. All characterizations are based on a series of past experiences pointing in the same direction. The habitual reading is thus a consequence of the hearer's own inferences – it is an implicature. If one wants to assign habituality to a certain construction in English, it should be the construction 'to be used to', not the simple form itself.

7. Summing up

The basic properties of the grammar just outlined makes it not only natural for people to create such a category, but also natural for children to learn it quickly and easily without violating the grammar itself. The basic properties are moreover capable of explaining non-standard uses of the ing-form – uses which can be regarded as the outcome of the pressure from the original unequivocal system based on the prominent role of unstable pictures. This pressure has been so strong that the possibilities of the system have been exploited to the outmost. The grammar proposed, however, has another advantage since it is in accordance with the typological grammar of English. It does not violate the leading principle of the English language which views reality as an internal representation in mind – it rather stresses the existence of such a principle. Thus both forms are based on an internal frame of reference. The simple form has a mental frame of reference – it refers to a mental situation corresponding to an inference based on the speaker's internalized experiences of situations in reality. The propositional content described by an utterance involving a simple form is true of the speaker's world. The progressive form has a visual (or mental screen-like) frame of reference – it directly refers to a picture being received, and only indirectly to the situation giving rise to the picture. The utterance gets access to reality via the picture. That the propositions created by verbs involving ING-forms can be said to be true with respect to certain situations in reality is therefore due to the fact that the received pictures are icons of situations in reality.

It should be pointed out that the proposed theory seems to be supported by evidence from a test conducted by Cynthia Johnson (1985). She had small children attend a puppet show and asked them to tell a story against this background. The children told their story in a way which was not anticipated by the author of the article. To the investigator's surprise the children widely used the progressive aspect of the present perfect tense form. What the children did was, however, what Johnson specifically said in her instruction to them: "Tell me what you have been seeing".

References

Andersen, J. E. et al. (1978). Pragmatics of the simple and expanded present. A speech act analysis. In G. Caie et al. (eds) *Occasional Papers 1976-1977*, Copenhagen: Akademisk forlag, 12-63.

Anderson, J. M. (1971). *An essay concerning aspect* (= Janua Linguarum, 167). The Hague: Mouton.

Bache, C. (1985). *Verbal aspect: a general theory and its application to present-day English.* Odense: Odense University Press.

Bache, C. (1995). *The study of aspect, tense and action. Towards a theory of the semantics of grammatical categories.* Frankfurt am Main: Peter Lang.

Bloom, L. M., K. Liffer & J. Haffitz (1980). Semantics of verbs and the development of verb inflections in child language. *Language* 56, 386-412.

Brinton, L. J. (1987). The aspectual nature of states and habits. *Folia Linguistica* 21, 195-214.

Brinton, L. J. (1988). *The development of English aspectual systems* (= Cambridge Studies in Linguistics, 49). Cambridge: Cambridge University Press.

Brown, R. (1973). *A first language. The early stages.* London: Allen & Unwin.

Comrie, B. (1976). *Aspect. An introduction to the study of verbal aspect and related problems.* Cambridge: Cambridge University Press.

Conrad, B. & S. Schousboe (1989). *Meaning and English grammar.* Copenhagen: University of Copenhagen.

Dahl, Ö. (1985). *Tense and aspect systems.* Oxford: Basil Blackwell.

Davidsen-Nielsen, N. (1990). *Tense and mood in English. A comparison with Danish.* Berlin & New York: Mouton de Gruyter.

Durst-Andersen, P. (1984). The acquisition of tense in Danish: Strategies and cognitive capacities. *Proceedings from Child Language Symposium*, Lund, May 17-19, Lund: Lund University, 18-29.

Durst-Andersen, P. (1992). *Mental grammar. Russian aspect and related issues.* Columbus, Ohio: Slavica.

Fletcher, P. (1985). *A child's learning of English.* Oxford: Basil Blackwell.

Freed, A. F. (1979). *The semantics of English aspectual complementation*. Dordrect: Reidel.

Friedrich, P. (1974). On aspect theory and homeric aspect. *International Journal of American Linguistics, memoir 28*.

Gathercole, V. C. (1986). The acquisition of the present perfect: explaining differences in the speech of Scottish and American children. *Journal of Child Language* 13, 537-60.

Givón, T. (1984). *Syntax. A functional-typological introduction. Vol. I*. Amsterdam: John Benjamins.

Goldsmith, J. & E. Woisetschlaeger (1982). The logic of the progressive aspect. *Linguistic Inquiry* 13, 79-89.

Gvozdev, A. N. (1949). *Formirovanie u rebenka grammatičeskogo stroja russkogo jazyka. Čast' pervaja i vtoraja*. Moskva: Izd. Akademii pedagogičeskich nauk RSFSR.

Hatcher, A. G. (1951). The use of the progressive form in English: a new approach. *Language* 27, 254-80.

Hockett, C. F. (1958). *A course in modern linguistics*. New York: Macmillan Publishing CO.

Jespersen, O. (1924). *The philosophy of grammar*. New York: H. Holt.

Jespersen, O. (1931). *A modern English grammar on historical principles*. Part IV. London: Allen & Unwin.

Johnson, C. J. (1985). The emergence of present perfect verb forms: semantic influences on selective imitation. *Journal of Child Language* 12, 325-52.

Johnson, M. R. (1981). A unified temporal theory of tense and aspect. In P. Tedeschi & A. Zaenen (eds) *Tense and aspect* (= Syntax and Semantics, 14), New York: Academic Press, 145-75.

Kuczaj, S. (1978). Why do children fail to over-generalize the progressive inflection? *Journal of Child Language* 5, 167-71.

Lyons, J. (1977). *Semantics Vol. 2*. Cambridge: Cambridge University Press.

Mapstone, E. R. & P. L. Harris (1985). Is the English present progressive unique? *Journal of Child Language* 12, 433-41.

Mufwene, S. S. (1984). *Stativity and the progressive*. Bloomington: Indiana University Linguistics Club.

Reichenbach, H. (1947). *Elements of symbolic logic*. New York: The Free Press.

Rispoli, M. & L. Bloom (1985). *Incomplete and continuing: theoretical issues in the acquisition of tense and aspect*. Journal of Child Language 12, 471-74.

Saurer, W. (1984). *A formal semantics of tense, aspect and aktionsarten*. Bloomington: Indiana University Linguistics Club.

Slobin, D. I. (1977). Language change in the childbook and in history. In J. Macnamara (ed) *Language learning and thought*. New York: Academic Press, 185-214.

Smith, C. S. (1983). A theory of aspectual choice. *Language* 59, 479-501.

Smith, C. S. (1991). *The parameter of aspect*. Dordrecht: Kluwer Academic Press.

Vendler, Z. (1967). *Linguistics in Philosophy*. Ithaca, New York: Cornell University Press.

Verkuyl, H. J. (1972). *On the compositional nature of the aspects.* Dordrecht: Reidel.

Vlach, F. (1981). The semantics of the progressive. In P. Tedeschi & A. Zaenen (eds) *Tense and aspect* (= Syntax and Semantics, 14), New York: Academic Press, 271-91.

Weisstein, N. & E. Wong. (1986). Figure-ground organization and the spatial and temporal responses of the visual system. In E. C. Schwab & H. C. Nusbaum (eds) *Pattern recognition by humans and machines. Vol. 2: Visual perception,* New York: Academic Press, 31-64.

Woisetschlaeger, E. F. (1985) [1976]. *A semantic theory of the English auxiliary system.* New York & London: Garland Publishing, Inc.

Remarks on *if, when* and *where*

Dorrit Faber and Finn Sørensen

1. Introduction

Embedded clauses containing *if, when* and *where* as complementizers are used frequently in legal texts. A sample of such use is given in (1):

(1) **Where** a person has entered into a contract after a misrepresentation has been made to him otherwise than fraudulently, and he would be entitled by reason of the misrepresentation, to rescind the contract, then **if** it is claimed, ..., that the contract ought to be or has been rescinded the court may declare the contract subsisting and award damages in lieu of rescission, **if** of opinion that it would be equitable to do so ... (From: Misrepresentation Act 1967, s 2(2)).

Each use of such a sentence expresses a circumstantial condition on possible state-of-affairs within the domain regulated by the statute in question. But what does it mean to say that an embedded clause is used to convey 'circumstantial conditions' on the state-of-affairs described by the embedding sentence? Even though the use of *if, when* and *where* points to a rather simple distinction between conditions as such, temporal conditions, and locational conditions, it is easy to find examples where the use of either *if, when* or *where* seems to result in very closely related circumstantial conditions, cf. the following versions which are based on (1):

(2) The court may declare a contract subsisting and award damages in lieu of rescission
    (a) when it is claimed that the contract ought to be or has been rescinded.
    (b) where it is claimed that the contract ought to be or has been rescinded.
    (c) if it is claimed that the contract ought to be or has been rescinded.

Why are (2a) - (2c) almost synonymous, which we think they are, the court's power to uphold the contract and award damages being the same irrespective of the choice of either *if, when* or *where*? So in spite of the intuition about the kind of circumstances introduced by the three complementizers it is not quite easy to discern the difference between them in certain contexts. This paradox between on the one hand the intuitively clear difference in lexical content between the three complementizers and on the other the semantic affinity in certain contexts between clauses containing them is the central topic of this article. While some authors seem to adopt a solution to this paradox which allows *if, when* and *where* to be synonymous in certain contexts, cf. the discussion in section 2, we shall argue in favour of a solution where *if, when* and *where* preserve their lexical properties in all contexts[1]. To do this we will make clear what we think are the relevant contexts and the functions of the three types of embedded sentences, cf. section 3. On the basis of the background presented in section 2 and the outline of a solution put forward in section 3, we conclude in section 4.

2. The neutralization thesis

With respect to the paradox introduced in section 1. Quirk et al. (1985: 1086ff) claim that the distinctive value of *if, when* and *where* can be 'neutralized' in certain contexts and that in such contexts they express "a more abstract notion of recurrent or habitual contingency".

According to Quirk et al. this claim can be illustrated by examples (3a-c) and (4a-c)

(3a) *When* there's smoke, there's fire.

(3b) *If* there's smoke, there's fire.

(3c) *Where* there's smoke, there's fire.

(4)   She always wrote an encouraging remark, even

    (4a) *when* the essay paper was poor.

    (4b) *if* the essay paper was poor.

    (4c) *where* the essay paper was poor.

In (3a-c) and (4a-c) the neutralization is shown by the possibility of replacing and rephrasing the complementizers by PPs like: *in cases when* or *in circumstances where*.

Although the remarks of Quirk et al. point in the same direction as our own discussion above in connection with (2), i.e. that it is difficult to differentiate between certain uses of *if, when* and *where,* we are not convinced that (3a-c) and (4a-c) are in fact examples of neutralization, nor that "recurrent or habitual contingency" is the value of the presumed neutralization. It is even highly doubtful that this value adequately describes the examples concerned.

The idea of a neutralization between *if, when* and *where* implies a feature analysis in which the feature [recurrent or habitual contingency] is part of the defining properties of the three complementizers, and in which the distinctive features [condition], [temporal] and [locational] can be neutralized in certain contexts. Apart from the fact that Quirk et al. do not make clear what the relevant contexts are, see our section 3, the proposed neutralization does not work.

Consider the following examples:

---

[1] In modern linguistics many authors talk about either an atemporal or a conditional *when*, see Carlson 1979, ter Meulen 1995, and Kratzer 1995.

(5a)   When he arrives (this afternoon), I'll leave you for a moment.
(5b)   If he arrives (this afternoon), I'll leave you for a moment.
(5c)   Where I am now, it is raining.

These sentences cannot be described in terms of a feature saying that they convey information about something which is either habitual or recurrent. And (5c) cannot be said to convey contingency. It states a simple fact. For these reasons the claim about neutralization as it is formulated in Quirk et al. is empirically inadequate, a fact that implies the empirical inadequacy of the notion of recurrent or habitual contingency as a defining property of both *if, when* and *where*. Notice, however, that we did not say that recurrent or habitual contingency, or something along those lines, is not pertinent for the description of sentences containing one of the three complementizers. But if it is pertinent, it is not because of the complementizers. This is what we claim to have demonstrated. For a more detailed refutation of the neutralization thesis expressed in Quirk et al., see Faber and Sørensen 1996.

3. An outline of the solution

While we do agree with Quirk et al. (1985) when they say that the sentences in (3) or (4) have approximately the same meaning, we do not agree with their solution to the paradox we introduced in section 1. In order to prepare the way for our solution to this problem, we will now present our analysis of the three complementizers. It concerns on the one hand the contexts in which the circumstantial conditions introduced by *if, when* and *where* respectively seem to be identical, and on the other, the functions of the embedded clauses with the three complementizers within the utterances which they are part of. We start out with an outline of the solution.

3.1. The core

An utterance of the sentence (6):

(6)   Contracts are indivisible.

is a categorial and unrestricted statement in the sense that the property of being indivisible is predicated to hold without restrictions of the kind of things which in legal contexts are called contracts.

Example (6) may be followed by either of the clauses (7a) - (7c):

(7a)   if the consideration is one and entire.
(7b)   when the consideration is one and entire.
(7c)   where the consideration is one and entire.

and thus give rise to three new sentences, (8a) - (8c) respectively, which may all be used in different appropriate legal contexts:

(8a)   Contracts are indivisible if the consideration is one and entire.

(8b)   Contracts are indivisible when the consideration is one and entire.

(8c)   Contracts are indivisible where the consideration is one and entire.

(8a) - (8c) are still categorial in the sense given above, i.e. the indivisibility is predicated of contracts. But the predication is no longer unrestricted. It is restricted so as to hold only in circumstances where the consideration is one and entire. So a first point of our analysis of (8a) - (8c) is that we take the embedded clauses, which we have isolated in (7a) - (7c), to be restrictors in relation to the predication expressed by the embedding clause[2], which is given in isolation in (6). But to say that (7a) - (7c) are used as restrictors in relation to (6) when someone uses (8a) - (8c) does not necessarily mean that the restrictors are identical in meaning or that the restrictions restrict in the same way. In fact we think that the restrictors in question are different and restrict in different ways, which is the second point of our analysis. These particular points of our analysis can be illustrated by way of the following paraphrase:

(9)   An utterance of (8a), (8b) or (8c) conveys the information that:

   contracts indicate indivisibility

either

(i)   in situations where the consideration is one and entire. (=(8a))

or

(ii)   in time intervals where the consideration is one and entire. (=(8b))

or

(iii)   in spaces where the consideration is one and entire. (=(8c))

Notice first that *if*, *when* and *where* are differentiated at the lexical level by the use in (9) of *situations, time intervals* and *spaces* respectively. These items thus have different properties in the proposal made in (9). Notice next that the three embedded circumstantial conditions in (9) are all seen as restrictions on something which is part of or identical to the predication expressed by the embedding clause. This part of the analysis makes the circumstantial conditions functionally similar, and we think that this similarity is what Quirk et al. (1985) wrongly interpret as a case of semantic neutralization, cf. the discussion in section 2. Notice finally that (9) does not state which item in (8a) - (8c) is being restricted. This undesirable aspect of (9)

---

[2]*If* is normally seen as a unit associated with a relation, cf. Barwise 1989 and Sandford 1989. *When* and *where* are normally considered to be wh-elements, and thus a kind of operator or quantifier, cf. Kratcher 1995.

is due to the fact that PPs of the form *in NP where* do not explicitly mention or mark in any way which item is said to be in the spaces determined by the PPs. For the time being we just want to say that our guess is that the clauses containing *if, when* and *where* restrict situations, time intervals and spaces, respectively.

3.2. Utterance types

In sentences such as (10) and (11):

(10)   When Peter arrived, I left.

(11)   Where Peter is now, it is raining.

when and *where* are used to create a common temporal space and a ditto locational space, respectively, within which two situations become related by the mere fact of being part of the same space. We call such utterances episodic utterances because they concern (or describe) one particular situation and because they are about a single state-of-affairs[3]. A clear example of an episodic utterance is (12):

(12)   The plaintiff, M. A. Jones, is claiming damages under clause 10 of the contract.

In cases where *when* and *where* are used in episodic utterances they thus denote a single temporal or locational space. This is not the case in general utterances. A general utterance involves some kind of plurality of state-of-affairs, each instance being of the same type. Consider (13):

(13)   The present Lord Chancellor sits in on these cases.

(13) does not describe a single state-of-affairs which can be localized in a specific space-time region, but a whole set of occasions where the same person sits in on a specific type of case. If *when* and *where* are used in the context of a general utterance they cannot denote a specific time or space region respectively. In such contexts they denote a set of temporal or locational spaces, each of which is described in the same way, i.e. in the way indicated by the embedded clause[4].

3.3. Modification

The lexical content associated with *if, when* and *where*, respectively, has a low degree of descriptive power. According to our way of looking at this problem *if* describes a condition, *when* describes a temporal space, and *where* describes a locational space, see our paraphrases in (9). But the overall impact of using an embedded clause with either *if, when* or *where* does not stem solely from the

---

[3]For a detailed compositional treatment of *when*-clauses, see Moens 1987.
[4]Note that the senses we are talking about involve either one or more entities of the same kind, not two unrelated meanings.

denotational properties of the complementizers. It also stems from the function of the embedded clause within the utterance it is part of. We assume that the three types of embedded clauses function as modifiers in relation to the embedding clause just as adjective phrases function as modifiers in relation to a noun, cf. *red house*, or as adverb phrases modify a verb phrase, cf. *speaks Danish quite well*. The general idea behind this conception of the embedded clauses is that their content makes explicit different kinds of circumstances under which the state-of-affairs described by the embedding clause is or can be realized. We have argued for this conception in Sørensen and Faber 1996, and therefore we shall not go into details at this point. But we want to illustrate one of its consequences by reference to an example given in Carlson 1979, an example Carlson analyses in a way which supports the point of view presented in Quirk et al 1985. Consider (14):

(14)   Cats are intelligent when they have blue eyes.

For Carlson the *when*-clause in (14) expresses an atemporal condition on the predication expressed by *cats are intelligent*, the embedding clause. We would say that the embedding clause describes a state and does not explicitly express the temporal frame of the state. The effect of using the *when*-clause is a restriction on the temporal frame which it narrows down to those temporal intervals in which cats also have blue eyes[5]. Notice that this analysis allows us to have only one *when*, to obtain approximately the same semantic effect as Carlson, and, a more coherent explanatory framework. For the time being we just wanted to present and illustrate the way in which we apply the modifier analysis to *if, when* or *where*. For the rest of this paper we assume this analysis to be correct.

4. Conclusion

We have now prepared the ground for a solution of the paradox we presented in section 1. Recall that the central issue was the apparent contradiction between the lexical properties of *if, when* and *where* and their use in what we now call general utterances, cf. section 3.2. The analysis we present is a solution to this paradox in the sense that we claim that such notions as 'condition', 'temporal space' and 'locational space' are part of any use of *if, when* and *where*. This results in the disappearance of the paradox. But we also allow for a certain degree of vagueness which makes the difference between *if, when* and *where* less marked. What we have in mind is this. We work with a universe having three kinds of entities: situations, times, and spaces. From an ontological point of view these kinds of entities are

---

[5]The strongly felt causal relation between the property of having blue eyes and being intelligent is an effect of the mere fact of putting together the two situations, and not derivable from the lexical content of *when*.

different. But in general utterances where the speaker only implicitly makes reference to times and places, the perception of the distinction becomes blurred. Note that a perceptual difficulty does not necessarily imply indistinctness.

With this in mind we apply our solution to the paradox by dealing with one complementizer at a time.

In some sense *if* does not directly contribute to the paradox, because it is associated with the same meaning whether it is used in an episodic utterance or a general utterance. But *if*-clauses and the value of *if*-clauses are often said to function as the pattern taken over by *when*-clauses and *where*-clauses.

Our discussion of the three complementizers will be based on the following type of example:

(15)   A contract is concluded if acceptance is received by the offeror.

Example (15) is a general utterance, and it clearly states that a contract is concluded (=Sit_1) only in the circumstances described by the embedded clause (=Sit_2). And Sit_2 is presented, through the choice of *if*, as a condition. Notice that in order to examine whether a particular situation is an instance of Sit_1 it is necessary to check whether there is a relevant instance of Sit_2.

The utterance in (15) can be rephrased as in (16):

(15)   A contract is concluded when acceptance is received by the offeror.

The only difference is that *when* has taken the place of *if*. Notice now that *when* can be paraphrased by *at the time*, not by *in circumstances where*. The use of *when* indicates that the point at issue here is the time of conclusion of the contract, which has legal consequences. So *when* is used with a temporal meaning. It is also clear that according to (16) a true instance of Sit_1 requires a true instance of Sit_2 at a particular time.

Our final example is (17):

(17)   A contract is concluded where acceptance is received by the offeror.

Example (17) is just like (16) and (15) except for the use of *where*. As was the case with (16) the content of (17) cannot be rephrased by 'in circumstances where' or 'in cases when' as legal consequences e.g. in connection with applicable law follow from precisely the place of conclusion of the contract. So even though (17) is a general utterance, *where* does refer to a locational space. From the remarks given above in relation to (15), (16) and (17) it follows that these utterances are not identical in meaning, because *if*, *when* and *where* denote different entities. Notice also that the truth conditions of (17) and (16) are more restrictive than those of (15). So there are cases falling under (15) which are covered by either (17) nor (16). But this situation is 'normal' given our proposal.

Examples (15) - (17) illustrate the fact that general utterances may have non-synonymous uses of *if, when* and *where*. And we think that this pattern is the general one. But why are the embedded clauses in (8a) - (8c) felt to be, if not synonymous, then closely related? Our answer is, as indicated above, that the perception of the relevant distinctions becomes blurred and even insignificant because situations, times and locations all serve as 'spaces' in relation to which state-of-affairs may be located and because the utterances in question describe unspecific 'spaces' of the kind just mentioned.

We therefore think that we are closer to an appropriate description of *if, when* and *where* than Quirk et al. (1985) and linguists working with conditional uses of *when* and *where*.

References

Barwise, I. (1989). *The Situation in Logic*. Standford: CSLI.

Carlson, G. N. (1979). Generics and Atemporal 'when'. *Linguistics and Philosophy* 3, 49-98.

Carlson, G. N. & F. J. Pelletier (eds) (1995). *The Generic Book*. Chicago & London: The University of Chicago Press.

Faber, D. & F. Sørensen (1995). Betingelser og lign. *KLIMT* 1, 23-34. Handelshøjskolen i København.

Kratzer, A. (1995). Stage-Level and Individual-Level Predicates. In Carlson & Pelletier 1995, 125-175.

Moens, M. (1987). *Tense, Aspect and Temporal Reference*. Centre for Cognitive Science, University of Edinburgh.

Quirk, R., S. Greenbaum, G. Leech & J. Svartvik (1985). *A Comprehensive Grammar of the English Language*. London: Longman.

Sandford, H. (1989). *If P, Then Q. Conditionals and the Foundations of Reasoning*. London & New York: Routledge.

Sørensen, F. & D. Faber (1996). En parentes. Om modifikation, steder og ytringstyper. *KLIMT* 2, 53-71. Handelshøjskolen i København.

ter Meulen, A. G. B. (1995). *Representing Time in Natural Language. The Dynamic Interpretation of Tense and Aspect*. Cambridge Massachusetts: The MIT Press.

Futurity in English: A Case for Messy Structure

Peter Harder

1. Introduction

In the past ten to fifteen years, a remarkable resurgence of interest in grammatical categories has occurred, after a period dominated by syntax, with generative grammar as the central force. The most obvious strand in this development is perhaps grammaticalization theory, which has reset the agenda within linguistics in several respects; apart from shifting the focus away from clause structure towards grammatical elements, it has reopened the issue of the relationship between synchrony and diachrony and posed the question of the relationship between form and substance – or, as I shall say, between structure and substance (in order to avoid the ambiguity of the word *form,* which is used as a contrast to both *meaning* and *substance).* The driving force in this movement has been a recognition that in grammatical morphemes we have a class of elements that are interesting both from a semantic and a structure-oriented perspective, and which offer possibilities of interesting cross-linguistic generalizations.

In this reorientation, the focus of international – i.e., in practice American – attention has returned to what has always been central to European linguistics, both in the era of traditional grammar and in European structuralism, including the Danish tradition. However, the thrust of the new approach jars against some of the basic assumptions in the European tradition: the emphasis on semantic substance as opposed to structural contrast (cf. Bybee 1988); the emphasis on cross-linguistic regularities as opposed to the 'immanent structure' of the language system; and the priority of diachrony over synchrony. The issues raised by this conflict of orientation and interest have not yet been clarified – in particular, the question of how the grammatical system of a particular language can be described in a modern perspective, has no pat answer at the present time.

A number of Danish grammarians were early birds in taking up the status of grammatical categories from the modern perspective; and Niels Davidsen-Nielsen was one of these. In his work, which was the starting point for my own interest in the field, he also tackled the difficult issue of how to handle elements with less than clear-cut structural properties. The question I am going to focus on is the status of the future in English and Danish; and the following may be regarded as the latest instalment in a long-standing debate from which I have derived a great deal of pleasure as well as benefit.

2. Three ways of looking at the future

If we simplify the issue slightly, there are three perfectly natural and logical ways of providing a simple answer to the question of whether a language like English or Danish has a future tense. First of all, within the approach of the Latin-oriented grammatical tradition, the description of any category would be based on an implicit assumption that the grammar of Latin provided a model for the description of the lesser, modern languages. Even if there was no exact equivalent of the inflected future form in Latin, the most obvious translation equivalent would have to serve. When English was approached in this way, certain types of use of the modal verbs *will* and *shall* naturally acquired the status of 'future forms', most directly by being used to translate the Latin inflectional paradigms, and by implication also in grammatical descriptions of English. As long as "real" grammar means "Latin grammar", this is clearly the best English can do to live up to the classical standard: it may be a poor future, but it's the best we've got.

This pattern of reasoning became problematic already in the generation before structuralism became the accepted scientific paradigm in linguistics, as the vernacular languages began to struggle free of classical domination in the era of the national philologies. Jespersen's critique of squinting grammar made the point forcefully, not only in relation to Latin but also in relation to the artificial preservation on older historical stages in descriptions of modern languages. With the structuralist revolution, this position was elevated to a basic dogma. In terms of the structural agenda, paradigmatic contrast became the chief criterion of category membership, and from that point of view there is clearly no room for a future tense in English. Not only is present and past alone in their paradigm (nothing else can go in the same slot), but the *will* and *shall* forms used to indicate the future are clearly modal verbs with other senses beside futurity, standing in a paradigmatic contrast with other modal verbs (a view argued by Palmer (e.g. 1986)).

But in the course of the 1980s the wheel made another turn. Once again the semantic substance, i.e. the type of meaning conveyed, came into focus as criterial for the choice of linguistic description, and the cross-linguistic perspective was seen as taking precedence over the details of language-specific organization. In Comrie's monographs on tense and aspect the test for admission into a grammatical category of a particular kind was a cross-classification of a "grammaticity" criterion (I use the word instead of grammaticality to indicate grammatical as opposed to purely lexical status) and a semantic criterion. In the case of tense, the criterion for membership of the tense category was "grammaticalized location in time", cf. Comrie 1985: 9; and as noted in Davidsen-Nielsen 1988, according to this criterion the English way of expressing the future becomes interesting once again, making the rejection of the future by modern English grammarians like Palmer less than obviously motivated. In the article that raises the question, he proposes a number of distributional and semantic criteria whereby the use of *will* to indicate futurity can be kept distinct from the other uses of the modal verb, proving that modern English has indeed carved out a well-defined place for a real, grammaticalized future. As grammaticalization theory got under way, the patterns of grammatical categories and their diachronic trajectories emerged in more concrete form, and the Danish and English modal verbs come to be seen as having a cross-linguistically regular and predictable place in the evolution of grammaticalized location in future time.

Among the merits of Davidsen-Nielsen's analysis I would like to mention, on the semantic side, the case he presents against the wholesale relegation of futurity to the province of modality (represented among others, by Lyons). Davidsen-Nielsen singles out the key criterion of categorical commitment: unlike what is the case with modalized statements like *it may be so, he must have done it,* statements with future *will* commit the speaker unequivocally to the (future) truth of his claim.

On the distributional side, the criteria of auxiliary status he employs filter out the epistemically used modals together with future *will* as constituting a natural class, showing clearly that they have a privileged degree of 'grammaticity" in the language. The natural conclusion is that there is every reason to recognize a future form as part of the grammar of English. Yet in my account of the future (Harder 1996), which on many points takes over the analysis proposed in Davidsen-Nielsen 1990, the ultimate answer to the question of whether the grammar of English should recognize a future tense is less clear than Davidsen-Nielsen's own emphatic affirmative. Is this simply "pussyfooting" (Davidsen-Nielsen 1996), or can some principled defence be established for this less than resounding acceptance of the future in English?

3. The relation between meaning and structure

Before I go into the details of my own position I would like to look at the principles involved in the account presented by Davidsen-Nielsen. As indicated above, the basic principle, which is congruent with that of Comrie and grammaticalization theory, is one according to which two properties are criterial. The first criterion is 'grammatical status"; the second criterion is semantic ("location in time"). What I want to look at now is the difference between investigating a particular language as part of a cross-linguistic investigation ("does language X have something of the kind we are looking for?") and writing a grammar of language X. If one is writing about futures generally, *will* and *going to* forms have a natural place in the story – just as the Danish *vil* form has; but Davidsen-Nielsen's description does not stop at this point. The aim is clearly the much more ambitious one of giving a description of this area of the grammar of English (and the grammar of Danish). In realizing this aim, Davidsen-Nielsen uses a notion of 'grammatical category' that is inherited from European linguistics, instead of (in the typical manner of American linguistics) simply enumerating the 'forms' of the language. In the description that ensues, the category of tense emerges as having eight members in both English and Danish (1990: 55):

In English as well as Danish tense is assumed to have the following eight members: *present, present perfect, past, past perfect, future, future perfect, future of the past, future perfect of the past*. If we disregard progressive forms, passive forms, and forms with modal auxiliaries, these members are – in regular verbs – implemented in the following way:

English

Present	V + -*s*/Ø
Present Perfect	*has/have* + V + *-(e)d*
Past	V + *-(e)d*
Past Perfect	*had* + V + *-(e)d*
Future	*will* + V
Future Perfect	*will* + *have* + *-(e)d* [sic]
Future of the Past	*would* + V
Future Perfect of the Past	*would* + *have* + V + *-(e)d*

On the expression side, as will be evident, the analysis is fairly messy, since the morphological markings associated with present and past are fused into one system together with the *have* associated with the perfect and the *will* associated with the future – all presented as forming one grammatical category. Davidsen-Nielsen compares this analysis with the one that keeps the three sets of elements apart and argues (pp. 68f) for keeping them together in one category. The way in which he argues for this conclusion is interesting for the principles it instantiates.

Both for the future and the perfect, the arguments are basically semantic, with an admixture of distribution. In the case of *will*, the two arguments have already been mentioned above: *will* as indicating future is semantically as well as distributionally distinct from modal *will*. In the case of the perfect, the argument against seeing the perfect as an aspect is semantic (the perfect tells us nothing about internal temporal contour); in the case of the assignment of the perfect to a wholly separate category of "phase" the argument is in terms of paradigmatic contrast: the distribution of present perfect vs. simple past should be describable in terms of direct contrast with respect to their shared semantic domain (past time reference), rather than via a paradigmatic contrast in two categories simultaneously: present vs. past tense and perfect vs. current phase.

Let me begin by saying that I think all these arguments are important and any theory needs to take them seriously. However, if they were to be taken as definitive, they would collectively imply a purely semantic definition of what a grammatical category is, once grammatical status is established: if grammatical forms are in the same semantic domain, they constitute one category. The distributional aspects of the argument are only designed to ensure that the grammatical forms are indeed grammatically distinguishable (in the case of the future) and directly contrastive (in the case of the present perfect and the simple past). Even if the usefulness of such a notion is clear, especially in the case of pedagogically oriented contrastive analysis, it still raises some questions of principle about the architecture of grammatical description. What is missing, the way I see it, is a precise discussion of the relation between meaning and structure, and of the structural criteria that need to be fulfilled in order to take the step from recognizing the existence of a particular grammatical morpheme to speaking about several morphemes as constituting a category. Central in this respect is the notion of a paradigm.

Although the notion of paradigmatic contrast may appear to be perfectly clear-cut, on closer inspection it turns out that it can be dissolved into a number of different relation types, cf. also Heltoft 1996. Oldest among them is the notion inherited from traditional grammar, that of the morphological paradigm consisting of all the forms of a word. In such paradigms, what is kept constant is the lexeme, and what varies is the 'accidental' modification – regardless of the syntactic potential of the different forms. In structuralist terms, therefore, the morphological modifications are not all on the same footing: the contrast in terms of person agreement is different from the contrast in terms of tense, and both are distinct from the contrast between participles and infinitive forms, etc. This is where the classical notion of a grammatical category received its structural reinterpretation: different sets of morphological modifications must belong to different categories if they entered into different structural relations. Paradigmatic contrast is not the only possible type of structural criterion for establishing categories; Hjelmslev (1938) proposed a definition of the different categories on the basis of their dependence relations – thus tense was defined on the basis of its role in governing *consecutio temporum*, etc.

However, the basic assumption was that a grammatical category consisted in a set of contrasting forms within a given semantic domain (which gave the category its name: tense, aspect, gender, number ...) – and at this point the clarification more or less stopped within the structural tradition. Thus it never became quite clear how to narrow down the precise type of paradigmatic contrast that warranted speaking of a category, and in what way the expression side and the content side needed to collaborate in order for a set of contrasts to constitute a category. As an example, the well-established category of case can be seen to encompass two different paradigms, if the content criterion is taken seriously (cf. Heltoft 1996: 482). The situation that tends to be presupposed is the very tidy case that is more or less exemplified by number in English: it has two semantically well-defined members; it operates only in one place (after the noun stem), designates an invariant meaning difference, and has (with very few exceptions) a predictable form.

But far from all the staple example of grammatical categories are as well-behaved as that. As an example of a less than tidy categorial contrast, we may take the paradigmatic contrast between perfective and imperfective in Russian. Aspect in Russian operates on the one hand with an unpredictable choice between derivational prefixes, but can also be indicated by suffixes (i.e. in a different formal slot); and some prefixes carry an unpredictable element of lexical modification with them. No clear-cut definitions and criteria appear to offer themselves readily.

Responding to the lack of clarity in this area, Bache (1995) presents a thoroughgoing analysis of the notion of grammatical category, and goes a long way towards reconciling the conflicting aims of having a tidy theory and having something that can account for messy situations in actual languages. Avoiding the pitfall of relying on a tidy set of universals, Bache explicitly opts for an *ad hoc* metalinguistic level of analysis, designed to be the repository of a maximum of simplicity and neatness, showing how one can use the simple calculus to make sense of messy data. A major element in this account is the careful demonstration of how the interplay between different semantic factors creates complexities that need not be attributed to categorial contrasts per se.

In terms of Bache's picture, it becomes clear how one can meaningfully operate with sets of clear-cut paradigmatic choices among semantically well-defined contrasting options, without attributing this simplicity to actual language forms. With a well-defined metacategory of (e.g.) aspect, one can look at particular language-specific sets of choices, such as the Russian prefixes and the English progressive and be precise about the extent to which the contrasts they signal are instantiations of the metacategory.

Nevertheless, it appears to me that there is still something missing in the picture of precision vs. messiness in language description that is presented. The main objection is to do with the way in which choice is structured in the individual language. Bache is aware of the complexities of language-specific categories (cf. especially the discussion pp. 147ff); and there is nothing in his theory that blocks a full clarification – but there is a difference between permitting and ensuring language-specific clarity. What is still underestimated in the picture is the extent to which the structural relation between language-specific grammatical meanings may defy attempts to capture them in terms of neat, clear-cut oppositions within well-defined semantic domains.

Returning to the problem at hand, the problem may be instantiated in relation to the future in English. As far as I can see, Bache's discussion of the future as a tense on the meta-level (1995: 266f) offers a general rationale within which Davidsen-Nielsen's specific arguments for recognizing a future tense in English would fit unproblematically. Hence, from a structural point of view, the problem that has not been addressed is the same that was raised above: once a form is recognized as being part of the grammar, the criterion for whether it belongs in a given category is purely semantic; the way in which the English language offers the choice of futurity to the speaker is not part of the picture.

The problem is raised by Bache in the shape of the 'minimal factor criterion' (1995: 160) according to which only one formal (expression) parameter may be involved at a time. Without rejecting this criterion, Bache points out two problems with it: it reduces all oppositions to pairs (corresponding to presence vs. absence of a given expression marker), and it rules out the direct comparison of forms that differ in more than one respect on the expression side – a clear example being the relation between the present perfect and the past that was also taken up by Davidsen-Nielsen: in terms of the 'minimal factor criterion' a comparison between these two forms would have to be in terms of both the contrast between present and past and the contrast between perfect and non-perfect, thus ruling out the natural question: what is the division of labour between the simple past and the present perfect in referring to past events?

Both these objections, however, could be answered in a way that would supplement the perspective offered by the idealized metacategories. The 'minimal factor criterion' could be revised so as to permit non-paired opposites, simply by seeing the relevant unit not as the expression parameter, but as the substitutional slot in itself. In that case, nothing prevents there being more than two members. In languages with a dual number, it goes into the same structural slot as the singular and the plural, yielding three members according to what may be called the 'minimal substitutional criterion'. The possibility of direct comparison between forms in non-minimal contrast can be accommodated by recognizing the co-existence, in actual language use, between multiple domains of choice. Selecting at random, we can say that the speaker has to choose between making an utterance and remaining silent; between different topics and different comments; between different auxiliary complexes – and, within the auxiliary component, between different minimal substitutional elements. The full structural description would then involve all the minimal as well as the constructional choice relations, specifying the degree of independent choice at each level; and the present perfect would then be a good case of a complex form that needed to be carefully described both at the minimal and the constructional level (cf. also Harder 1996: 327). In addition to this extra level of structural precision in the paradigmatic dimension, there would also be a corresponding need for precision in the syntagmatic dimension: precisely where do the choices in a given category go into the syntagmatic chain of meanings? With respect to the ideal metacategories, these two considerations imply that we do not get a grammatical description of a specific language simply by applying metacategories to it: we need to ask both how many members the category has in the language in question, and also whether the substitutional relations fit directly into those envisioned by the metacategory.

4. The English future: towards a messy theory

The theory I present of the future is designed to reflect the emphasis I have defended above on the way individual languages structure the semantic choices. The emphasis on minimal substitutional choices means that the ideal tense category is not one with a three-way contrast between present, past and future – perhaps not even from a cross-linguistic point of view. As pointed out by Vet (1981), the familiar examples of futures are not in direct substitutional relation with present and past; rather, the future is added to the choice of either present or past. This does not mean that there could not be a language with a direct, three-way contrast (languages may be permitted to structure themselves in many different ways, and stranger paradigms have been found) – but I have yet to see a convincing example of this. (I asked Joan Bybee if she could find such a language in the data base that she and her collaborators have constructed (cf. Bybee, Perkins and Pagliuca 1994); but direct substitutional contrast could not be unambiguously picked out).

In relation to English, it is reasonably clear that future *will* collaborates syntagmatically with present and past tense (as well as with the perfect forms). This does not prevent us from seeking an account in terms of an overall tense system, with a syntagmatic as well as a paradigmatic dimension. But it means that the English tense system, seen as including the future, will not correspond to the neat list of members in a paradigm of the kind that is everybody's prototype; or, at least, it means that the paradigm will be a constructional paradigm decomposable into minimal substitutional pairs.

What about minimal substitution? Viewed in terms of the tense theory alone, the natural answer would be to say that the future contrasts with non-future only. But when the question is the status of the future in English, the structural relation between the grammatical morphemes of English must be taken into account. We therefore have to look at the actual substitution relation between future *will* and other forms of the language. Here the structurally well-defined paradigm of modal verbs in English necessarily asserts itself. In English, *will* as indicator of pure futurity is one choice, first among the full paradigm of modal verbs, secondly in terms of the "internal paradigm" (Harder 1996: 207) of variant meanings associated with *will*. In terms of the paradigmatic structure of English, there is therefore little doubt that the *will* future must be understood as a semantically deviant option in the modal slot.

However, there is one further property of grammatical paradigms that now needs to be explored. Grammaticalization theory, as described above, does not have a fully developed theory of grammatical structure. This is natural in the sense that its core area is the diachronic processes whereby lexical elements gradually acquire grammatical properties, so that a cut-and-dried distinction between grammatical structure and the lexicon would run counter to the nature of the phenomena investigated in the theory. On the other hand, by its very nature, the development towards increasingly grammatical status would be easier to capture if the theory had a clear picture of what the prototype of a fully grammaticalized element was. I would like to discuss one of the criteria traditionally associated with grammatical status, i.e. obligatoriness.

Obligatoriness points up the essential difference between grammatical and lexical properties of a language. Lexical choice is by definition open, reflecting ideally the full variety of human experience and permitting combination of lexical items constrained only by the limitations of performance power and pragmatic meaningfulness. In the case of obligatory grammatical categories, the nature of linguistic choice is quite different; here the language forces you to make a specification that may not be communicatively important. As pointed out by Boas and Jakobson, languages differ less with respect to what they can express than with respect to what they must express. To take a celebrated case, in declarative and interrogative clauses, the choice between present and past tense is obligatory in English (and other Standard Average European languages); when selecting verb forms there is no way round it. By anybody's criterion this is a fact that needs to be stated about the grammar of those languages.

However, obligatoriness is not criterial for grammatical status. No-one would doubt that English modal verbs are highly grammaticalized, yet it is not obligatory to choose one out of the verbs in the modal paradigm in the same sense that it is obligatory to choose a tense out of the present/past paradigm. This intuitively accords with the mixture of "lexicality" and "grammaticity" that is a generally recognized feature of the modal verbs.

In the case of the future, the issue of obligatoriness offers an interesting avenue towards being precise about its messy status in English. Let us begin by noting that the question of obligatoriness does not arise if grammatical elements are viewed one at a time, as in the approach that is most natural within grammaticalization theory. In that perspective, what happens is typically that a lexical element (such as a verb of movement or intention) gradually becomes generalized as indicator of futurity. This is not to say that grammaticalization theorists have ignored the issue; Dahl (1985) explicitly mentions it as the hallmark of grammatical difference between languages. But obligatoriness is necessarily the property of a category, not of a 'gram' – at least unless it is semantically empty: an obligatory single gram would have to be meaningless.

If it is the choice (rather than the gram itself) that is obligatory, we need to specify what choice we are talking about. As indicated above, I think the most revealing way to look at it in the case of the future from a cross-linguistic perspective, is in terms of the binary ('minimal substitution') choice of future vs. non-future. Interestingly enough, I think this is also a good way to describe the case in English (cf. also Harder 1996: 373), so that this binary choice is superimposed upon the choice between English present and past tense. The central case in which this choice is relevant, however, is clearly in the domain of the present tense, i.e. in the case where the issue is: simple present vs. (present) future. The reason why this is something that needs to be described in the grammar of English comes out clearly when English is compared with Danish. As described in Davidsen-Nielsen 1990: 123, Danish uses only the future *vil* in cases where the temporal address is not indicated in other ways. If we ignore the grey areas, this means that the choice of plus or minus futurity in the verb phrase is obligatory in English, whereas it is optional in Danish. But in accepting this distinction, it may be asked, are we not forced simultaneously to accept that the future is a full-blown member of the verb system of English? Is there any scope left for pussyfooting at all?

The answer to this question provides a clear-cut example of messy structure. If we return to the status of the *will* future as part of the modal paradigm in English, there seems to be a contradiction here somewhere. How can *will* be in a pairwise contrast with non-futurity and yet be one among the multiple members of the modal paradigm? The resolution of this conflict has to do with the balance between arbitrariness and motivation in linguistic structure. The way I see it is that the obligatory paradigmatic choice in English is not grammatically narrowed down to an ideal, unambiguous pair such as singular/plural in nouns. It is not so that the English language forces an unambiguous choice between *will* and zero on its speakers. Rather, the speakers have an open-ended set of alternative indicators of futurity to choose from, ranging from the very grammaticalized and specifically future-indicating *will* via modalized ways of speaking about the future as coded by the other modal verbs, via the less grammaticalized *be going to,* and idiomatic constructions like *be on the point of,* to fully lexical expressions with an element of futurity in them such as *want* or *plan.* So if the speaker does not want to make a statement claiming that something is true at the present time, he has a range of alternative options open to him, compare (1) and (2):

(1)   I work hard.

(2a)   I will work hard.

(2b)   I may work hard.

(2c)   I am going to work hard.

(2d)   I am on the point of working hard.

(2e)   I plan to work hard.

The problem that is involved here has to do with the status of zero forms in the grammar. A natural assumption would be that zero only makes sense as one member of a well-defined obligatory paradigm. As an open choice, it is difficult to see how zero would be distinct from nothing at all, hence zero requires a clear-cut linguistic paradigm; yet here I present an open-ended choice with lexical members involved.

The situation I am trying to define for the English future is somewhere between this position and the one outlined in Bybee 1994. In this article, specifically devoted to the role of zero forms, Bybee discusses the interaction between grams, pointing out that as a new grammatical element arises, it will affect the division of labour between grammatical forms within the field; thus, the rise of the progressive form in English endowed the simple present with the role of indicating habituality. But the tendency of her account is to emphasize the similarity between zero grams and other grams: they stand for parts of the same semantic territory that the positively defined forms belong in, simply occupying areas that other forms happen to have left over.

Without denying the existence of this similarity, it seems to me that the relationship between forms, i.e. paradigmatic contrast, must have a special status in the case of zero: unlike a positively defined form, a zero form can only have positively defined meaning to the extent that it is unambiguously defined as an alternative to something else. However, in contrast to the argument that would entail a full-fledged grammatical paradigm, I think it is perfectly possible for a paradigmatic choice to exist in which there is a basic two-way contrast between a zero and a positive member, but no single unrivalled form to occupy the role of positive member. The basic paradigmatic choice is between 'nothing' and 'something', but in the role of 'something' there are several options, as it were.

In the light of this possibility, let me discuss the objections that Davidsen-Nielsen advances against my unclear position. I described the future in English as a sort of "squatter in the modal paradigm" (1996: 369). Davidsen-Nielsen (1996) points out that this description does not resolve the issue of where the future belongs: position in the modal paradigm does not entail modal status, since both the dynamic interpretation of *can* and the volitional interpretation of *will* must be understood as belonging outside the category of modality proper – they, too, are "squatters". Since we have to operate with deviant elements in this paradigm anyway, why not be forthright about this in the case of the future – since my tense system in fact operates with futurity as a member?

I have to begin by admitting that there is indeed an unclarity in my position (which was pointed out in Bache's opposition at the public defense of my dessertation): I have offered no answer for the question of what my criterion is for admitting a given form to my tense category. The reason I failed to make that clear was that I did not think it was possible to be perfectly clear-cut about it in relation to a specific language – but this of course is no excuse for not making the *issue* clear. As indicated above, I subscribe to the position defined by Bache, in terms of which the only road towards clarity is to define an *ad hoc* metalinguistic category which you then apply to the description of specific languages. In choosing an eight-tense system decomposable into three binary choices as my descriptive framework I have thereby implicitly committed myself to a position where I say, "these forms, organized in these paradigmatic relationships, constitute what shall be known as 'tense' within my theory". This contrasts with the three-tense system in which past, present and future constitute the ideal choices, on the metacategorial level. But in relation to English the difference lies in the importance I attach to the minimal substitutional criterion on the language-specific level, i.e. the precise type of choice imposed by the linguistic system itself.

As I have adumbrated above, the positions of both Bache and Davidsen-Nielsen strike me as having an element of semantic "a priori"-ness about them. Once the semantic oppositions defined in the metacategory have been established, the question that we need to answer in a language-specific category is basically whether we find paradigmatic choices that instantiate the properties that are selected as criterial in the definition of the meta-linguistic category. Whether those choices are embedded in a wider structural context that has properties not captured in the metacategory is not an issue that is automatically settled within this approach. As against that, I think the ultimate answer to the question of the status of a grammatical element such as futurity in a given language must depend more on the whole pattern of paradigmatic organization than on the selection of choices that is profiled by a matching operation where one term is a pre-defined metacategory.

Let me spell out what this entails in relation to the situation that I have described for the future. Davidsen-Nielsen's arguments for allowing the future to be something special (since other members are also deviant) are fully valid as arguments about the semantic qualification of *will* for status as indicator of futurity rather than modality, and I have based my own account on them. But they do not eliminate the structural pattern whereby future *will* as well as volitional *will* and dynamic *can* are forced by the straitjacket of English grammar into the same grammatical slot as the semantically more central members of the modal paradigm. In a grammatical description of English, we therefore have to say that past and present tense as structural categories collaborate with a whole range of more or less modal meanings, among which we find the future *will*.

If we combine this with the situation in which a zero member of a grammatical category can be paradigmatically opposed to a positive member that has a number of competing instantiations, the messy structure of the future in English grammar can be explicitly stated. It can be said without qualification that English has a grammaticalized non-future, which is a semantic property of all 'simple' forms. This non-future member does not exist in Danish: it is not so that by choosing simple forms, you automatically choose to indicate that the time of verifiability lies ahead; on this point English is clearly different in a way that any grammatical description must recognize. But the status in English of the positive contrast in the shape of the future form in itself is a bit like a black hole in the grammar: the grammatical role of futurity can be registered through its impact on the neighbouring simple forms, by the way it affects their behaviour, rather than from the direct observation of any unambiguous paradigmatically contrasting positive member.

This is where French offers an interesting contrasting picture. The French future form covers a territory which is very similar to that of the English *will* form, as pointed out by Davidsen-Nielsen. In terms of the picture I defend, the difference is that futurity in French has developed its own paradigmatic slot. This is familiar in the case of the morphological future that arose when the original postposed auxiliary coalesced with the verb stem, cf. Fleischman 1978. Less familiar is the fact that the French *go*-future goes into the same paradigm, as reflected in the impossibility of combining the two options: when combined with the morphological future, the verb *aller* loses its future sense and retains only its lexical sense (cf. Vet 1986); *j'irai le faire* cannot mean 'I will be going to do it', only 'I will/shall go and do it'. For varieties of French that have both futures, there is thus a special place in the grammatical structure where you can choose between two types of futurity and non-future.

The situation I have attempted to describe is one in which the grammatical status of grammatical forms such as the future is graded in terms of a set of criteria, of which I have attributed great weight to 'obligatory choice' and 'minimal paradigmatic contrast' in the appropriate semantic domain. In order to give a resounding affirmative answer to the question "has English a future?", the language would have to be able to offer both, as does French. Danish fails on both counts, so the grammatical status of the Danish future is fairly obviously weak. The peculiar status of English is that it passes the first test, but fails the second – a situation I have not seen described elsewhere.

This means that the question of whether a given language has a future can be asked in several ways, some of which can be answered in the affirmative, others in the negative. To begin with we may ask, "does the language have a grammaticalized form that as one of its variants can indicate pure, categorical future?" On this criterion, Danish, English and French all have a future. The next question could then be whether the choice of futurity is obligatory in the verbal system: on this test, English would have a future, while Danish would drop out. Finally one might ask whether there was an unambiguous paradigmatic opposition between positive and negative forms in a separate slot, and here only French would qualify.

A central point in the approach I defend is that structure presupposes substance, rather than the other way round as claimed by Hjelmslev. This means that structural criteria are superimposed upon semantic criteria; they do not render semantic substance distinctions irrelevant. An adequate structural description will therefore include a characterization of the substance domain associated with each linguistic form. Because of that, there will be no conflict between a description that reflects the structural organization of elements in the specific language and one that lends itself to cross-linguistic semantic generalization. What is more, I think the patient description of syntagmatic and paradigmatic relations, i.e. choices and combinations, in the individual languages is a necessary step towards useful cross-linguistic generalizations, including grammatical metacategories – as illustrated in the discussion above. Davidsen-Nielsen's own work on English and Danish is a model example of this kind of work; in differing with him with respect to the status of the future, I am taking issue with an aspect of the premises he has selected for his analysis – while benefiting from the descriptive results he has provided. In a theory in which meaning is basic, and structure can only be understood in relation to meaning, the relation remains transparent in the discussion, and the step from language-specific structural description to cross-linguistic semantic generalization can therefore be taken without requiring any special maneuvering. With respect to the issue that this article has been concerned with, the step can be described as follows:

Because of the obligatory choice between future and non-future in the verbal paradigm in English, the simple form has non-futurity as one of its semantic properties. If that implication is to be avoided in the case of a concrete utterance, the speaker must do something about it. Within the modal paradigm, he can then choose pure futurity as one option, realized (though unambiguously only in certain contexts) by *will* – which also carries a number of the properties associated with grammatical status. This enables the investigator of futurity on a semantic and/or cross-linguistic basis to put down English as a language with a grammaticalized future. So if that is the horizon of enquiry, let me end by saying without further qualifications that I do think English has a future!

References

Bache, C. (1995). *The Study of Aspect, Tense and Action. Towards a Theory of the semantics of Grammatical Categories.* Frankfurt am Main: Peter Lang.

Bybee, J. (1988). Semantic substance vs. contrast in the development of grammatical meaning. In S. Axmaker, A. Jaisser & H.Singmaster (eds) *Proceedings of the Fourteenth Annual Meeting of the Berkeley Linguistic Society. General session and parasession on grammaticalization.* Berkeley: Berkeley Linguistics Society, 247-264.

Bybee, J. (1994). The grammaticalization of zero. In W. Pagliuca (ed) *Perspectives on Grammaticalization.* Amsterdam & Philadelphia: John Benjamins.

Bybee, J., R. Perkins & W. Pagliuca (1994). *The evolution of grammar. Tense, aspect and modality in the languages of the world.* Chicago: University of Chicago Press.

Comrie, B. (1985). *Tense.* Cambridge: Cambridge University Press.

Davidsen-Nielsen, N. (1988). Has English a future? *Acta Linguistica Hafniensa* 21,1, 5-20

Davidsen-Nielsen, N. (1990). *Tense and Mood in English. A Comparison with Danish.* (Topics in English Linguistics 1). Berlin & New York: Mouton de Gruyter.

Davidsen-Nielsen, N. (1996). Opposition to Harder (1996), presented orally at the defence. MS, Copenhagen Business School.

Fleischman, S. (1982). *The future in thought and language. Diachronic evidence from Romance.* Cambridge: Cambridge University Press.

Harder, P. (1996). *Functional Semantics. A Theory of Meaning, Structure and Tense in English.* Berlin & New York: Mouton de Gruyter.

Hjelmslev, L. (1938). Essai d'une théorie des morphèmes. In L. Hjelmslev (1959) *Essais linguistiques* (Travaux du cercle linguistiques de Copenhague XII). København: Nordisk Sprog- og Kulturforlag, 152-164.

Lyons, J. (1977). *Semantics.* Vols I-II. Cambridge: Cambridge University Press.

Palmer, F. (1986). *Mood and Modality*. Cambridge: Cambridge University Press.

Vet, C. (1986). A Pragmatic Approach to Tense in Functional Grammar. *Working Papers in Functional Grammar* 16.

Predication and the Nominal Clause

Michael Herslund

0. Introduction

Verbless sentences are not common in English or in the Western European languages in general. They seem to occur exclusively in special registers such as headlines, inscriptions, aphorisms and the like (cf. also Jespersen 1937: 30f). In different languages newspaper headlines such as the following are found:

(1)   *English*
        Seven wounded in Hebron attack (Financial Times 2.1.97, 1)

(2)   *French*
        L'Iran en panne de Coke (Express 26.10.95, 17)
        'Iran in Coke break-down'

(3)   *German*
        Europa unter Schnee und Eis (Frankfurter Allgemeine 31.12.96, 1)
        'Europe under snow and ice'

(4)   *Danish*
        Nyrup klar til politisk offensiv (Politiken 1.1.97, 1)
        'Nyrup ready for political offensive'
        Nyrups offensiv i ruiner (Politiken 4.1.97, 1)
        'Nyrup's offensive in ruins'

And when England won the 1966 Football World Championship, a special edition of the commemorative stamps issued at the occasion bore the inscription:

(5)   England winners

What is common to all these examples is that they are bipartite: they are easily interpreted as consisting of a subject and a predicate, the subject denoting some entity of which some property is predicated:

(5')   *England*   –   *winners*
        Entity/Subject   –   Property/Predicate

Another common feature of the examples of (1) to (5) is that they denote states resulting from some previous activity. But since there is no verb to express the kind of state or the finer details of it, the meaning of such sentences is hardly paraphrasable by other verbs than the maximally general verb BE, or some idiomatic variant of BE easily inferable from the collocation in question. In these cases the traditional analysis states that a form of the verb BE can be supplied. But the question is whether the traditional analysis of examples such as these as elliptical is really well-founded.

French and German for instance favour such structures more than either English or Danish: in certain circumstances, in addition to their use in headlines, they use verbless sentences, viz. either as (aphoristic) statements or as some kind of exclamative utterances. Such sentences occur with the sequence Predicate – Subject; the opposite order with the subject preceding the predicate would in fact be impossible. And this marked word order and the absence of BE could be indicative of a special status for such clauses, cf. the following from (Biblical) French and German:

(6) Heureux les simples d'esprit.
 'Blessed (are) the simple-minded'

(7) Charmante, cette fille.
 'Charming (is) that girl'

(8) Vorbei die Zeit des unnatürlichen Bundes (Behr & Quintin 1995)
 'Gone (is) the time of the unnatural alliance'

(9) Ein netter Kerl der Peter (ib.)
 'A decent chap (is) the Peter'

1. Verbal and nominal clauses

In most languages of the more familiar European type, as is well known, the concept of predication, and hence that of a sentence, presupposes the explicit presence of a finite verb. This element has a threefold function: 1) it denotes the relations between some entities (its lexical content including its argument structure); 2) it links the sentence to the surrounding reality by inscribing the denoted situation in time and reality relative to the utterance (tense, mood and modality); 3) it asserts this linguistic material of the situation referred to. This third function is, strictly speaking, the predicative function, i.e. the combination of the finite verb with a subject, which is partly independent of the other two. As we shall see, it can, under certain conditions, be performed without the others (cf. Benveniste 1950: 154f).

Now, the existence of *nominal clauses*[1] in many languages around the world represents a challenge to the universality of the verbal way of instantiating the

---

[1] I use this term as a translation of the French 'phrase nominale'. Such structures seem to have received no name in the Anglo-Saxon linguistic tradition: Jespersen calls them 'nominal sentences' (1937: 30f) and Bloomfield (1933: 173) distinguishes between *narrative* and *equational* predications, the latter being exemplified by e.g. Russian *ot'ec doma* 'father (is) at home'.

predication. In some languages all or a subset of BE-sentences are quite regularly constructed as verbless sentences, as nominal clauses in a very strict sense, where there seems to be no reason to insert, or understand, a verb BE. The procedure is widespread in many "exotic" languages (see e.g. Hjelmslev 1948: 191ff, Benveniste 1950: 151, Tesnière 1959: 155ff), but it is not necessary to search too far away, because it is also common in the older Indo-European languages, especially in Greek, less so in Latin. Such clauses, where there is no finite verb, and where the predicate, i.e. what is asserted of the subject, has the shape of a nominal element, viz. an adjective or a noun, can be exemplified by Latin:

(10) Omnia praeclara rara.

'All things marvellous (are) rare'

One feature distinguishes crucially the examples of (1) through (9) above from (10): the latter is general or generic – maybe even analytic – whereas the former can be general as well as particular, i.e. asserted as valid for some particular individual at some particular point of time.

2. The structure of the nominal clause

With regard to the three functions of the verb the nominal clause only retains the most general features: 1) the situation denoted is simply a state; 2) it is tenseless, i.e. it is not inscribed in any particular time interval, and it is of the most general modality; 3) the predicative function seems to be the only function shared by the nominal and the verbal clause: "L'assertion aura ce caractère propre d'être intemporelle, impersonnelle, non modale, bref de porter sur un terme réduit à son seul contenu sémantique" (Benveniste 1950: 159). The presence of a predicative relation is what Hjelmslev identifies as a verbal characteristic without a verbal base, hence his claim: "L'interprétation que nous proposons est donc celle qui consiste à considérer le zéro de la phrase nominale du latin comme l'expression du relief bas excessif de la prédication, et *sans que le contenu de la phrase comporte une base verbale*" (1948: 187). His analysis claims that two of the three verbal functions identified above are present in the nominal clause – aspect/tense/mood and predication – and the point he wishes to make is that "verbal morphemes" aren't verbal at all, they are properties of the sentence!

Since one of the three functions of the verb is to denote different kinds of relations between entities, the absence of a verb ought to correspond to just one kind of relation. Now the relation expressed and asserted by the simple juxtaposition of two nominals could only be some very simple relation. And this simple relation could hardly be anything else than a state – which is probably the simplest situation imaginable. And when the predicate is realised as a nominal element, a noun or an adjective, this state could hardly be anything but an equation, i.e. the identification of two entities, or the ascription of some property to an entity. Hence the label *equative clause* for such structures. Owing to this character of the predication it is essential to distinguish between nominal and copular clauses because the latter are verbal, even when the copula under certain conditions is suppressed, as is e.g. the case in Russian, see section 2.1 below. As stated by Emile Benveniste in his seminal analysis of the nominal clause in Indo-European: "Il y a bien opposition entre *omnis homo mortalis* et *omnis homo mortalis est*; mais elle est de nature, non de degré" (1950: 159). But as pointed out by Humbert (1960: 65ff), the distinction is often subtle and can be difficult to draw with precision in languages which have both verbal, with or without ellipsis, and nominal (non-elliptical) equative clauses.

The nominal clause is, as mentioned, not particularly widespread in Latin, but one finds examples such as:

(11) Summum ius, summa iniuria.

'Supreme justice (is) supreme injustice' (Cicero, Blatt 1946: 25)

(12) Quid peius muliere?

'what (is) worse than a woman?' (Plautus, Ernout & Thomas 1964: 146)

(13) Amor omnibus idem.

'love (is) to all the same' (Virgil, ib.)

In most nominal clauses in Greek the predicate is an adjective, as in the Latin example (10) above, or a noun:

(14) **áriston** húdōr

best-Nom water-Nom

'the best thing is water' (Humbert 1960: 65)

(15) *turannìs* **khrēma sphalerón**

tyranny-Nom thing-Nom shocking-Nom

'tyranny is a shocking thing' (Herodotus, ib. 66)

(16) **makárioi** hoi penthoũntes

blessed-Nom Def-Nom grieving-Nom

'blessed are those who grieve' (Matthew 5,4, ib. 68)[2]

(17) **pēma** kakòs geítōn

calamity-Nom bad-Nom neighbour-Nom

'a bad neighbour is a calamity' (Hesiodus, Benveniste 1950: 163)

(18) éntha gár sophíēs deĩ, bíēs érgon **oudén**

where for sagacity-Gen is-needed violence-Gen effect-Nom nothing-Nom

'for where sagacity is needed, violence is of no avail' (Herodotus, ib. 163)

---

[2] The Latin text retains the nominal clause: *Beati, qui lugent*, with a relative clause as its predicate.

(19)   **skiãs   ónar**   *ánthrōpos*
       shadow-Gen dream-Nom man-Nom
       'man is the dream of a shadow' (Pindarus, ib. 162)

What is remarkable is, however, that also structures where the predicate is instantiated by a noun in the dative or by a prepositional phrase – sometimes reduced to the preposition alone – are attested:

(20)   **soi**   tò   géras   polù   meîzon
       thou-Dat Def   booty-Nom   much   bigger-Nom
       'thine is the largest booty' (Il. 1.167, Benveniste 1950: 165)

(21)   **soi   d' épi** mèn morphē   epéōn,   **éni** dè phrénes   esthlaí ...
       thou-Dat Prt in   Prt form-Nom   words-Gen in   Prt mind-Nom   noble-Nom
       'In you (is) beauty of speech, therein (is) noble sentiment' (Od. 11.367, Seiler 1996)

(22)   **énth'éni** mèn philotēs, **én** d' hímeros, **én** d'   oaristús
       inside in Prt love-Nom in Prt desire-Nom in   Prt seduction
       'Therein (in the coat of Aphrodite) (is) love, therein (is) desire, therein (is) amorous conversation' (Il.14.216, ib.)

A comparable example from Latin could be the motto: *Officium ante omnia* 'Duty before everything'.

The total picture of the structural schemata of the Indo-European nominal clause, then, is the following:

(23)   NP – Adj
       NP – N$_{nom}$
       NP – N$_{dat}$
       NP – PP

This identification of a structural pattern coextensive with what is commonly found in subject complement position in BE-clauses has two consequences. On the one hand, it is at the root of the very widespread deletion analysis (section 2.1), on the other it adduces corroborating evidence in favour of the "adject"-analysis (section 2.2) proposed by the present author in collaboration with Finn Sørensen (see e.g. Herslund & Sørensen 1993, 1994, 1996, Davidsen-Nielsen 1996). At the same time this analysis sheds some new light on the analysis of the nominal clause.

2.1. The nominal clause as a reduced BE-clause

Most scholars seem to have analysed the nominal clause as a copulative clause from which a form of BE has been deleted (see e.g. the survey in Hjelmslev 1948). But in Benveniste's (1950) view this is a misrepresentation of the true nature of the nominal clause. Whereas the deletion analysis makes the equation of (24a), Benveniste sees this as a false analogy and the true analogy as (24b):

(24a)   Omnia praeclara Ø rara. = Omnia praeclara **sunt** rara.

'All things marvellous (are) rare'

(24b)   Omnia praeclara **rara**. = Omnia praeclara **pereunt**.

'All things marvellous (are) rare/decay'

The consequence of this view is of course that the nominal clause is something different from the copulative clause and that its nominal predicate is a predicate on a par with a finite verb, but – and this is the crucial point of Benveniste's interpretation – this predicate is, as already mentioned, due to its nominal character, unable to express the verbal categories of mood and tense, and so the nominal clause is limited to asserting general, generic or even analytic sentences. When some specific situation is described, the nominal clause is no longer possible and to the prepositional examples (20) to (22) correspond clauses with the (lone) preposition prefixed to the verb BE (Seiler 1996):

(25)   idōmetha ...   hóssos   khrūsós   te   kaì   árguros   askōi   **énestin**

look-1pl-Med how-much gold-Nom Prt and silver-Nom sack-Dat in-is-3sg

'Let's look ... how much gold and silver is in the sack' (Od. 10.45)

If one accepts the analysis of (24b), it follows that verbless clauses, as are well-known from e.g. Russian, such as (26) and (27):

(26)   Ivan – soldat.

'Ivan (is) (a) soldier'

(27)   Dom – nov.

'(The) house (is) new'

are not nominal clauses, strictly speaking. They are in fact not limited to expressing general statements and they can be inflected e.g. in the past tense, in which case the copula reappears. If they were analysed as genuine nominal clauses, one would have to say that equative clauses are nominal in the present, but copular in the past:

(28)   Ivan byl soldat/soldatom.

'Ivan was (a) soldier'

(29)   Dom byl nov.
         '(The) house was new'

A verbless clause of a language which otherwise has a copula verb can only be analysed as a nominal clause if there is some corresponding copular clause with a slightly different meaning. Now in Russian there is hardly any alternative way of expressing *dom – nov*, so it doesn't qualify as a nominal clause (cf. also Durst-Andersen 1995).

It is in fact also characteristic that languages which have such verbless equative clauses, i.e. clauses where the copula is omitted in the present, always have a means of distinguishing these from the sequence noun – adjective constituting an NP with which they would otherwise be homonymous. In Arabic and Hungarian (Hjelmslev 1948: 194), as well as in Greek, the definite article, and word order, serves this purpose (cf. also the French and German examples (6) to (9) above):

(30)   *Arabic*
         el-bēt 'ālī
         'the house (is) big'
         el-bēt el-'ālī
         'the big house'

(31)   *Hungarian*
         a ház magas / magas a ház
         'the house (is) big'
         a magas ház
         'the big house'

In Russian, which has no article, the two different forms of the adjective serve this purpose:

(32)   Dom – nov
         'The house (is) new'
         novyj dom / dom novyj
         '(the/a) new house'

This might well be one reason why Latin, which has none of these devices, does not really favour the nominal clause (cf. Hjelmslev 1948: 194): it is in fact impossible to differentiate *domus nova* 'the house (is) new' from *domus nova* 'the new house'.

One might then distinguish two types of clauses with nominal predicatives, the copular clause and the nominal clause. In the first case the *predicative* (the complement) is nominal, in the second it is the *predicate* which is nominal:

Clause	Subject	Predicate	Complement
Copular	*dom* *domus*	*Ø/byl* *est*	*nov* *nova*
Nominal	*domus*	*nova*	

Table 1.

Within the copular clause type different languages draw different distinctions: some languages only express the copula outside the present tense (e.g. Russian), some always express it (e.g. English), some, finally, distinguish between different copulae (e.g. Spanish). Such languages seem to (re)create, within the verbal clause, a distinction reminiscent of the nominal-verbal clause distinction of Indo-European insofar as one BE-verb (viz. *ser*) states general and essential properties, whereas the other (viz. *estar*) expresses the temporary and accidental being. But the copular clause is fundamentally different from the nominal because it, as the verbal clause it is, expresses the verbal categories that are denied the nominal clause:

	Copular	Nominal
± Copula	*Dom Ø/byl nov*	*Omnia praeclara rara*
+ Copula	*The house is new*	
ser/estar	*La casa es/está nueva*[3]	

Table 2.

Superficially, then, the first type is identical with the nominal clause, but this syntactic neutralisation should not lead to the conclusion that they are identical. They are not. The first is a verbal, i.e. a copular clause, the second a nominal clause. Some caution is needed, however. There seems in fact to be some terminological confusion in the usage of the concept of 'nominal clause': whereas Benveniste uses it constantly and consistently only of genuinely verbless structures such as (10), other linguists have used the term, or rather its French equivalent, 'phrase nominale', of genuine nominal and copular clauses alike. This is, for example, the case with Meillet (1920: 179f).

---

[3] On the distinction *ser/estar* and the adjective *nuevo* in Spanish, see e.g. Fogsgaard (1989: 215).

2.2. The nominal clause and the notion of 'adject'

In what precedes I have argued, following Benveniste (1950), that the nominal clause is an autonomous construction not resulting from the deletion of anything. Its special build-up, i.e. a nominal element predicated immediately of another nominal element, has the consequence that in languages which use a copula to express tensed and modalised equative clauses (just like all other verbal predications) the nominal clause is restricted to general or even generic/analytic statements: because of the tenselessness of the clause, the predication, i.e. the assertion of the ascription of some property or state, is presented as absolutely valid (cf. Benveniste 1950: 160: "Une assertion nominale complète en soi, pose l'énoncé hors de toute localisation temporelle ou modale et hors de la subjectivité du locuteur"), hence its use in aphoristic and maxim-like statements. One might in fact assume that Greek continues the Indo-European situation where the finite verb, in the present as well as in other tenses, necessarily inscribes the predication in time and therefore is not capable of expressing universally valid equations, hence the retention of the nominal clause in such cases (cf. Benveniste 1950: 167). The crucial factor to notice is then that the nominal predication is not actualised by any verbal morpheme, only by the assertion of it itself. In this respect the nominal clause is reminiscent of the kind of (secondary) predication assumed by the analysis of certain structures as adject constructions (cf. Herslund & Sørensen 1993, 1994, 1996, and Davidsen-Nielsen 1996).

The basis of the adject-analysis is the assumption of the existence of a secondary predication in trivalent structures. So a clause like (33a) has the analysis of (33b):

(33a) She put the lamp on the table.

(33b) She put the lamp on the table
$$\underbrace{\phantom{\text{She put the lamp on the table}}}_{\displaystyle 1.}\;\;\underbrace{\phantom{\text{the lamp on the table}}}_{\displaystyle 2.}$$

where there is a secondary predication between *the lamp* and *on the table*. Generalising this view, it is suggested that trivalent structures always introduce secondary predications between their object and some prepositional phrase, or some noun or adjective phrase (the adject) as in (34) and (35):

(34) They elected him *president*.[4]

(35) They painted it *red*.

---

[4]The observation that the copula is more easily absent in embedded than in independent clauses has often been made, cf. Jespersen 1937: 122 or Riegel 1985: 46.

and that the same is true of bivalent clauses where the adject relation obtains between the intransitive subject and the adject, as in (36) and (37):

(36)　He became *president*.

(37)　It became *red*.

The striking thing to observe is now that the structural schemata characteristic of the nominal clause identified in (23) are coextensive with the structures found in adject positions. Furthermore, the secondary predication assumed in order to account for a great number of otherwise obscure and unrelated facts (cf. Herslund & Sørensen 1993, 1994, 1996) has the nature of a "sleeping" predication, i.e. it is only brought to life, as it were (cf. Jespersen's metaphor)[5], via the primary predication of the finite verb: by itself it states something very general, only related to the reality depicted by way of the primary predication. It has in other words all the characteristics of a nominal clause, except the assertive power. Whence the idea that the nominal clause, in the languages where it is found, is nothing else than a secondary predication promoted to the rank of primary predication. Languages which have genuine nominal clauses are languages which have so to speak the power of promoting their secondary predications to primary and assert them directly.

The idea of a secondary predication linking the subject and the adject (e.g. the subject complement) is in fact well-known and more or less explicitly propounded in "traditional" grammar. One exponent of this view is Jespersen, who gives the following diagram of his nexus combinations (1937: 121):

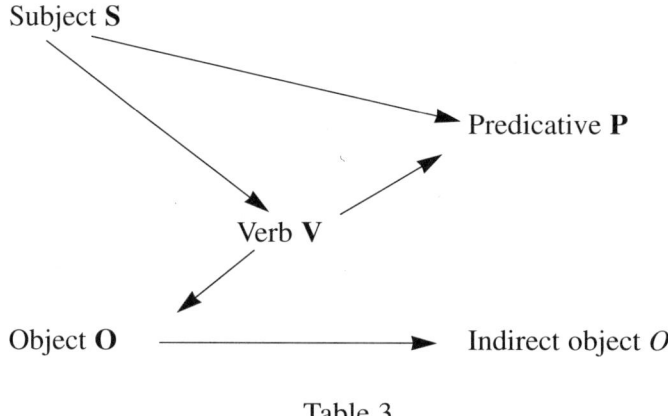

Table 3.

---

[5] "... in a junction we add one dead piece to another, as bricks are placed on top of and by the side of one another to build a house. But in a nexus we get life and movement" (1937: 120f).

The arrows connecting **S** and **P**, and **O** and *O* correspond to our secondary predications.

Something very similar is found in Tesnière (1959: 158ff), especially as illustrated by his stemma 157:

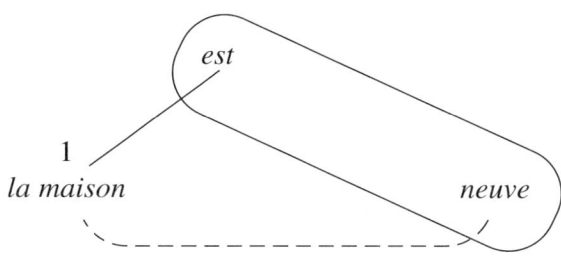

Table 4.

In Tesnière's view, the copular clause is structurally a verbal, but semantically a nominal clause, which is expressed by the dotted line.

2.3. The nominal clause as a promoted secondary predication

How does this proposal fit in with e.g. the analysis of the Latin stock example *Omnia praeclara rara*? Rather well, insofar as the copular clause, *Omnia praeclara rara sunt*, has the following analysis:

(38)   2.
   _____
   Omnia praeclara rara sunt.
   _____
         1.

where the chunk *omnia praeclara – rara*, i.e. the secondary predication, has exactly the shape and the structure of the nominal clause as depicted in Table 1. Structurally then, the nominal clause is indistinguishable from the secondary predication under the adject analysis. The predication has just been made autonomous.

Furthermore Humbert speaks explicitly of an embedded nominal clause in the case of other copular verbs than BE (*in casu* the verb *eidō* 'see, Med. seem'): "Enfin on admet ordinairement l'existence de phrases *nominales-verbales*, dans lesquelles le prédicat, qui est un *verbe*, comporte une qualité et contient comme *implicitement* une phrase *nominale*: par exemple Ξ 472 *ou mén moi kakós eídetai* "il ne me semble pas (= il n'est pas pour moi) de basse naissance"'" (1960: 65). So what Humbert sees as embedded under the verb SEEM is a nominal clause as a secondary predication:

(39)   2.
        ─────────────────────────────────
        Ø kakós moi   ou   eídetai
        he bad   me-Dat   not seem-3sg-Med-Pres-Ind
        ─────────────────────────────────
            1.

exactly the same analysis as the one assumed in (38) above. And as pointed out by Benveniste (1950: 160) there is every reason to treat the verb BE as any other copular verb.

3. Conclusion

We then get the following classification of languages according to the way they instantiate equative sentences: all equative clauses are nominal (e.g. Turkish, cf. Tesnière 1959: 155), some equative sentences are nominal (Greek), all equative sentences are verbal, the copula being omitted in the present (Russian), and all equative sentences are verbal with an expressed copula (English). This can be depicted in the following table:

	Nominal	Verbal
Turkish	all	
Greek	general	particular
English		all

Table 5.

But this classification brings us back to the examples of the introductory section and the question raised there: what about such structures? Are they really elliptical or are they genuine examples of nominal clauses?

Let us return to example (5), *England winners*. If this sentence is elliptical, what is then the full expression? According to the simplest analysis it should be *England are winners*, but that does not seem to render the exact value of the expression at all. The point is namely that the fact that England has won the world championship is not simply being stated, but that the assertion has been promoted to the status of inscription. Assertions can be promoted to the status of inscription by being carved in stone, translated into Latin, or by being rendered by a nominal clause. So my proposal is that *England winners* is in fact a nominal clause, that the modern Western European languages do have nominal clauses, but that these are confined to special uses, as inscriptions, emblems, mottos, maxims and the like. The use of nominal clauses in mottos are well-known, e.g. in Danish:

(40)   Folkets kærlighed, min styrke.
       'The people's love, my strength'

And the best known use of the nominal expression, viz. in newspaper headlines can be seen as a variant of this: by using a nominal clause the important and indeed emblematic function of the headline is emphasised. As seen in (1) to (4), such examples exhibit the same structures as the Indo-European nominal clause – with the possible exception of the morphological dative – cf. (23) and the following structures from French with an adjective, an NP and a PP as predicatives, respectively (Riegel 1985: 47):

(41)   L'équipe de France victorieuse.
       'The French team winners'
(42)   L'équipe de France championne du monde.
       'The French team world champions'
(43)   L'équipe de France en finale.
       'The French team in finals'

The nominal construction promotes the entire expression into something absolute which the reader should imperatively retain. In fact headlines are often conclusions rather than premises or simple introductions to the following text. And this accords well, apart from the special atemporal feature of the Greek nominal clause, with the general character of the nominal clause as described by Benveniste: "La phrase nominale vise à convaincre en énonçant une "vérité générale"; elle suppose le discours et le dialogue; elle ne communique pas une donnée de fait, mais pose un rapport intemporel et permanent qui agit comme un argument d'autorité" (1950: 162). Or: "Etant apte à des assertions absolues, la phrase nominale a valeur d'argument, de preuve, de référence. On l'introduit dans le discours pour agir et convaincre, non pour informer" (1950: 165). The function of the headline seems indeed to be argumentative rather than informative. And the same is true of the exclamative-like nominal clauses of French and German, as in (6) to (9)[6]: they render the utterer's unreserved and unqualified opinion. Hence these uses of the nominal clause, as in ancient Greek, instead of the normal copular clause.

---

[6]The French constructions are discussed in Riegel 1985, cf. also Forsgren 1987. In Riegel's analysis, however, a copula is deleted and, with it, "la localisation temporelle, modale et aspectuelle du rapport énonciatif" (1985: 141). This analysis is a hybrid between the two analyses discussed in the present article, the deletion analysis (section 2.1) and the "nominal clause proper *cum* adject promotion" analysis (sections 2.2 and 2.3).

References

Behr, I. & H. Quintin (1995). De la phrase nominale à l'énoncé non verbal. Paper read at the *Colloque Benveniste*, Cerisy-la-Salle, 12-19 August 1995.

Benveniste, E. (1950). La phrase nominale. In *Problèmes de linguistique générale*, Paris: Gallimard [1966], 151-167.

Blatt, F. (1946). *Latinsk Syntaks i Hovedtræk*. København: Gyldendal.

Bloomfield, L. (1933). *Language*. London: Allen & Unwin [1969].

Davidsen-Nielsen, N., ed. (1996). *Sentence Analysis, Valency, and the Concept of Adject*. Copenhagen Studies in Language 19.

Durst-Andersen, P. (1995). De to syntaktiske systemer i russisk. In P. Durst-Andersen & J. Nørgård-Sørensen (eds) *Ny forskning i grammatik* 2, Odense: Odense University Press, 91-114.

Ernout, A. & F. Thomas (1964). *Syntaxe latine*. Paris: Klincksieck.

Fogsgaard, L. (1989). *SER/ESTAR og udsigelsen*. Copenhagen: Basilisk.

Forsgren, M. (1987). Attribut et prédication. A propos de Martin Riegel: *L'adjectif attribut*. *Revue Romane* 22, 264-278.

Herslund, M. & F. Sørensen. (1993). Valence Theory. An Introduction to the Danish Project. In M. Herslund & F. Sørensen (eds) *The Nordlex Project. Lexical Studies in the Scandinavian Languages. LAMBDA* 18, 1-22.

Herslund, M. & F. Sørensen. (1994). A Valence Based Theory of Grammatical Relations. In E. Engberg-Pedersen et al. (eds) *Function and Expression in Functional Grammar*, Berlin & New York: Mouton de Gruyter, 81-95.

Herslund, M. & F. Sørensen (1996). Introduction. Discussion. In N. Davidsen-Nielsen (ed) 1996, 9-13, 143-157.

Hjelmslev, L. (1948). Le verbe et la phrase nominale. In *Essais linguistiques*, Paris: Editions de Minuit [1971], 174-200.

Humbert, J. (1960). *Syntaxe grecque*. Paris: Klincksieck.

Jespersen, O. (1937). *Analytic Syntax*. New York: Holt, Rinehart & Winston [1969].

Meillet, A. (1920). Sur les caractères du verbe. In *Linguistique historique et linguistique générale*, Paris: Klincksieck [1965], 175-198.

Riegel, M. (1985). *L'adjectif attribut*. Paris: PUF.

Seiler, H. (1996). Localisation et prédication. Paper read at the *Colloque: Typologie et diversité des langues*, Paris 8-9 November 1996.

Tesnière, L. (1959). *Eléments de syntaxe structurale*. Paris: Klincksieck.

On the Use of Mood and Modal Verbs in Italian and Danish[1]

Bente Lihn Jensen

1. Introduction

The purpose of this article is to illustrate some basic differences in the use of mood and modal verbs in Italian and Danish, and in the light of these differences to discuss how the categories may most appropriately be described in a grammar such as the one currently being prepared by the working group for Italian under the research project Lingvistik og fremmedsprog[2] (Linguistics and Foreign Languages).

Our view of mood and modal verbs as constituting two grammatical categories is based on Italian, in which the modal verbs may appear in different moods, as shown below in (1a) - (1d). This means that the modal verbs cannot be ascribed to the category of mood, in which context they would function as auxiliary verbs of so-called analytic mood, though this is quite possible in English and Danish (cf. Davidsen-Nielsen 1990[3] and Bostrup 1991).

(1a)   Il tetto *deve* essere riparato.   (*deve*: present I[4] of *dovere*)
       the roof – modal verb[+ necessity] – be repared
(1b)   Il tetto *dovrà* essere riparato.   (*dovrà*: simple future of *dovere*)
(1c)   Il tetto *dovrebbe* essere riparato.   (*dovrebbe*: simple conditional of *dovere*)
(1d)   Temeva che il tetto *dovesse* essere riparato. (*dovesse*: imperfect S[5] of *dovere*)
       feared[3rd.pers.sg.] – that ...

---

[1] I am indebted to Martin Aitken for kindly having translated the present article from the Danish manuscript.
[2] In 1993 the Danish Research Council for the Humanities initiated 5 five-year grammar-writing projects in the following languages: English, French, German, Russian and Italian. The working group for Italian comprises, besides the present author, project leader Gunver Skytte, University of Copenhagen, and Iørn Korzen, Copenhagen Business School. The project is described in detail in e.g. Skytte 1993.
[3] The difference between English and Italian in this respect is also mentioned in Davidsen-Nielsen 1990: 48.
[4] 'I' denotes indicative.
[5] 'S' denotes subjunctive.

By way of introduction it can be said that not only do the individual moods and modal verbs differ as to their use in the two languages, they also differ in their expression in that Danish has more modal verbs at its disposal than Italian, which in turn has more, particularly finite, moods than Danish, as will be evident from Figure 1.

Figure 1   Moods and modal verbs in Danish and Italian

	DANISH	ITALIAN
MOODS, FINITE	Indicative	Indicative
	Imperative	Imperative
	(Subjunctive)[6]	Subjunctive
MOODS, NON-FINITE	Infinitive	Infinitive
	Participle	Participle
	Past	Past
	Present	Present
	Gerund	
MODAL VERBS	*behøve*	*potere*
	burde	*dovere*
	kunne	*volere*
	måtte	
	skulle	
	ville[7]	

For the sake of comparison it may be mentioned that according to Bergenholtz (1989) the three most frequent modal verbs in Danish are *kunne*, *skulle* and *ville*, which occupy 20th, 28th and 30th places respectively on the frequency list with a total of 15 864, 9 466 and 8 942 occurrences in a corpus of 2 million running words sampled from newspapers, weekly magazines and novels. In contrast, the three Italian modal verbs *potere*, *volere* and *dovere* as they appear in (i) *LIF* (1971) comprising written material sampled from the following five areas: theatre, novels, film, newspapers & weekly magazines and text books and (ii) *LIP* (1993) comprising exclusively spoken language sampled from five different discourse situations in the areas Milan, Florence, Rome and Naples occupy 32nd/31st, 35th and 38th/36th places respectively. The two dictionaries are each based on material comprising 500 000 words. However, multiplying to obtain directly comparable

---

[6]The parentheses denote that the form, as noted by Rask (1995: 72), is no longer productive.
[7]The actual number is greater, but those indicated are (i) the most central and (ii) of greatest interest in the present context.

quantities results in frequencies for the *LIF/LIP* material of 6 849.2/9 100 occurrences in the case of *potere*, 5 672.36/8 212 for *volere*, and 5 189.56/7 972 in the case of *dovere*. The disparity between the number of occurrences in the two frequency dictionaries may theoretically be attributed to more frequent use of modal verbs in the spoken medium than in the written and/or a development in the language away from the synthetic towards the analytic. (While it is beyond the scope of the present article to pursue this aspect further, it may be noted that both tendencies are observable in modern Italian).

In order to impart to the reader an impression of the distribution of the various moods in Italian, two frequency lists taken from Voghera 1992 are shown below in Figure 2. Both are based on the same spoken corpora and indicate the percentage distribution of moods in main and subordinate clauses (finite and non-finite) respectively.

Figure 2 Percentage distribution of verb forms according to mood in main and subordinate clauses. Figures from Voghera (1992: 213 & 236)[8].

	MAIN CLAUSE	SUBORDINATE CLAUSE
INDICATIVE	88.1%(91.4)	62.9%
IMPERATIVE	4.1%	-
SUBJUNCTIVE	0.4%	4.5%[9]
FUTURE	3.3%	unspecified (included under Indicative)
CONDITIONAL	4.0%	0.7%[10]
INFINITIVE	0.1%	22.9%
PARTICIPLE	-	5.4%
GERUND	-	3.6%

---

[8]In Voghera the future is included under the indicative. The figure in parentheses for the indicative in main clauses indicates the incidence of the indicative inclusive of the future, whereas the non-bracketed figure indicates the incidence according to the classification used in the present article. The figure in parentheses is included here for reasons of comparability. Since in Voghera the data pertaining to the various verb forms in subordinate clauses are less detailed than those relating to verb forms occurring in main clauses, it has not been possible to specify the future's share of the total incidence.

[9]The marked difference in the incidence of the subjunctive in main and subordinate clauses is explained by the fact that the subjunctive is a mood most often found in the latter clause type. On the occasion of J. Schmitt Jensen's defence of thesis (see Jensen 1970), one of the official opponents concluded that according to Schmitt Jensen's theory the title on the front cover of the book could have been "Subjonctif est hypotaxe en italien" and not, as is the case, "Subjonctif et hypotaxe en italien". The subjunctive in main clauses functions almost entirely as a request in formal language, i.e. the hearer is addressed by means of *Lei* rather than *tu*, corresponding to *De* and *du* respectively in Danish.

[10]The marked difference is explained here by the fact that the conditional is primarily used in conditional constructions, the mood of the main clause being conditional, that of the subordinate clause subjunctive. The subordinate clause will, however, often remain unarticulated. Furthermore, the conditional is often used as a polite form of the type *Vorrei un caffè* (= I would like a cup of coffee), some linguists believing the notion of possibility being implicit, others taking the converse view. Regardless of which view one subscribes to, the occurrence of the subordinate clause of the type in question in such utterances is extremely rare.

2. Modality

Mood and the modal verbs comprise two grammaticalized ways in which the two languages may express modality, i.e. the speaker's intention with the utterance, his commitment to the propositional content of the utterance, and his attitude towards the hearer as expressed in the linguistic manifestation[11].

In other words, modality is inextricably linked with the concept of speech acts (see Searle 1975) in that representatives, as will be evident from section 2.1., always express epistemic modality, whereas directives and commissives express deontic modality[12]. It should be noted, however, that representatives may in addition to epistemic modality express other forms of modality such as alethic modality, i.e. concerning physical necessity/possibility. The concept of alethic modality will not be treated further in the present article.

2.1. Epistemic modality

The concept of epistemic modality is invoked here in a broad sense as being practically synonymous with evidentiality as invoked by Chafe & Nichols (1986). However, while the latter authors in their Introduction state that "We do not wish, for the moment at least, to suggest what the boundaries of evidentiality in the broad sense are" (1986: vii), the title of the work defines the concept as "the linguistic coding of epistemology", the term being further employed by Chafe in his own contribution "to cover any linguistic expression of attitudes toward knowledge" (1986: 271).

The same article operates with, for English, four so-called modes of knowing: (i) belief, (ii) induction, (iii) hearsay, (iv) deduction, each of which based on a different source of knowledge: (i) ?? [sic], (ii) evidence, (iii) language, (iv) hypothesis (1986: 263).

While our knowledge of English is insufficient to enable us to fruitfully discuss the division from the point of view of English, we note that since Italian, and ostensibly Danish too, distinguishes between conclusions drawn on a logical basis and those on a non-logical basis, it would seem natural to consider the former type of knowledge as comprising a category of its own: if conclusions are drawn on a logical basis, it would seem correct to assume that other individuals besides the speaker should be able to draw the same conclusions; for this reason we shall refer to this type of knowledge as *objective evidence*, as opposed to *subjective evidence*, which indicates that it is the speaker's viewpoint only which is passed on. This means that we in the Italian project operate with the following four sources (the Italian project does not

---

[11]See Jensen *forthcoming* for a more detailed treatment of this subject.
[12]Concerning 'reported deontic modality' see 2.2.1.

distinguish between 'source of knowledge' and 'mode of knowing'): (i) subjective evidence, (ii) objective evidence, (iii) hearsay, (iv) hypothesis.

For each source the speaker may express varying degrees of commitment to the truth-value of the proposition. Bybee (1985: 180), here quoting Steele (1975), operates with the following degrees of commitment: (i) certainty, (ii) almost certainty, (iii) probability, (iv) possibility, (v) weak possibility, all of which recur in Italian, albeit not for each individual source.

Chafe does not include factual knowledge under the heading of evidentiality, but since the speaker may present his knowledge as something to which he himself can subscribe, either because it concerns something he has seen, heard or otherwise experienced, or because he believes what he has put forward to be the case, we find it natural to distinguish between that to which a truth-value may be assigned and that to which no such value may be assigned. In linguistic terms what is distinguished is factual and non-factual knowledge.

Since any state of affairs (SoA) is temporally located in relation to the moment of speech (MoS), and possibly also to another SoA, we must in the case of epistemic modality operate with three parameters: (i) source of knowledge, (ii) degree of commitment, (iii) temporal location. The latter is of peripherical interest in the present context and will therefore henceforth only be referred to where this is necessary for purposes of understanding (see e.g. Figure 5 in section 4).

The various knowledge sources are exemplified below:

1. Subjective evidence

A: degree of commitment: certainty = factuality

(2a)   Laura *er* i øjeblikket i London.   Adesso Laura *è* a Londra.

(2b)   Laura *er ikke* i London i øjeblikket.   Adesso Laura *non è* a Londra.

B: degree of commitment: non-factuality

(3)   Laura *er vist* i London i øjeblikket.   Adesso Laura *sarà* a Londra.

2. Objective evidence

A: degree of commitment: factuality

(4)   To og to *er* fire.   Due più due *fanno* quattro.

B: degree of commitment: non-factuality: almost certainty/probability

(5)   Laura *må være* i London.   Laura *dev'essere* a Londra.

C: degree of commitment: non-factuality: possibility

(6)   Laura *kan være* i London.   Laura *può essere* a Londra.

3. Hearsay

In grammaticalized form it is expressed in Italian by means of the conditional. In contrast, Danish uses the modal *skulle*, which may occur in either the present or the past tense:

(7)   Laura *skal/skulle (efter sigende)* være i London i øjeblikket.   Adesso Laura *sarebbe* a Londra.

(8)   Mauro *skal/skulle (efter sigende) være på vej* til Frankrig.   Mauro *starebbe per andare* in Francia.

4. Hypothesis

(9)   Hvis jeg vinder, *køber* jeg hus i Italien.   Se vinco/vincerò, *compro/comprerò* una casa in Italia.

(10) Hvis jeg skulle vinde/vandt, *ville købe/købte* jeg hus i Italien.   Se vincessi, *comprerei* una casa in Italia.

Although the speaker *inter alia* has the two indicated choices available to him in both languages, the two options differ in use in that the Danish example in (9) may be considered the unmarked form, whereas the unmarked choice in Italian would be (10), the mood here being subjunctive in the subordinate clause and conditional in the main clause. The use of the present/future – as in the Italian example in (9) above – automatically signals that the speaker presents the future realization of the condition as probable.

2.2. Deontic modality

Deontic modality exists where a person is given permission to or is obliged to/compelled to act. Typically, the Danish speaker will use the imperative in order to express what in Bybee & Fleischman 1995: 6 is called subject-oriented modality, while the modals included in Figure 1 are used to express what is termed agent-oriented modality (op.cit.).

In Italian, subject-oriented deontic modality is implemented by means of either the imperative or the subjunctive[13], whereas agent-oriented modality will typically

---

[13]The choice between the imperative and the subjunctive is dependent on the number of hearers (cf. addressees), as well as on the degree of formality. In the case of more than one hearer, the imperative (*Venite! Accomodatevi!*) is most often used in both registers, whereas the imperative is used in informal register in the case of one hearer (*Vieni! Accomodati!*) and the subjunctive is used in the formal register (*Venga. Si acomodi.*). In the case of prohibition, *non* + infinitive (*Non ci andare!*) is used when addressing one hearer only in the informal register, *non* + subjunctive (*Non ci vada.*) occurring in the formal register, whereas *non* + imperative (*Non andateci!*) occurs where the number of hearers exceeds one.

be implemented by the modals *dovere* and *potere*, although *volere*, too, is very frequently selected. The latter case involves a change in perspective in relation to the *dovere/potere* construction (cf. (15) in section 2.2.1 and (26) in Figure 3, section 3).

As is well-known, Danish differentiates within deontic necessity with regard to the source of the obligation/compulsion: where the source is a social authority *skulle* is used; where the source is the speaker himself *måtte* is used, and where the source is a moral authority *burde* is used (cf. Hansen 1972).

(11)   Jeg *skal* ringe til Ole (det har han bedt mig om).
(12)   Jeg *må* ringe til Ole (ellers får jeg ikke en rolig time).
(13)   Jeg *bør* ringe til Ole (nu hvor han er syg).

This grammaticalized distinction does not exist in Italian, where as a general rule *dovere* is used in all instances. The example containing *burde* may, however, be rendered using *dovere* in the conditional, though it should be stressed that the speaker is unlikely to do so. In the case of the speaker wishing to make explicit the subtleties inherent in the Danish system, he must have recourse to lexical items:

(14)   Sento il dovere di farlo.

   feel[1.pers.sg.] – the obligation/duty to do-it   (= Danish: *må*).

2.2.1. Reported deontic modality

The deontic content may also be expressed by representatives such as (15) - (16). We can then refer to the concept of 'reported deontic modality', the overriding purpose of the utterance being to inform the hearer of some world-state:

(15)   *Ole må gerne gå i biografen.*   *Ole può andare al cinema*, dunque
       Må jeg så ikke også?   voglio andarci anche io.

(16)   Eva sagde at *jeg skulle ringe*.   Eva mi ha detto di *telefonarti*.

3. Some basic differences

3.1. One lexical item corresponds to several in the other language

3.1.1. One lexical item in Danish

As previously mentioned, Italian has at its disposal a greater number of finite moods than Danish, which in turn exhibits a greater number of modal verbs than Italian. This could indicate that the use of modals is more widespread in Danish than in Italian. That this is indeed the case may be seen from the above mentioned data taken fra Danish and Italian frequency dictionaries (see Introduction) and is further evident from Figure 3, which presents examples of the use of the Danish modal *skulle* and its equivalent expressions in Italian.

Figure 3   Examples of the use of *skulle* and its equivalents in Italian

(17)	– Hvad *skal* du *lave* på fredag? – Jeg *skal* til Århus.	– Venerdì cosa *fai*? – (Venerdì) *vado* a Århus.	(present I) (present I)
(18)	Jeg *skal* til Århus på fredag, det *skal* jeg virkelig.	Venerdì *vado* a Århus, ci *devo andare*.	(present I) (*dovere*: present I)
(19)	På fredag *skal* Ole til Århus.	Venerdì Ole *andrà* a Århus.	(simple future)
(20)	Du *skal ringe* til kontoret.	*Devi chiamare* l'ufficio.	(*dovere*: present I)
(21)	Jeg fik at vide at jeg *skulle ringe* til kontoret.	Mi hanno detto... a. .. di *chiamare* l'ufficio. b. .. che *chiamassi* l'ufficio. c. .. che *dovevo chiamare* l'uff.	(infinitive) (imperfect S) (*dovere*: imp.I)
(22)	Han *skal* (efter sigende) *kunne* japansk.	*Saprebbe* il giapponese.	(conditional)
(23)	Han *skal kunne* japansk (for at få jobbet).	*Deve sapere* il giapponese (per ottenere il posto).	(*dovere*: present I)
(24)	De søger en medarbejder der *skal kunne* japansk.	Cercano un collaboratore che *sappia* il giapponese.	(present S)
(25)	Jeg *skal nok hjælpe* dig.	Ti *aiuterò* io.	(simple future)
(26)	*Skal* jeg *hjælpe* dig?	*Vuoi* che io ti *aiuti*?	(*volere*: present I subject_hearer)
(27)	Du *skal og må gøre* det.	*Non puoi fare* a meno di *far*lo.	(neg. + *potere*: present I + neg.)
(28)	Taget *skal repareres*.	a. Il tetto *dev'essere riparato*. b. Il tetto *sarà/verrà riparato*	(*dovere*: present I) (simple future passive)
(29)	Taget *skal blive repareret*.	Il tetto *sarà/verrà riparato*.	(simple future passive)
(30)	Hvad *skal* jeg *gøre*?	Cosa *fare*?	(infinitive)
(31)	Eva fortalte at hun *skulle* til Rom.	Eva mi disse... a. .. che *sarebbe andata* a Roma. b. .. che *andava* a Roma. c. .. che *doveva andare* a R.	(compound Cond.) (imperfect I) (*dovere*: imperfect I)

Here, the modal *skulle* is used:

– in directives (excluding questions)	((18.2), (20), (27), (28) corresponding to (28a))
– in questions	((17.1), (26), (30))
– in commissives	((25), (29))
– in representatives	
– indicating subjective evidence	((17.2), (18.1), (19), (28) corresponding to (28b))
– indicating hearsay	((22))
– containing reported deontic modality	((21), (23), (24), (31) corresponding to (31c))
– containing reported epistemic modality	((31) corresponding (31a-b))

As can be seen, Italian makes use of all of 11 different expressions. Besides *dovere* (see (18.2), (20), (21c), (23), (28a), (31c)), which like *skulle* is a modal including within its semantics the value [+necessity], making it the most immediately salient rendering for many Danes[14], the possible selections are as follows:

– present indicative of main verb	((17), (18.1))
– future of main verb	((19), (25), (28b), (29))
– simple conditional of main verb	((22))
– compound conditional of main verb	((31a))
– imperfect indicative of main verb	((31b))
– present subjunctive of main verb	((24))
– imperfect subjunctive of main verb	((21b))
– subject$_{hearer}$ + *volere* + subordinate clause	((26))
– negation + modal verb *potere* – negation	((27))
– infinitive	((21a), (30))

Although the number of equivalent forms listed in Figure 3 is probably close to the maximum, a corresponding pattern would emerge if we were to examine the other Danish modals in a similar way.

---

[14]Cf. "*Dobbiamo al cinema stasera?*", the title of a student's compendium (Thygesen 1995) dealing with modal expressions in Danish and Italian, clearly indicates the Danish point of departure, cf. "*Skal vi i biografen i aften?*". For the benefit of readers unfamiliar with Italian, the title is incomprehensible to an Italian, who would say either "*Andiamo al cinema stasera?/Stasera andiamo al cinema?*" or "*Stasera dobbiamo andare al cinema?*" (where the latter example stresses necessity/obligation).

3.1.2. One lexical item in Italian

In the same way as one and the same modal verb in Danish equates to several expressions in Italian, one single item in Italian, e.g. the future[15], may correspond to several in Danish, as shown in Figure 4:

Figure 4   Examples of the use of the future and its equivalents in Danish

(32)   Venerdì Ugo *andrà* a Parigi.   a. Ugo *tager* til Paris på fredag.
                                       b. Ugo *skal* til Paris på fredag.

(33)   – Che ore sono?   – Hvad er klokken?
       – *Saranno* le 17.   – Den *er vist/nok* 17.

(34)   Domani a quest'ora *sarò* a Roma.   I morgen ved denne tid ...
                                           a. ... *er* jeg i Rom.
                                           b. ... *vil* jeg *være* i Rom.

(35)   "*Vi divertirete* molto."[16]   a. "I *kommer til at more jer* meget."
                                       b. "I *skal more jer* meget."/"*Mor jer* meget."

(36)   Ti *aiuterò* io.   Jeg *skal nok hjælpe* dig.

Here the Italian future is used:

– in representatives
    – indicating subjective non-factual evidence
        – SoA simultaneous with MoS   ((33))
        – SoA posterior to MoS   ((32), (34), (35) corresponding to (35a))
– in directives   ((35) corresponding to (35b))
– in commisives   ((36))

3.2. The role of syntax

Another general difference concerns the influence syntax can bring to bear on the choice of modal expression. As a case in point, Italian often exhibits different linguistic manifestations according to whether the semantic content is presented in a main clause or in a subordinate clause, as shown in (20) vs (21) and (23) vs (24) in Figure 3.

---

[15]Here, as in Jensen 1994: 29, we assume that verbal inflections are to be considered as lexical units.
[16]The quote is from a literary example given to me by my colleague Svend Bach. The literary text, the origin of which is regrettably unknown, continues as follows: *i due giovani non capirono se questo fosse detto in tono di previsione o di ordine* (= the two youngsters did not understand whether it was uttered as a prediction or as an order).

Typically, the subjunctive will feature in the subordinate clause, whereas the imperative or a construction containing a modal verb will occur in the main clause.

While modifications of this kind are far more seldom in Danish, they do nevertheless occur, as can be seen from examples (38b) and (38c):

(37) Jeg *skal nok hjælpe* dig.

(38) Jeg lover at
    a. ... jeg *nok skal hjælpe* dig.
    b. ... jeg *vil hjælpe* dig.
    c. ... *ville hjælpe* dig.

Where the subordinate clause in Italian allows a choice of constructions, as is the case in for example (21), which for convenience is reproduced below, the selection of the infinitive construction is generally to be recommended, partly because due to the relative brevity of expression this will be regarded as the most elegant choice, and partly because the construction is the most neutral (cf. Figure 2, which shows that 22.9% of all verb forms in subordinate clauses are infinitive). If we consider (21a), (21b) and (21c), the b-variant will in all cases be regarded as belonging to the domain of the written language, while the c-variant is considered characteristic of the spoken language. The a-variant may in contradistinction be used in both registers.

(21) Jeg fik at vide at jeg *skulle ringe* til kontoret.
    Mi hanno detto ...
    a. .. di *chiamare* l'ufficio. (infinitive)
    b. .. che *chiamassi* l'ufficio. (imperfect S)
    c. .. che *dovevo chiamare* l'uff. (*dovere*: imp.I)

Similarly, in constructions containing verbs such as *sperare* (= to hope) the subjunctive, future, or indicative may in theory be used in the subsequent subordinate clause, as shown in (39) and (40), though with a resulting change in meaning such that the subjunctive generally expresses uncertainty as to the realization of the situation (cf. Vanvolsem 1995), the future indicates that the situation in all probability will be realized, whereas the indicative, besides theoretically being able to present the situation as a fact, first and foremost signals informal language use, acceptable primarily in communion with family and friends.

(39a) Spero che lei mi *perdoni*. (*perdoni*: present subjunctive)
      I hope that you_formal me foregive_subj.

(39b) Spero che lei mi *perdonerà*. (*perdonerà*: simple future)

(39c) Spero che lei mi *perdona*. (*perdona*: present indicative)

Depending on the content of the subordinate clause, the use now of the subjunctive, now of the future, now of the indicative may be perceived as the most polite or acceptable form. In the above example, the b-variant will thus typically be the most acceptable, at least as far as the utterance is put forward in writing, in that the hearer will not feel obliged to reply immediately to the speaker's supplication in the affirmative. Of course, the nature of the speaker's lapse also plays a role: the more serious the aberration, the more difficult the speaker must expect it to be for the hearer to offer his forgiveness. This latter aspect inclines towards the use of the subjunctive.

In (40), on the other hand, the a-variant would probably be considered the most polite in that the utterance is presented in the formal register. In the case of the speaker electing to use the informal register, however, the c- or b-variant would typically be the most adequate.

(40a) Spero che *venga* anche lei./ (*venga*: present subjunctive)
 I hope that come[subj.] too you[formal].

(40b) Spero che *verrà* anche lei. (*verrai*: simple future)

(40c) Spero che *viene* anche lei. (*vieni*: present indicative)

In order to avoid such problems, an infinitive construction may be selected, as shown in (21a). However, there is a catch involved in that the use of the infinitive construction is not always possible, this particular choice presupposing that the superordinate clause contains a linguistic item referring to the item which logically functions as subject of the infinitive, typically in the form of subject or dative, as is the case in (21a) in which *mi* is the dative object.

This condition, however, is not met in (39) and (40), though this may be achieved either by changing the verb form from active to passive, as in (39d), or by replacing it with a verb demanding a different type of construction, as in (40d):

(39d) Spero di *essere perdonata*.
 I hope to be forgiven.

(40d) Spero di *veder*la sabato.
 I hope to see-you[formal] Saturday.

4. Reflections on how the use of mood and modal verbs in Italian may most appropriately be described in a usage grammar for Danes

As is evident from the examples of the use of mood and modal verbs in Italian and Danish given in section 3 above, the two languages exhibit important differences as to the areas treated. These differences must be explained typologically.

As the author of a usage grammar of the reference-grammar type where the aim is partly to offer a description of Italian with regard to both system and use and partly to enable the user of the grammar to (i) produce correct and meaningful uterancces in Italian and (ii) interpret Italian utterances correctly, one must inevitably pose the question of how this aim may best be achieved. It should be noted, however, that it is beyond the scope of this paper to propose definitive solutions, the objective here being merely to provide pointers as to which directions we regard as appropriate and which we regard as inappropriate.

Taking the latter first, in most existing grammars the question of the use of the modal verbs in Italian is either not treated at all or else the individual modals are treated *back-to-front*, by which we mean that the grammars in question take Danish as their point of departure. This is the case in both Plum 1978 and Bach & Schmitt Jensen 1990: 459. The following quotation rendered from Plum will suffice to illustrate our point:

> § 282 The modal verbs indicate the prerequisite of the action contained in the main verb ... In Danish, "skulle" and "ville" are often used to form the future tense: "han skal rejse til Amerika om et par uger"; "der vil gå lang tid". Here, Italian naturally employs the future form: "partirà per l'America"; "passerà molto tempo" (1978: 179)

The shift in viewpoint from Italian to Danish is in our opinion unfortunate. Although we concur with the view that it is important for the writer of the grammar always to take Danish into account in writing for a Danish audience, this does not imply that Danish should be taken as one's starting point. On the contrary, the description should be language-specific. Therefore, we would prefer in treating the future tense to make the reader aware of the fact that under certain conditions the future form equates to Danish *skal* or *vil* (+ infinitive)[17] (to say nothing of the present indicative!), the aim necessarily being to ensure that the guidelines offered be as exact as possible without at the same time getting lost in detail.

As far as we can see it is not only appropriate but also necessary to relate the use of mood and modal verbs to the semantico-pragmatic category of speech acts[18]. As to whether the speech-act model should be presented prior to the individual moods/modals, as is the case for example in Allan, Holmes & Lundskær-Nielsen 1995, or whether the manifestation rules concerning the individual moods/modals are indicated in connection with the various speech-act types, this is in our opinion

---

[17]The parentheses indicate that the two forms will not always be followed by the infinitive. If movement is indicated, a directional construction, rather than the infinitive, will occur (cf. example (19) in Figure 3).
[18]The Italian usage grammar currently being prepared builds on Searle's five-point taxonomy. The reader is referred to Jensen forthcoming for further details.

of minor consideration, the important issue being that the subject be treated within the framework in question.

This said, it should be stressed that we do not consider the speech-act model in the form in which it has been presented by Searle to be sufficiently fine-meshed. As far as Italian is concerned, little benefit would be had of retaining the type of speech act referred to as representatives without further subdivision, since with the exception of the imperative and the modal *volere* all Italian moods and modals can be used to express epistemic content. Subdivision would therefore be requisite, and in this respect the classification outlined in the section on epistemic modality would in our opinion be useful.

Moreover, there is the issue of the speaker's degree of commitment, which on the face of it would seem to vary according to source, and, finally, the temporal location of the situation in relation to the moment of speech and possibly in relation to other situations[19].

In simplified form, the descriptive model may be illustrated as in Figure 5. It is important to stress, however, the purely illustrative nature of the outline, which in no way should be regarded as exhaustive. Comparison between Italian and Danish reveals that by employing the suggested description it is possible, at least in broad terms (and within the confines of the present article it is not possible to enter into further detail), to observe an approximate one-to-one relationship. However, it is important to point out that the two languages differ on several points as regards content and therefore do not employ the same linguistic forms of expression. This is for example the case with the Italian future, which semantically indicates PROBABILITY[20], a value which is grammaticalized differently in Danish (in the form of the particles *nok* and *vist*). In Italian the value is *inter alia* pertinent to future situations viewed by the speaker as non-factual. The speaker appears to have greater difficulty viewing a future state as factual as compared to a future action where the concern is the near future and where the subject of the utterance is himself. To the extent that the utterance concerns someone other than the speaker, however, there is a much greater tendency in both instances to use the future, cf. example (42).

(41) Domani *sarò* a Londra. >< Domani *vado* a Londra.
      tomorrow be$_{\text{fut 1st pers.sg}}$ -I in London   tomorrow go$_{\text{pres 1st pers.sg}}$ -I to London

(42) Domani Luca *sarà* a Londra. >< Domani Luca *andrà* a Londra.
      tomorrow Luca be $_{\text{fut 3rd.pers.sg}}$ in London   tomorrow Luca go$_{\text{fut 3rd.pers.sg}}$ to London.

---

[19]This issue is inextricably bound up with the concept of mood, not only in Italian, where verbal inflections at once indicate person, number, tense, mood and voice, but also in Danish.
[20]The word is capitalized in order to indicate semantic content.

Figure 5   Example of description of typical uses of mood/modals in representative speech acts in Italian and Danish (main clauses only)

	ITALIAN	DANISH
1. source of knowledge: subjective evidence		
A. degree of commitment: factuality	Indicative	Indicative
a. SoA simultaneous with MoS	present	present
b. SoA anterior to MoS	past	past
c. SoA posterior to MoS	present	present/*skal*
B. degree of commitment: non-factuality[21]		
a. SoA simultaneous with MoS	simple future	(present I + A[22])
b. SoA anterior to MoS	future of the past	(past I +A)
c. SoA posterior to MoS	future	(indicative +A)
2. source of knowledge: objective evidence		
A. degree of commitment: factuality	indicative	indicative
B. degree of commitment: probability[23]	*dovere*	*måtte*
C. degree of commitment: possibility	*potere*	*kunne*
3. source of knowledge: hearsay	conditional	*skulle*[24].

5. Concluding remarks

On the basis of the above, in which the problem complex is merely outlined, we may conclude that the two languages Danish and Italian exhibit important differences as to their use of mood and modal verbs. Broadly, we may assume that such disparity will render difficult the understanding and acquisition of the second language irrespective of whether we refer to Danes wishing to learn Italian or Italians wishing to learn Danish.

In view of the vital importance of the subject area to any communication situation, it is essential that the usage grammar provide a thorough treatment of the subject, particularly in consideration of the fact that the topic is (or at least has hitherto been treated as being) outside the scope of the dictionary. As outlined

---

[21] For Italian only the grammaticalized form, which is far from being the only form used, is given. Instead of the simple future, one often finds the present indicative, which co-occurs with adverbs of the type *forse* (= perhaps), *probabilmente* (= probably).

[22] 'A' in this connnection stands for adverb/adverbial, including the Danish modal particles of the type: *vist, nok*, but also adverbs such as *måske* (= perhaps) and *sandsynligvis* (= probably). Grammaticalization is the case in the first instance, though not of mood or modal verbs (hence the parentheses), but not in the second.

[23] The actual value, as mentioned in 2.1. above, is 'almost certainty/probability'.

[24] There is no grammaticalization of degrees of commitment in Italian. Danish, however, distinguishes between present and past of the modal *skulle*, the latter signalling that the speaker distances himself from what he has heard (cf. Davidsen-Nielsen 1990: 94f).

above, we consider speech act theory to be an appropriate descriptive model provided that the grammarian within the category of representatives distinguishes between different sources of knowledge and degrees of commitment as mentioned in section 2.

References

Allan, R., P. Holmes & T. Lundskær-Nielsen (1995). *Danish A Comprehensive Grammar*. London and New York: Routledge.

Bach, S. & J. Schmitt Jensen (1990). *Større Italiensk Grammatik*. København: Munksgaard.

Bergenholtz, H. (1989). *Frekvensordbog baseret på danske romaner ugeblade og aviser 1987-1988*. Handelshøjskolen i Århus.

Bortolini, U., C. Tagliavini & A. Zampolli (1971). *Lessico di frequenza della lingua italiana contemporanea (= LIF)*. Milano: Garzanti.

Bostrup, L. (1991). Modal Auxiliaries and Case. In K. M. & O. Lauridsen (eds) *Constrastive Linguistics. Papers from the CL-symposion at The Aarhus School of Business, 28-30 August 1989*, Handelshøjskolen i Århus, 1-17.

Bybee, J. (1985). *Morphology A Study of the Relation between Meaning and Form*. Amsterdam & Philadelphia: John Benjamins Publishing Company.

Bybee, J. & S. Fleischman (eds) (1995). *Modality in Grammar and Discourse*. Amsterdam & Philadelphia: John Benjamins Publishing Company.

Chafe, W. (1986). Evidentiality in English Conversation and Academic Writing. In W. L. Chafe & J. Nichols (eds) *Evidentiality: The Linguistic Coding of Epistemology*, Norwood, NJ: Ablex, 261-272.

Chafe, W. L. & J. Nichols (eds) (1986). *Evidentiality: The Linguistic Coding of Epistemology*. Norwood, NJ: Ablex.

Davidsen-Nielsen, N. (1990). *Tense and Mood in English. A Comparison with Danish*. TiEL 1. Berlin & New York: Mouton de Gruyter.

Davidsen-Nielsen, N. (1993). *Discourse Particles in Danish*. PEO 69 (= Prepublications of the English Department of Odense University. Odense: Odense Universitetsforlag.

De Mauro, T., F. Mancini, M. Vedovelli & M. Voghera (1993). *Lessico di frequenza dell'italiano parlato (= LIP)*. Milano: ETASLIBRI.

Hansen, E. (1972). Modal interessens. Nu bør det (komme) frem. *Danske Studier*, København: Akademisk Forlag, 5-36.

Jensen, B. L. (1994). Den italienske futurum og verden. In F. Sørensen (ed) *Leksikon og verden*, Ark 76, København: Handelshøjskolen i København, 29-45.

Jensen, B. L. Forthcoming. Om Modalitet. In L. Falster Jokobsen & G. Skytte (eds) *Ny forskning i grammatik* 4. Odense: Odense University Press.

Jensen, J. S. (1970). *Subjonctif et hypotaxe en italien*. Odense: Odense University Press.

LIF (see Bortolini et al. 1971).

LIP (see De Mauro et al. 1993).

Plum, M. (1978). *Italiensk grammatik*. København: Reitzel.

Rask, K. (1996). *Stilistik Sprogets former og litterære figurer*. København: Reitzels Forlag.

Searle, J. R. (1975). A Taxonomy of Illocutionary Acts. In K. Gunderson (ed) *Language, Mind and Knowledge*. Minneapolis: University of Minneapolis Press.

Skytte, G. (1993). Italiensk. Italiensk sprogbrug. Et referenceværk for danske specialister i italiensk sprog. In C. Bache (ed) *Ny forskning i grammatik Igangsat af Statens Humanistiske Forskningsråd*, Odense: Odense Universitetsforlag, 63-71.

Steele, S. (1975). Is it possible? *Working Papers on Language Universals* 18, 35-58.

Thygesen, H. (1995). *"Dobbiamo al cinema stasera?" Om brugen af modalverber i dansk og italiensk*. Københavns Universitet, Romansk Institut.

Vanvolsem, S. (1995). Il valore modale del congiuntivo. In H. Leth Andersen & G. Skytte (eds) *La subordination dans les langues romanes*. Etudes romanes 34, Copenhague: Munksgaard, 181-194.

Voghera, M. (1992). *Sintassi e intonazione nell'italiano parlato*. Bologna: Il Mulino.

On the Semantics of Agentive *af* in Danish

Per Anker Jensen

1. Once upon a time ...

It was a beautiful morning in the spring when I first came across *Aspects of The Theory of Syntax*. Studying professor Schibsbye's *English Grammar* for the grammar exam had aroused a keen interest in me for grammatical studies, and here I was with a book on syntactic theory which certainly had not been mentioned once in the classes I had attended on English grammar. The Chomskyan way of looking at grammar, English grammar, Danish grammar, any grammar of any natural language, seemed to me to be quite unrelated to studying English grammar in the English Department at the University of Copenhagen. What is most surprising about this state of affairs is perhaps not so much that books on linguistic theory were not properly introduced as background or supplementary reading in the grammar classes, but rather that some 15 years of research in English syntax had been carried out in the framework of transformational grammar without giving rise to even the briefest mention in those grammar classes.

In all fairness, however, not all staff in the English Department shared this rather standoffish attitude towards generative linguistics. One exception immediately comes to mind: Niels Davidsen-Nielsen was the name.

The earliest course offered in the English Department in the generative framework was in the autumn semester of 1970 under the title: '*Indføring i moderne engelsk transformationsgrammatik for særligt interesserede.*' Between the autumn semester of 1970 and the autumn semester of 1973, four courses in the generative framework were offered in the department. Two of them were introductory courses on English syntax, viz. autumn 1970 and autumn 1972, the 1972 one with a whiff of generative phonology added at the end. As amply documented by authentic course plans excavated in my loft, this introductory course was based mainly on Jacobs & Rosenbaum's well-known 1968-book, supplemented with Langacker's *Language and its Structure*, rule excerpts from M. K. Burt's popular 1971-introduction, *From Deep to Surface Structure*, and Davidsen-Nielsen's partly hand-written, partly typewritten, pedagogical 'baby-grammars' of English, which served as the basis for innumerable memorable exercises in English syntax at home and in class. The two other courses dealt with generative phonology and morphophonology (spring 1971 and autumn 1973). As I recall, the former course was based on Sanford Schane's work and work in progress by Eli Fischer-Jørgensen, and the latter on Fudge's 1973-anthology *Phonology*. Each of these four courses was taught by Davidsen-Nielsen, and depended entirely on his presence in the Department, which is apparent from the absence of generative courses in the autumn of 1971, when he was exchange professor at Tufts University, Mass.

At the time, Davidsen-Nielsen was working mostly in the areas of phonetics and phonology. As is well-known, he later moved into syntax and murkier areas of semantics, always with a view to contrasting English and Danish, most notably in his excellent book *Tense and Mood in English: A Comparison with Danish* (Davidsen-Nielsen 1990). In view of this early and well-documented interest in generative syntax, his wish to 'move on' from phonology and phonetics into syntax and beyond may very well have been sparked off several years before he actually started publishing in these fields.

2. Goal

Having enjoyed working in generative frameworks ever since the early 70's, in this paper I will be pursuing some more recent trends in generative grammar, taking us out of the Chomskyan transformational framework into non-transformational, feature-based, head-driven generative grammar, which puts a fair amount of energy into wondering how to get a compositional semantics to work on top of a lexically derived syntactic structure. More specifically, I will report on work in progress[1] involving some problems in the lexical semantics of the 'agent expression' in passives like (1) and its semantic relation to agent-modified nominal constructions like the subject of (2), its corresponding predicative construction in (3), and genitive constructions like (4) with their predicative counterpart, illustrated in (5):

(1) Den bog der er skrevet af Bo er ny.
     'the book that is written by Bo is new'

(2) Bogen af Bo er ny.
     'book-the by Bo is new'

(3) Bogen er af Bo.
     'book-the is by Bo'

(4) Bos bog er ny.
     'Bo's book is new'

(5) Bogen er Bos.
     'book-the is Bo's'

---

[1]For some years Carl Vikner and I have been working on the semantics of relation-requiring items like genitive *-s*, *have*, and noun-coumpounds. *Af* shares properties with those, and this paper is a first approximation to fitting *af* into the general outline of the semantics of relation-requiring items proposed in papers like Jensen and Vikner 1994, 1996a, and 1996b.

Finally, brief mention will be made of *have*-constructions in order to give a fuller picture of the complexity of the semantic field we are dealing with.

I will begin by going over and commenting on some related work carried out by Stockwell, Schachter and Partee on the genitive construction in the early 1970's, around the time when the generative approach first came to my attention.

3. Stockwell, Schachter & Partee: *The Major Syntactic Structures of English*

In 1973, Stockwell et al., following up on work especially by Lees and Jackendoff, dug into some of the problems connected with the syntax and semantics of the genitive construction. They came up with an interesting analysis couched in a novel Chomskyan-TG-cum-Fillmorean-case-grammar approach, trying to unify the syntactic strengths of transformational grammar with the semantic interests of deep case grammar. At the focus of our attention here is their treatment of examples of the type:

(6)   John's book

cf. (4) above, as opposed to examples like (7a-d):

(7a)   John's friend
(7b)   John's weight
(7c)   John's age
(7d)   John's portrait

Stockwell et al. (1973: 685) observe that the genitive constructions in (7) carry a similar meaning to constructions involving a head noun taking a PP-complement, cf. (8a-d):

(8a)   a friend of John
(8b)   the weight of John
(8c)   the age of John
(8d)   a portrait of John

Relational nouns like *friend*, *weight*, *age*, and *portrait* contain all the information required to determine the sense contributed by the genitive, hence the preposition is semantically empty and is conceived of as a NEUTRAL case marker on the noun. NEUTRAL case is defined as "the case most closely connected with the head itself and least interpretable independently of the head". This treatment is quite natural within their framework and neatly relates the genitive constructions in (7) to the complement constructions in (8).

They propose three criteria for positing a case source for genitives, summarized under A, B, and C below, cf. Stockwell et al. 1973: 686:

A) For a noun to carry a case marker, there has to be a paraphrase relation between a genitive+noun construction and a noun+complement construction, compare the following a and b-pairs:

   a *The child's age/size – The age/size of the child*
   b *The child's toy/book – *The toy/book of the child*

Since the Ab-pair cannot be paraphrases, cf. the ungrammaticality of the complement construction, the genitive in *the child's book* cannot be case-derived.

B) For case-carrying nouns no paraphrase relation can be established between the genitive+noun construction and a construction with a predicative genitive, compare:

   a *Mary's pencil – The pencil is Mary's*
   b *Mary's husband – *The husband is Mary's*

So, the absence of a predicative-genitive paraphrase in the Bb-pair is taken as evidence in favour of a deep-case source for the genitive, i.e. a NEUTRAL case marking on *husband*, whilst the possibility of a predicative genitive in the Ba-pair is taken as evidence against a case source for the genitive in *Mary's pencil*, i.e. *pencil* does not carry case.

C) This is a semantic checking criterion (Stockwell et al. 1973: 687): If a case source for a genitive is posited, the semantic relation between the genitive and the noun should be the appropriate one for the postulated case.

While it seems clear that *John's* in *John's portrait* in the sense 'the portrait of John' receives a NEUTRAL case marking from *portrait* due to the interpretation which *portrait* imposes on *John* as the object portrayed, there could be no case marking corresponding to the ownership sense of that same phrase, since *portrait* implies no sense of ownership. Later on the authors reject restrictive relative clauses containing the transitive verb *have* as the source of genitives with non-relational nouns like *book, pencil*, etc., e.g. *John's book* ⇐ *the book that John has*. So, they end up having no account of what they call the 'ownership' sense of genitives, a fact of which they are themselves well aware, cf. (1973: 702).

In sum, then, the analysis they propose for (6), *John's book*, is that, by criteria A, B, and C, the genitive in that construction cannot be derived from a case source. The criteria show the following picture:

(9) A *a book of John
     B the book is John's
     C a book by John

Interestingly, however, *John's book* is rather less clear cut on the C-criterion than on the A and B ones. That is, (9C) would seem to make it quite plausible to posit a deep-case source on *book* for the genitive in (6), as the meaning of *a book by John* coincides neatly with one possible reading of *John's book*. They reject this analysis, however, on the following grounds:

1. The relation between *John* and *John's book* is undetermined by the meaning of *book*:

    "At most, the meaning of *book* (and what we know about books from various sources) sets vague limits to the association. John may own or have borrowed the book. He may have played some part in writing, illustrating, printing, distributing or selling the book, or he may simply have it in his hand, or have been assigned the task of reporting, summarizing or attacking it. In none of these examples, then, does the interpretation of the genitive correspond to the usual interpretation of a case ... " (Stockwell et al. 1973: 694).

It's quite true that (6) may take on all the interpretations mentioned, and indeed an infinite number of others. The important point is, however, that not all readings one may come up with are equally 'natural', or equally far fetched, if you like. While in a concrete situation (6) may refer to a book that John has been asked to summarize, this certainly is not an interpretation that independently asked subjects will come up with if asked to paraphrase the meaning of the phrase *John's book*. More than likely, agreement would centre around a very limited number of 'natural' readings, I would suggest two: either 'the book John owns' or 'the book that John has written'. Following Pustejovsky (1991: 429-33), I will distinguish between, on the one hand, lexical or default readings, and on the other, pragmatic readings. The two readings I have suggested here count as the lexical ones, and all the others are purely pragmatic. The basis for making this distinction comes from data involving the interpretation of NPs as complements of proposition-requiring verbs like *enjoy* and *begin*, to which we return below.

2. The problem of how to give a uniform account of *John's book* and *John's chair* if only the former allows the agentive reading:

    "... it does not seem to be possible to propose any general derivation from Agentives of those genitives whose semantic relation to the head noun is creator-to-created, cf. *Chippendale's chair* – ?*The chair by Chippendale* and *Charlie's chair* – **the chair by Charlie*. Apparently, then, we cannot derive [such] genitives from deep structure Agentives, since we cannot state the conditions under which genitivalization of the Agentive is obligatory." (Stockwell et al. 1973: 695).

Stockwell et al. seem to make it purely a question about world knowledge whether an agentive reading of *Chippendale's chair* – A *chair by Chippendale*, is judged acceptable, i.e. that which counts is whether the hearer knows or does not know that Chippendale was a famous designer of furniture, and I agree that there seems to be a problem here with the interpretation of the data. Even though I have no explanation for the relative oddness of *the chair/building/knife by John* as compared to *the book/article/paper by John*, I will opt for the more general treatment allowing default agentive readings for all of them.

The proposal by Stockwell et al. is to derive constructions like (6), with non-relational nouns, from predicative genitives, thus:

(10)   *John's book* ⇐ *the book that is John's*

They claim to find support for their position in that:

> "... the derivation of preposed genitives in constructions like *John's book*, where the interpretations may include John's having written, illustrated, printed or published the book, etc., poses no particular problem if preposed genitives are derived from predicative genitives, since the predicative genitives themselves allow all of these interpretations." (Stockwell et al. 1973: 701).

I find that this statement is simply wrong. The predicative genitive cannot get the agentive interpretation, which the preposed genitive allows. So, on this account they simply cannot explain the fact that *John's book* has an agentive reading at all. The predicative genitive only establishes what Jensen and Vikner (1996a: 27) call a 'control'-relation between *John* and *the book*.

If we compare predicative genitives with *have* constructions, the striking fact is that they are very similar semantically in not allowing the agentive interpretation, i.e. *John has a book* cannot mean that 'there is a book that John has written'. They are also similar in that both construction types may be further specified by relation-requiring items and thereby be coerced into assuming an agentive reading, cf. <u>have</u>: *John has an article* (non-agentive) vs. *John has an article in Language* (agentive); <u>Predicative genitive</u>: *The book is John's* (non-agentive) vs. *That book is John's best* (agentive). So, in such cases the locative PP and the superlative, respectively, seem capable of bringing out the covert agentive potential of *article* and *book*.

There are, then, a couple of places where it seems worth looking for improvements of the proposal by Stockwell et al. (1973). First, their treatment of the predicative genitive, which they accord a very central position in making it the basis of the derivation of preposed genitives with non-relational nouns. They thereby fail to account for the agentive reading of examples like (6), since predicative genitives do not allow this reading on their own. The effect of the Stockwell et al. proposal, then, is to rank the agentive reading on a par with all other, pragmatic, readings. Secondly, on their account there is no systematic relation between the agentive interpretation of the preposed genitive in (6), *John's book*, and the agentive PP in *a book by John*. In their approach this relation could only be established given that the non-relational noun *book* was marked as having AGENTIVE case. Thirdly, they offer no account of the relation of *have* constructions to predicative genitives.

So, I would like to have an account relating the meaning potential of *have* to the predicative genitive, while separating the interpretation of agentive *af* from both of these, and then have *af* related to the agentive reading of the preposed genitive, which, in its turn, is related to the non-agentive meaning of *have*. Graphically it may be depicted provisionally as (11):

(11)

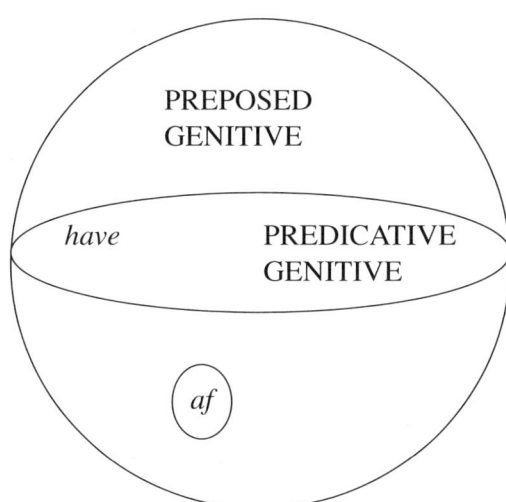

What this says is that the meaning potential of preposed genitives includes that of predicate genitives, *have* constructions, and *af*, being able to take on all default senses of those items. *Have* is sense related to predicative genitives, and *af* shares sense potential neither with *have* nor with predicative genitives.

Let's return now to the examples given initially in (1) - (5).

4. A preliminary semantic lexicon

As indicated in (11), *af* has the simplest semantics of the items considered. Indeed, if the passive example in (1), *Den bog der er skrevet af Bo er ny*, is considered in isolation, there would seem to be little reason to assume that *af* has any independent semantic content at all, that is, all the relevant semantic content seems to be retrievable from other meaning-bearing words in the sentence, viz. *den*, *bog*, *skrevet*, *Bo*, and *ny*. On this assumption we might accord some preliminary semantic representations to the lexical items in (1)-(5), giving a lexicon such as (12):

(12) PRELIMINARY LEXICON

Danish	Gloss	Semantic representation
den:	'the'	**the'(y,‖N'‖, ‖VP'‖)**
bog:	'book'	**bog'(y)**
bogen:	'book-the'	**the'(y, bog'(y), ‖VP'‖)**
der:	'which'	-
er:	'is'	-
skrevet:	'written'	**skrive'(x,y)**
af:	'by'	-
Bo:	'Bo'	**Bo'**
ny:	'new'	**ny'(y)**

By way of explanation, the format of formulas like those for *den* and *bogen* is given in the quantifier structure (13):[2]

(13)   QUANTIFIER(VARIABLE, RESTRICTION, ASSERTION)

that is, the quantifier is a functor taking three arguments: the variable quantified over, a restriction, and an assertion. The restriction bears its name because it places a restriction on the individuals in the domain which are relevant when evaluating the formula. That means, for instance, if we take an example like (1), we are not talking about cars, babies, lovers, or mermaids, but about books written by the individual called *Bo*. The assertion, in turn, represents the information predicated in the sentence of that set of individuals which is pointed out as relevant by the restriction. Both the restriction and the assertion must be well-formed formulas for a quantifier structure to be well-formed, that is, they are either quantifier structures or predicate structures, where a predicate structure consists of a predicate followed by zero or more arguments, cf. (14):

(14)   PRED(ARG1, ..., ARG$_n$)

Examples of predicate structures are found in the semantic representations for *bog*, *skrevet* and *ny* in (12).

Now, the lexical entries in (12) are intended to convey, respectively, that the semantics of *den*, is represented as establishing a relation between whatever is the denotation of the nominal expression determined by *den* (written as ‖**N'**‖ in the formula and corresponding to the semantic contribution of the construction *bog der er skrevet af Bo* in (1)), and whatever is denoted by the VP of the sentence (represented as ‖**VP'**‖ in the formula corresponding to the semantic contribution of the construction *er ny*). The semantics of *bog* is represented as a 1-place predicate, whilst the definite

---

[2] For a more elaborate explanation of restricted quantification, see Jensen and Vikner 1996c: 41ff.

noun, *bogen*, which may function as a full NP, is represented much like *den* because of the morphological definite article, but the root morpheme *bog-* places a restriction on the variable quantified over to apply only to objects that are books, cf. the explanation given above, and the assertion slot is left open for a formula to represent the VP-meaning. *Skrevet* is represented as a 2-place relation, and *ny* as a 1-place predicate structure, a property. The meaning of the proper name *Bo* is represented here simply as an individual constant in order to avoid unnecessary complication.[3]

Throughout I shall simply be assuming suitable syntactic structures on which to base a compositional semantics, even though I do not consider it a trivial matter to establish these. Combining the semantic contributions of the individual words and constituents of the sentence, it now seems possible to compose a semantic representation for (1), cf. (15):

(15) **the'(y, and(bog'(y), skrive'(Bo',y)), ny'(y))**

So, in (15) *den* provides the skeleton of the semantic representation in the shape of a quantifier structure with the quantifier slot filled by **the'**, a variable, and two empty slots to be filled out by the contributions of the constructions *bog der er skrevet af Bo*, 'book which has been written by Bo', and *er ny*, 'is new', respectively. The relative construction *bog der er skrevet af Bo* yields two formulae originating in the head noun and the relative clause, respectively. These two formulae are combined by the functor **and**[4] to give **and(bog'(y), skrive' (Bo',y))**, which fills the restriction slot in (15). The assertion slot, in turn, is filled by the semantic contribution of the predicate *er ny*, which, ignoring the representation of tense here, equals the contribution of *ny*, i.e. the formula **ny'(y)**.

Now, for the NP in (16) the representation in (15) commits us to the representation in (17):

(16) Den bog der er skrevet af Bo

(17) **the'(y, and(bog'(y), skrive'(Bo',y)), ||VP'||)**

Under the plausible assumption that (16) is synonymous with the NP in (18),

(18) Bogen af Bo

'book-the by Bo'

which functions as the subject in example (2) above, it follows that (16) and (18) should end up both having the semantic representation given in (17), since this is the only way we can be absolutely certain that they will get identical interpretations in an NLP-system, for instance.

---

[3] For the proper representation of proper names, see Jensen and Vikner (1996c: 87ff), who follow Thomsen (forthcoming).
[4] For an account of the introduction of the **and**-functor in Danish relative constructions, see Jensen and Vikner (1996c: 177f).

This immediately causes a problem for the lexical account we have proposed in (12) and applied in the semantic analysis of (1) shown in (15). Consider once more the lexical entries for *bogen*, *af*, and *Bo*, repeated in (19):

(19) *bogen*:   **the'(y, bog'(y), ||VP'||)**
      af: -
      Bo: **Bo'**

To put it bluntly: This won't work! There is no room for **Bo'** anywhere in the quantifier structure introduced by *bogen*, no relation in which **Bo'** can act as an argument. The missing relation here is the write-relation, represented as **skrive'(x,y)**, which in the semantic analysis of (1) was provided directly by the passive participle, cf. the entry in (12) for *skrevet*, but which is not available from any other semantic representation proposed in (12). Clearly, we would encounter precisely the same problem when trying to compose semantic representations for *Bogen er af Bo* in (3), and *Bos bog* in (4) in the sense 'the book that Bo has written'.

How to deal with this problem?

5. Qualia structure in a 'generative lexicon'

Over the past few years an interesting proposal has been put forth by James Pustejovsky (Pustejovsky 1991 and 1995) in favour of augmenting the semantic description of nouns considerably. Under the slogan "Spread the semantic load!", he argues that it is insufficient to concentrate on verbal semantics if one wants to capture the dynamic nature of lexical semantics, in particular what he calls the logical polysemy of words. Pustejovsky's theory, among several other things, involves adding a 'qualia structure' to the noun semantics. The qualia structure contains a representation of the essential attributes of an object as defined by the lexical item in question. The attributes are encoded in four roles, each representing one essential attribute of a typical referent of the lexical item described. The definitions of the four qualia roles are rendered in somewhat abbreviated form in (20), but cf. Pustejovsky 1995: 76ff, 85ff for a thorough discussion:

(20) Qualia roles:

CONSTITUTIVE ROLE:	The relation between an object and its constituents or proper parts.
FORMAL ROLE:	That which distinguishes the object in a larger domain, its material.
TELIC ROLE:	The purpose or function of the object.
AGENTIVE ROLE:	Factors involved in the origin or "bringing about" of an object.

Concentrating here on the AGENTIVE and TELIC roles, we might propose a lexical entry for *bog* like (21):

(21)

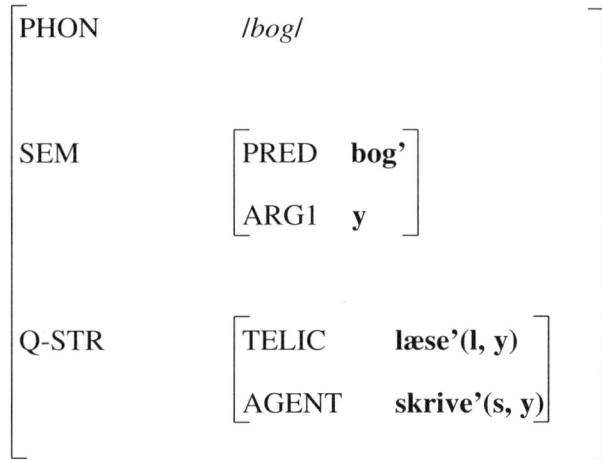

This partial feature structure for the lexical item *bog* tries to capture the intuition that there is more to the semantics of this word than the simple fact that it is a non-relational noun. This information is certainly still relevant, and is represented as the value of the SEM-feature, which is the feature-structural equivalent of the predicate logic notation **bog'(y)**. In other words, the SEM-specification corresponds to the representation proposed for *bog* in the preliminary lexicon in (12).

Pustejovsky proposes that in addition to that lexical knowledge, as native speakers we also have knowledge of potential alternative readings that a certain lexical item may assume under certain well-defined (we hope) circumstances. Such alternative readings may involve a completely different semantic type from the one that is usually connected with the word in question. For example, an individual-denoting noun may be 'coerced' into denoting an event.

If we look again at (21), the feature Q-STR introduces in its value the two qualia roles we have decided to concentrate on here, viz. the TELIC and the AGENTIVE ones. In the entry at hand these two roles represent essential knowledge we have about a typical referent of the word *bog*. The information given in the qualia structure of a certain noun delimits the range of default interpretations this word can bring to bear in a sentence given certain triggering circumstances. It is very important to note that the qualia roles are intended to be restricted to our lexical knowledge of the noun in question, and definitely not to let the qualia structure introduce just any old piece of world knowledge we might each of us happen to associate with the noun. There is no denying that this statement of intention subtracts nothing from the severe methodological problem of separating common sense world knowledge from purely lexical knowledge. Basically, what can properly be accorded status as lexical knowledge, and by that token be introduced into the qualia structure, depends on what can be argued on purely linguistic grounds, i.e. without recourse to knowledge solely conditioned by the non-linguistic context of a specific utterance. Pustejovsky has provided some illustrative examples, which work for Danish as well as English. Consider (22) and (23):

(22) Bo *nød* den bog
 'Bo enjoyed that book'
(23) Bo er lige *begyndt på* en ny bog
 'Bo has just begun a new book'

It is certainly possible that in a concrete situation in which someone utters (22), it could be interpreted as 'Bo enjoyed translating that book', or 'Bo enjoyed looking at that book', or even, if Bo were a dog, 'Bo enjoyed eating that book', etc. But clearly, such interpretations would hinge entirely on the hearer's knowledge in that situation that Bo had translated the book, looked at it affectionately, or eaten it, respectively. The first thing to wonder about here is how events like 'translate a book', 'look at a book', 'eat a book' are possible interpretations at all. What is going on here is that the normal denotation potential of NPs, which includes reference to individuals, masses, or groups, may change so radically as to even include event denotation. Secondly, it seems clear that the suggested interpretations, translating, looking at, and eating, are completely situation-dependent rather than founded on any purely lexical knowledge of the individual words constituting the sentence. The lexical semantics of the words involved here would much sooner elicit what we refer to as the default interpretation of (22), viz. that 'Bo enjoyed reading the book', i.e. another event, but an event with a completely different status linguistically than those previously mentioned. Exactly the same holds for (23), except that the verb cluster *begynde på* may activate an agentive interpretation of this sentence in addition to the telic one, which seems to be the only role accessible to the verb *nyde*, 'enjoy'.

The crucial point for our purposes here is that native speakers can agree on a finite, small number of context-independent interpretations for such cases as (22) and (23), and that is what justifies bringing into the lexical semantics of *bog* relational predicates like **læse'**, 'read', and **skrive'**,'write', rather than spurious ones like **oversætte'**, 'translate'', **se_på'**, 'look_at'', **spise'**, 'eat'', or representations of other strictly situation-bound possibilities of interpretation.

6. The semantics of *af* revisited

Let us now re-address the question of how to compose reasonable and consistent semantic representations for the sentences in (1) - (3), which all contain an occurrence of *af*.

The augmented representation of the lexical semantics of *bog* still leaves us the possibility of composing the semantic representation in (15), **the'(y, and(bog'(y), skrive'(Bo',y)), ny'(y))**, for (1), which is as it should be. The predicate **skrive'(x,y)** in (15) is contributed by the passive participle *skrevet* as before, and there is no need to access the event-semantics available in the qualia structure of *bog*. So, presumably, in (1) only the SEM-specification of *bog* in (21) is activated to supply the relevant part of the restriction.

As regards the examples (2) and (3), the situation after the introduction of the qualia structure in the semantic representation of nouns has changed in that there is now somewhere to go looking for the relation which was missing in our earlier account, that is, the write-relation. We now know that in the AGENTIVE role of the qualia structure of the noun *bog* this relation can be accessed, given the right circumstances for a semantic type shift of the noun. Since the default interpretation of both (2) and (3) supposedly incorporates a reading event, the right circumstances must be present in those examples. The pertinent questions now are: how is the relational, event-denoting sense in the AGENTIVE role of *bog* activated, and how is the non-relational sense of *bog* ignored, as it were, in the process of creating the semantic representations for (2) and (3). I would suggest that the answers involve the dynamic semantics of *af*.

Semantically, predicative and non-predicative constructions sometimes differ quite dramatically. Compare, for instance, (24) and (25):

(24)   A teacher was killed.

(25)   Kim is a teacher.

In (24) the subject NP gets a quantified interpretation, i.e. 'for some individual who is a teacher, that individual was killed', whereas the predicative NP in the latter doesn't, i.e. the latter sentence does not mean 'there exists a teacher that Kim is'. A comparable situation is found with PPs. In non-predicative use we find PPs as complements of relational nouns, cf. (26):

(26)   Bo er medlem af bestyrelsen.
       'Bo is member of the board of directors'

The PP *af bestyrelsen* cannot be made into a predicative of its governing noun, *medlem*, cf. (27):

(27)   *medlemmet er af bestyrelsen.
       'member-the is of the board of directors'

As illustrated in (3), the agentive PP does not share this property with complement PPs, since agentive PPs may freely occur in predicative position:

(3)   Bogen er af Bo.
       'book-the is by Bo'

Whereas (26) has *af* as a purely syntactic connective device, whose presence is totally determined by its governing noun, cf. the role of *of* in Stockwell et al.'s examples in (8), (3) shows the predicative and, semantically speaking, highly active preposition *af*, which I assume is identical to the one found in the passive sentence in (1). My proposal is that *af* should be accorded a semantic representation which is able to bring out the relation in the AGENTIVE role of the noun it modifies in examples like (2) and (3), and which is, at the same time, able to ignore the non-relational meaning of the noun, i.e. it should concentrate on getting at the value of the Q-STR-path of the noun it modifies and ignore the value of the SEM-path of that noun.

As a first approximation, let's assume a partial lexical entry for *af* such as (28):

(28)

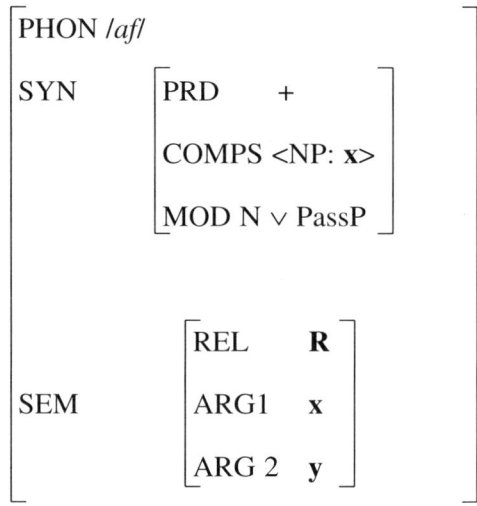

This says that *af* is predicative and takes a NP-complement whose referential index is bound to the first argument of an unspecified 2-place relation, **R(x,y)**, in the semantic representation. Syntactically I assume that *af* has a MOD-feature, which indicates that it can head a PP modifying either a noun as in (2) or (3), or a passive participle as in (1). Assuming now that the semantic representation of *Bo* is still the individual constant **Bo'**, the composition of *af* and *Bo* in the PP *af Bo* would result in the first argument of the relation **R** becoming instantiated to **Bo'** as shown in (29):

(29)

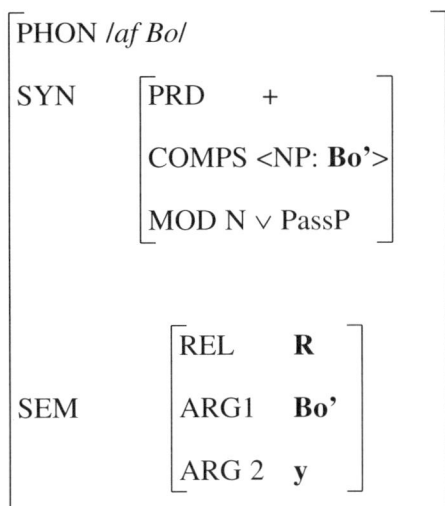

The representations in (28) and (29) explain why *af* does not activate the non-relational reading, i.e. the value of the SEM-path in the lexical entry for *bog*. That is because the 1-place predicate **bog'(y)** cannot unify with, i.e. is not compatible with, the 2-place predicate that *af* requires according to the present account.

We still need a tool that will allow us to get at the AGENTIVE role of the modified noun, so that we get an instantiation of the predicate variable **R**. This is what I have been referring to as the dynamic semantics of *af*: it requires the instantiation of a 2-place predicate, enforcing or 'coercing', as it is in the lingo, a shift of the semantic type of nouns like *bog*, which it modifies, and which are basically non-relational. Furthermore, not just any relation will be a possible instantiation of **R**. The relation has to denote a certain event type involving an individual that can act as the agent of the process, be it a natural force or an animate being of some sort.

The coercion device we need for *af* has to be incorporated directly in the lexical entry for *af*. It is not enough to just specify the **event**-type restriction on **R**, since this would also be compatible with the event specified in the TELIC role, **læse'**, '**read**'', which would amount to a prediction that *Bogen af Bo* could mean 'the book that Bo has read', which is not the case. Thus we actually have to point to the specific qualia role that *af* is able to access. This is done by incorporating a semantic typeshifter in the lexical entry for *af*. What the typeshifter does, then, is state explicitly that *af* requires a relation from the AGENTIVE role of the noun it modifies, cf. (30):

(30)

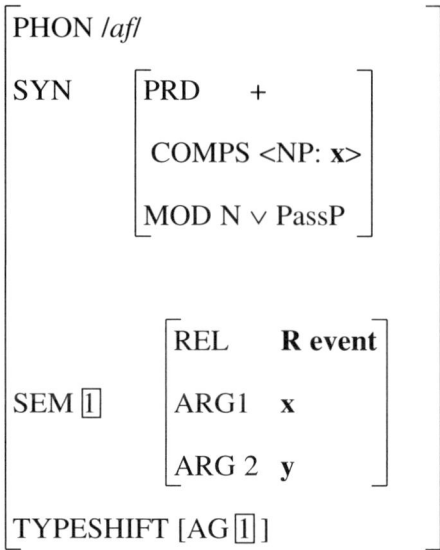

The path TYPESHIFT|AG serves as the starting point for the hunt for the relation in the AGENTIVE role of the noun modified by PP[*af*]. The tag [1] in front of the values of both the TYPESHIFT|AG-path and the SEM-path indicates that these paths will share whatever value the TYPESHIFT|AG-path comes up with. This means that at a certain stage in the semantic composition of (2), viz. when the full subject NP, *Bogen af Bo*, has been analyzed, *af* will have the instantiation shown in (31):

(31)

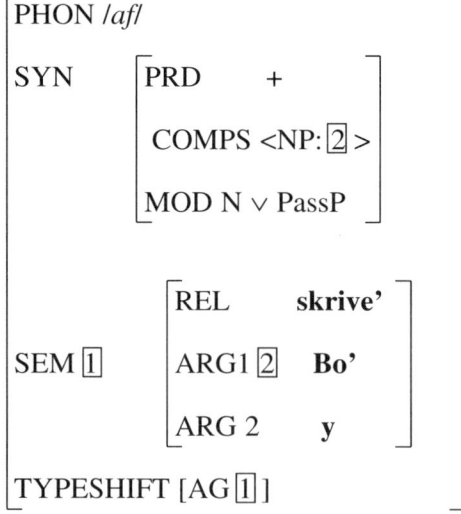

The typeshifter has picked up the relation **skrive'(x,y)** from the qualia structure of *bogen*, cf. (21), and the first argument of the relation has been instantiated to **Bo'** from the syntactic complement of *af*, and, finally, the variable occupying the position of the second argument of the **skrive'**-relation, **y**, is bound to the variable representing the referent of *bogen* in (2), cf. the semantic representation of the subject NP of example (2) shown in (32):[5]

(32) **the'(y, and(bog'(y), skrive'(Bo',y)), ||VP'||)**

We have to address an important question here, namely: What evidence is there that we actually need to incorporate the semantic representation from the AGENTIVE role of the noun in the lexical entry of *af*? Good evidence in favour of this treatment comes from (3):

(3) Bogen er af Bo.
     'book-the is by Bo'

The predicate in example (3) consists simply of the VP *er af Bo*, 'is by Bo', which, if nothing else is done, will contribute only the semantic representation accorded to *Bo*, i.e. the individual constant **Bo'**, since both *er* and *af* are semantically empty. This is precisely what forces us to let some element in the predicate 'import' the necessary agentive meaning from somewhere else, *af* being the obvious candidate for taking care of this 'import'. Hence, in the semantic analysis of (3), we get the very peculiar situation that the subject NP, *bogen*, actually contributes semantic content at two different positions in the sentence, both in the subject, i.e. the grammatical function it fills itself, and via *af* in the predicate, as illustrated in (33):

(33) Bogen er af Bo.

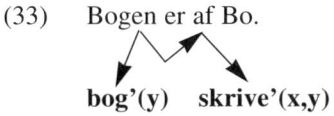

   bog'(y)   skrive'(x,y)

This is how we get the semantic representation in (34) for (3):

(34) **the'(y, bog'(y), skrive'(Bo',y))**

Further, the interpretation of predicative constructions like (3) seems to provide very interesting corroborative evidence in favour of the concept of qualia structure as a necessary part of the lexical semantics of nouns alongside their 'normal' referential semantics, since, clearly, the SEM-specification in the lexical entry for *bog* in (12) would not by itself suffice to account for the meaning of (3).

---

[5]For reasons of space, I will ignore the technical details of establishing this variable binding by reentrancies in feature structures and stick to the logical notation whenever possible.

This concludes our treatment of the semantics of agentive *af* in examples (1) - (3). Next we consider its relation to the genitive examples in (4) and (5).

7. The genitives

Our story about the agentive reading of (4), *Bos bog er ny*, 'Bo's book is new', is much like that of (3), *Bogen af Bo er ny*. That is, genitive *-s* is accorded a semantic representation which is not identical to, but overlaps that of *af* in that genitive *-s*, too, must be able to access the AGENTIVE role of the head noun of the genitive construction. But, clearly, (4) has an additional reading which *af* doesn't, viz. the reading that relates the semantics of preposed genitives to that of *have* constructions. This reading is referred to by Jensen and Vikner (1996b) as the 'dispositional' sense of the genitive, and they represent it by a semantic 2-place predicate, **control'**. Following their proposal we get a lexical entry for *-s* like (35):

(35)

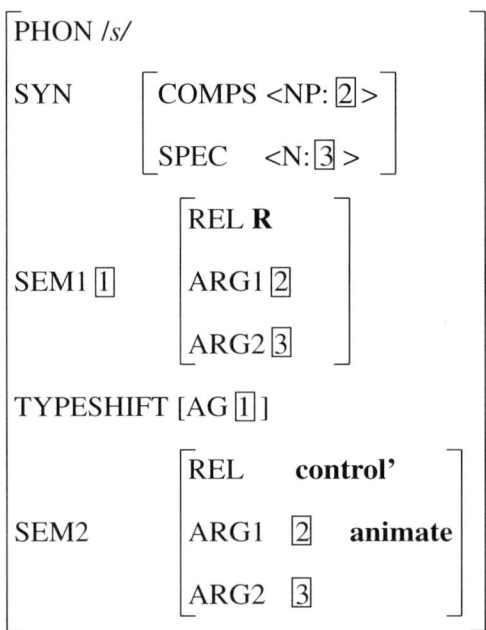

What this means is that *-s* takes a NP complement, that is *Bo* in (4), and it specifies a nominal, i.e. *bog* in (4). Semantically the complement serves as the first argument, whilst the specified nominal delivers the second argument of the relation. So, on this account (4) will get two readings, one rendering it synonymous with (2) by instantiating **R** to the **skrive'**-relation via the typeshifter, and another which says that Bo has the book in question at his disposal. The latter reading makes (4) synonymous with (36):

(36)   Den bog Bo har er ny.
        'the book Bo has is new'

Thus, for (4) we get the semantic representations in (37) and (38):

(37)   **the'(x, and(bog'(x), skrive'(Bo',x)), ny(x))**
(38)   **the'(x, and(bog'(x), control'(Bo',x)), ny(x))**

In most cases genitive and *have* constructions exhibit the same potential for interpretation, that is, if it is possible to use a genitive construction of the form *X's Y*, then there will most likely be a corresponding well-formed and true sentence of the form *X has a Y* and vice versa. But even though *have* is semantically closely related to preposed genitives both in terms of being relation-requiring and in terms of allowing a **control'** interpretation, it is unrelated to *af* as far as the possible instantiation of the relation variable **R** is concerned.

Finally, we have to face the problem of predicative genitives like (5):

(5)   Bogen er Bos.
        'book-the is Bo's'

This sentence allows only the **control'** reading, not the agentive one. Furthermore, it is remarkable that even with nouns which must contain appropriate relations in their qualia structure, for instance *næse*, 'nose', which presumably specifies a part-whole relation in its CONSTITUENT role, it seems difficult to get that relational reading when we have a predicative genitive, cf. (39):

(39)   Næsen er Bos.
        'nose-the is Bo's'

I think the only natural reading of (39) is the **control'** reading, and not the reading on which the nose mentioned is or used to be a part of Bo. In terms of lexical description this leads me to assume that we need two separate entries for predicative and preposed genitives. Hence, in (35) a specification like [SYN|PRD -] must be added to indicate that this entry covers only preposed genitives, and an additional entry must be formed containing a corresponding positive value in the specification [SYN|PRD +], and only the SEM2-part of (35) should be included in this entry, cf. (40):

(40)

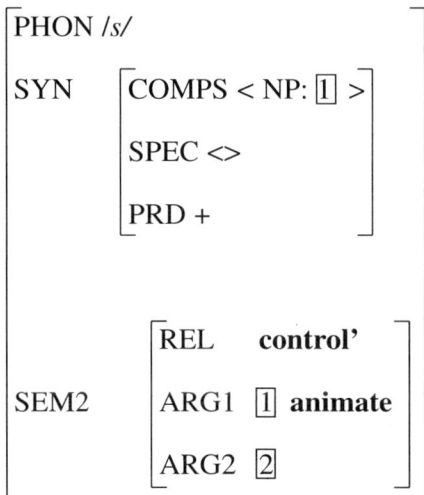

If this is correct, we might supplement the figure in (11) by the one in (41), which shows three sets, one containing the lexical items and constructions that are compatible with a **control'** reading, i.e. both of the genitives plus *have*, a second set which contains the items that are compatible with the relational reading, i.e. the preposed genitive and *have*, and a third set including items that are compatible with an agentive reading, and which contains only the preposed genitive and *af*:

(41)

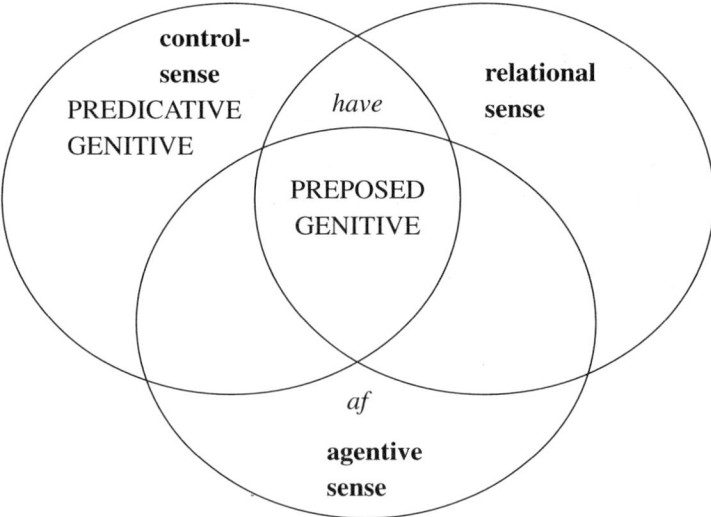

With a lexical entry for *have* like (42), the intersecting sets in (41) come out as a partial overlap in the semantics of the lexical entries for *af*, *-s*, and *have*, compare (30), (35), and (40) with (42):

(42)

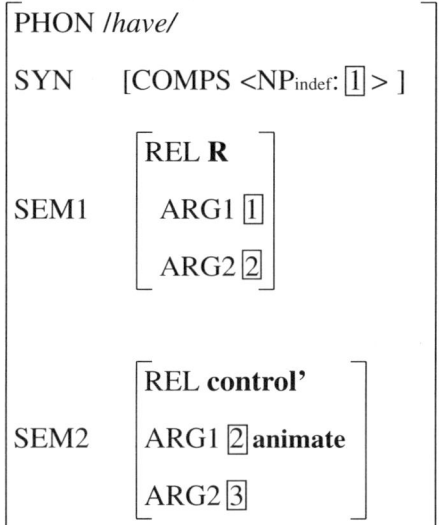

8. Summary

In rather informal terms I have sketched a formal approach to the semantic analysis of agentive *af* in Danish. My approach is much influenced by earlier work by Jensen and Vikner on issues concerning genitive *-s*, the transitive full verb *have*, and certain compound nouns. My goal has been to investigate similarities between those constructions and the semantics of Danish *af*. I have shown how the semantics of *af* overlaps with the semantics of preposed genitives, but not predicative genitives, and how *af* is related to *have* only in being relation-requiring, but not in its actual possibilities for instantiation of the relation variable **R**. How the sense overlaps might be expressed has been indicated in the rough lexical entries given in the paper.

References

Burt, M. K. (1971). *From Deep to Surface Structure*. New York: Harper & Row.

Chomsky, N. A. (1965). *Aspects of The Theory of Syntax*. Cambridge, Mass.: The MIT Press.

Davidsen-Nielsen, N. (1990). *Tense and Mood in English. A Comparison with Danish*. Berlin & New York: Mouton de Gruyter.

Fudge, E. C. (ed) (1973). *Phonology*. Harmondsworth. Penguin Books.

Jacobs, R. A. & P. S. Rosenbaum (1968). *English Transformational Grammar*. Waltham, Mass.: Blaisdell Publishing Co.

Jensen, P. A. (1992). Genitive Phrases in Danish. *Copenhagen Studies in Language* 17, 47-92. Samfundslitteratur.

Jensen, P. A. & C. Vikner (1996a). The Double Nature of the Verb *have*. *LAMBDA* 21, 25-37. Copenhagen Business School.

Jensen, P. A. & C. Vikner (1996b). "Genitiv og *have*-konstruktioner på dansk". Paper read at the 'Fagling-workshop: Possessive strukturer i dansk'. Copenhagen Business School, 30-31 May, 1996.

Jensen, P. A. & C. Vikner (1996c). *Natursprogsbehandling og unifikationsgrammatik* II. Handelshøjskolens forlag. Copenhagen.

Langacker, R. W. (1968). *Language and its Structure*. New York: Harcourt, Brace & World.

Pustejovsky, J. (1991). "The Generative Lexicon". *Computational Linguistics* 17, 409-441.

Pustejovsky, J. (1995). *The Generative Lexicon*. Cambridge, Mass.: The MIT Press.

Schibsbye, K. (1966-67). *Engelsk Grammatik* I-IV. Naturmetodens Sproginstitut. Copenhagen.

Stockwell, R., P. Schachter & B. H. Partee (1973). *The Major Syntactic Structures of English*. New York: Holt, Rinehart & Winston Inc.

Thomsen, H. E. (forthcoming). On the Proper Treatment of Proper Names. *Nordic Journal of Linguistics* 1997.

Some Norwegian Discourse Particles and their English Correspondences

Stig Johansson and Berit Løken

1. Background

In a recent paper Niels Davidsen-Nielsen (1996) discusses the characteristics of nine Danish discourse particles, showing both the features shared by these particles and the ways in which they differ from each other. A broad distinction is made between modal particles (*nok, vel, vist*) and categorical particles (*da, dog, jo, nu, skam*). The discussion of the former provided the starting-point for this paper.[1]

2. Danish modal particles

The Danish modal particles *nok, vel,* and *vist* are orientated towards the speaker, i.e. 'they reflect the speaker's conception of, or attitude to, his own knowledge of the state of affairs referred to' (Davidsen-Nielsen 1996: 285):

(1)   John er *nok/vel/vist* i London.

        John is ____ in London.

Nok reflects an evaluation by the speaker alone, *vel* and *vist* are 'polyphonic': *vel* includes the hearer in the assessment, *vist* informs the hearer that there are others who believe that the situation referred to is true. Davidsen-Nielsen suggests the following labels to capture the basic meaning of the particles:

   nok   'assumptive'
   vel   'confirmation-seeking'
   vist   'putative'

Although he mentions that the Danish discourse particles 'are notoriously difficult to translate' (p. 312), Davidsen-Nielsen does not deal with crosslinguistic correspondences beyond providing English glosses for his examples and pointing out (p. 287) that in a comprehensive Danish-English dictionary *nok, vel,* and *vist* are translated into comment clauses with *I* (*I suppose, I dare say, I think, I believe*).

---

[1]This paper was produced within the contrastive linguistic project at the Centre for Advanced Study, Norwegian Academy of Science and Letters, 1996-1997.

3. Norwegian modal particles and their correspondences

The Danish modal particles *nok, vel,* and *vist* have close formal equivalents in Norwegian (*nok, vel, visst*), and the characterization provided for Danish appears to fit the Norwegian particles as well. The purpose of this paper is, however, not to compare Danish and Norwegian, but to examine the three Norwegian particles from the point of view of their English correspondences. These are some questions to be raised:

- How are the Norwegian particles dealt with by English translators? How do the correspondences compare with the translations in bilingual dictionaries?

- What are the sources of the particles in English texts translated into Norwegian? Are there differences in the form and range of correspondences depending upon the direction of translation (from Norwegian to English vs. from English to Norwegian)?

- Are there notable differences in the distribution of the particles in Norwegian original vs. translated texts?

- How do the particles included in the study differ with respect to the form, meaning, and range of their correspondences?

- To what extent does the crosslinguistic perspective illuminate the meaning and discourse function of the particles?

These questions will be studied in the light of material drawn from a parallel corpus of English and Norwegian texts (see Section 3.1).

In addition to the particles *nok, vel,* and *visst*, the study includes the epistemic use of the adverb *sikkert*, as in:[2]

(2) Det koster *sikkert* en liten formue i måneden å få bo der! (EG1.4.s51)

  Must cost a packet, living there.

Here *sikkert* is used in much the same way as the particle *nok*. The two words have even been found in the same context:

(3) Det gikk *nok sikkert* an å prøve seg der ... (KF2.1.3.s217)

  It'd probably be worthwhile having a go there ...

What is the relationship between *nok* and *sikkert*? To what extent do they differ with respect to their correspondences in English?

---

[2]Quotations from the corpus are given with reduced coding. The text identification code is only included for the original text. For an explanation of the encoding system, see Johansson *et al.* 1996. The identification codes for the texts are explained in Appendix 1.

3.1. Material

The study is based on material from the English-Norwegian Parallel Corpus (Johansson and Hofland 1994, Johansson and Ebeling 1996), more specifically 27 extracts of 10,000 to 15,000 words from Norwegian fiction texts and their translations, and the corresponding number of English original texts and their translations into Norwegian (see Appendix 1).

All instances of *nok, sikkert, vel*, and *visst* were drawn from the corpus. As all these forms have more than one use, the first task was to exclude irrelevant material. The main criteria are position and modification. A modal particle characteristically appears in medial position in the clause and does not enter into structures of modification. Accordingly, *nok* has been excluded in examples like *gammel nok, det er nok*, where it corresponds to English *enough. Sikkert* has been excluded where it is used as a manner adverbial (as in *vet du det så sikkert?*) or as an independent utterance corresponding to English *sure(ly)*. The same applies to *visst* in initial position and in the independent utterance *ja visst*, in both cases corresponding to English *certainly*. Among the instances of *vel* that have been excluded are those where it is used as a modifier in a numerical expression (as in *vel over seksti*) and as an utterance initiator or an independent utterance (corresponding to English *well*).

The positional criterion has been ignored in some instances of *vel*, which appears to have greater positional freedom than the other modal particles. The material includes some instances of *vel* in final position (4) as well as a few examples where it occurs twice, both medially and finally (5).

(4) Ikke noe alvorlig, *vel*? (EG1.3.s196)

  Nothing serious, I hope?

(5) I couldn't have asked her anything more, could I, Reg? (RR1.4.s403)

  Jeg kunne *vel* knapt ha spurt henne om mer, kunne jeg *vel*?

3.2. Classification of the correspondences

After the material had been sifted, all the English correspondences were identified and categorized according to their grammatical form. Correspondence is used both to describe the relation between element X in one language and element Y in the other language, and as a term for the elements that enter into this relation.[3] The categories are:

---

[3]Cf. the use of 'translation' both for the process and the product. 'Correspondent' was rejected as a term for corresponding element, as it is normally used about human beings.

A. Adverb

(6) Hun var *visst* ikke den sterkeste likevel. (THA1.49.s4)
Perhaps she was not the strongest, after all.

(7) Det er *vel* på sett og vis dømt til å mislykkes. (CL1.1.3.7.s5)
That's *probably* doomed to failure, when you come right down to it.

(8) De klarer *nok* å kjøpe seg til en behagelig død også. (BV2.2.1.s234)
They'll *no doubt* manage to buy themselves a comfortable death too.

The most typical English correspondences in this category are adverbs like *probably* and *surely*.

B. Verb construction

(9) He *must* be a brilliant teacher. (RD1.7.s101)
Han er *sikkert* en veldig flink lærer.

(10) Parents *seem to* have no control over children these days. (PDJ3.1.1.s48)
Foreldre har *visst* liten kontroll over barna sine nå for tiden.

(11) Han finner meg *nok*. (EHA1.2.1.s127)
He's *bound to* find me.

This category contains modal verbs like *must* and *might* (9), lexical verbs like *seem* (10), and a few instances of marginal auxiliary constructions like *be bound to* (11). In these cases there is a modification of the verb construction, but no new clause is inserted.

C. Tag question

(12) Det var *vel* ikke Panten? spør Herman. (LSC1.2.s49)
"It wasn't the Bottle Man, *was it?*" asks Herman.

(13) Jeg hindret deg ikke i å lese, *gjorde jeg vel*? (EG2.4.s74)
I never stood in your way, *did I?*

In (12) there is a tag question in English corresponding to the Norwegian particle. Instances where there are tags in both languages (as in (13)) are treated as zero correspondences (see G below).

D. Independent interrogative clause

(14) Du spyttet det *vel* ut igjen? (LSC1.3.s491)
"Didn't you spit it out?"

The category comprises those instances where a Norwegian declarative clause containing a particle corresponds to an English interrogative clause.

E. Clause with a first-person subject

(15) Det var jeg *vel* kanskje også, men ikke slik hun innbilte seg. (FC1.1.s269)

And perhaps I was too, *I suppose*, but not in the way she imagined.

(16) Det forstår De *sikkert*. (KA1.1.s209)

I'm sure you understand that.

The category contains both comment clauses (15) and examples where the Norwegian particle corresponds to a superordinate clause in the English text (16). Both will be referred to below as 'first-person' clauses.

F. Other clause

(17) De vet *nok* hva de der skal brukes til de middelskolejentene (KF2.1.3.s140)

"They know a thing or two about these, those grammar-school lasses, *you can bet your arse on it!*" he said.

(18) "The children in Little Weirwold have been quite spoilt, *it seems*," commented the Doctor. (MM1.3.s234)

Barna i Little Weirwold har *visst* vært bortskjemt, bemerket legen.

Instances of this kind contain an English declarative clause with a second (17) or a third person (18) subject.

G. Zero correspondence

(19) Guten er *visst* redd og vil ned! (KFL1.1.5.s67)

The boy is frightened and wants to be put down!

(20) Fool and joker he might be: king of the country he was. (FW1.4.s173)

Dumrian og tøysekopp kunne han *nok* være stedets herre var han.

Zero correspondences are the instances where there is no item in the English version that can be identified specifically as the rendering of the particle (see also example (13) above). However, there may be other elements in the context that express much the same meaning, as we shall see below in the discussion of zero correspondences (Section 4.2).

In addition to the categories above, there were a small number of more marginal types of correspondences (categorized as 'miscellaneous'). A full list of all the correspondences for each of the particles is given in Appendix 2. The categories and their frequencies are shown in Table 1, which distinguishes between English correspondences in translated texts and sources of the particles in English original texts translated into Norwegian. Where relevant, the former will be referred to as translations, the latter as sources.

Table 1. The types of correspondences of *nok, sikkert, vel,* and *visst* in original and translated text, expressed in per cent within each column.

Type of corresp	*nok*		*sikkert*		*vel*		*visst*	
	orig N=141	tra N=79	orig N=82	tra N=51	orig N=221	tra N=159	orig N=53	tra N=27
zero	31.2	64.6	11	11.8	29.9	42.8	26.4	14.8
adverb	46.1	10.1	57.3	43.1	33	11.9	28.3	11.1
verb constr	11.3	10.1	11	29.4	5	4.4	34	44.4
tag quest	0.7		1.2		9	10.1		
interrog cl					1.8	5		
1st p cl	5.7	6.3	17.1	11.8	14.9	23.9	9.4	22.2
other cl	2.8	3.8	2.4	3.9	5	1.3	1.9	7.4
misc	2.1	5.1			1.4	0.6		

A mere glance at Table 1 and Appendix 2 reveals that there is a great variety of English expressions corresponding to the Norwegian particles, far more than revealed in bilingual dictionaries. This is apparent from the survey below, which includes a comparison with the translations listed in a major Norwegian-English dictionary (Kirkeby 1986).[4] The survey focuses almost exclusively on translations of Norwegian original texts. Translations and sources are compared in Section 3.7.

3.3. Correspondences of *nok*

The translations of *nok* given in Kirkeby's dictionary are *probably, all right, be sure to, I see, indeed* and *well enough*. How have the translators of the corpus texts dealt with the particle *nok*? The main category is adverb, which accounts for close to half

---

[4] The translations given in Haugen (1984) have also been consulted, but will not be referred to, as they form a subset of the renderings listed in Kirkeby's dictionary. Unlike Kirkeby, Haugen has no entry for the epistemic use of *sikkert*.

of the instances. By far the most frequent of these is *probably*, which represents one fourth of all the correspondences of *nok*.

(21)   Hun er *nok* blant de mer velstående i distriktet. (TB1.4.s88)

    She is *probably* one of the more well-to-do people in the district.

Other recurrent items in this category include *no doubt*, *all right*, *surely*, *certainly* and *perhaps*.

The second most frequent category is zero correspondence, which represents close to a third of the instances:

(22)   Radioen vil *nok* gå greitt. (KF1.1.6.s5)

    The radio will be an easy job.

In (22) there is still an element of uncertainty in the English version because of the modal auxiliary. In many cases, however, the zero strategy results in a categorical statement corresponding to a modalized one, as in (23). The uncertainty, or reluctance to admit that something is the case, is lost in the English translation.

(23)   Eva og Martin hadde *nok* rett. (THA1.27.s35)

    Eva and Martin had been right.

Verb constructions represent about a tenth of the correspondences of *nok*. The most frequent single correspondence in this category is epistemic *must*, as in (24):

(24)   Etterpå gråter en av guttene, det er *nok* William. (BV2.1.1.s200)

    Afterwards one of the boys starts to cry, it *must* be William.

Other members of this category are *be bound to*, *seem to* and the modal verbs *could*, *might*, and *should*.

The clausal category is chiefly represented by first-person clauses expressing some degree of uncertainty and containing verbs like *suppose* and *think*. The 'miscellaneous' category is numerically insignificant, but formally interesting. In both original and translated texts there are instances where emphatic *do* corresponds to *nok* (25). There is also an instance of *nok* in a translated text corresponding to fronting in the English source text (26).

(25)   "Det klinger *nok* en bjelle et sted – langt borte – men jeg kan ikke plassere ham." (GS1.4.s181)

    "It *does* ring a bell somewhere – a distant one – but I can't place it."

(26)   "*Fun evening* this is going to be," was all he could think of to say. (FW1.4.s219)

    "Det blir *nok* en festlig aften," var alt han kunne komme på å si.

In (25) *nok* expresses concession; note the coordination with *but*.

Of the translations given in Kirkeby's dictionary, two (*I see* and *well enough*) are not found in the material. Two (*be sure to* and *indeed*) occur once. *All right* has three occurrences. *Probably* is thus the only one of the renderings given in the dictionary that occurs with any frequency. Recurrent instances which are conspicuously lacking in the dictionary are *must* and *no doubt*.

3.4. Correspondences of *sikkert*

The translations given in Kirkeby of the epistemic use of *sikkert* are *probably, very/most likely, no doubt, be likely to, stand to, I'm sure*, and *I suppose*. These represent the categories adverb, verb construction, and first-person clause. In the corpus material, the main type of correspondence is adverb, with over half of the instances. Four items (*probably, no doubt, certainly*, and *surely*) stand out in this group, accounting for the great majority of the instances. *Probably* and *no doubt* are straightforward and adequate renderings, conveying the lack of commitment expressed by *sikkert*:

(27) "De har *sikkert* vært på den samme pressekonferansen." (OEL1.4.s185)

"They've *no doubt* been to the same press conference."

Certainly and *surely*, on the other hand, seem to express nearly the opposite meaning of that expressed by *sikkert*, as in (28):

(28) Han var *sikkert* eldre. (THA1.75.s10)

He was *certainly* older.

Surely in initial position, however, functions better than in medial position. Compare:

(29) Plutselig går døren opp og en konstabel hinker ut, han kunne *sikkert* gå helt fint da han kom. (LSC1.4.s71)

Suddenly the door opens and a policeman hobbles out. *Surely* he was able to walk just fine when he came in.

(30) En skoleklasse med sju-åtteåringer kom syngende og skrikende bak meg, med ski over skuldrene og små sekker som *sikkert* var fulle av varm kakao, matpakker og appelsiner. (LSC2.5.s20)

A school class of seven- or eight-year-olds came singing and screaming behind me, with skis on their shoulders and little bags that were *surely* packed with hot cocoa, sandwiches and oranges.

The second most frequent type of correspondence is a first-person clause, most often *I'm sure*:

(31) Så lagar *sikkert* han bestefar ranglestav til deg. (KFL1.1.2.s10)

Then *I'm sure* Grandfather will carve you a hiking stick.

The other items in this category are *I think, I'm pretty sure*, and *I suppose*.

The two remaining categories that are of some importance are verb construction and zero correspondence. The most important item in the verb construction category is epistemic *must*:

(32) Det var uten vindu og hadde *sikkert* også vært uten lys. (JW1.1.2.s61)

It had no window and *must* also have been without lighting.

As regards zero correspondence, *sikkert* stands out from *nok, vel* and *visst* by having a much lower frequency (see Section 4.2).

Comparing the dictionary entry with the corpus data, we find that most of the translations given in the dictionary are also found in the corpus material. Of the items found most frequently in the corpus, two are missing as renderings of epistemic *sikkert* in the dictionary: *certainly* and *surely*. As pointed out above, these must probably be regarded as less felicitous translations.

3.5. Correspondences of *vel*

The translations of the uses of *vel* that are relevant for the study are collected under two subheadings in Kirkeby's dictionary: *formodentlig* ('presumably') and *forhåpentligvis* ('hopefully'). Under the first heading, we find *probably, presumably, I think*, and *I suppose*; under the second, *I hope, surely*, and tag question. These represent three of the types of correspondences in Table 1: adverb, first-person clause, and tag question. In the corpus material *vel* is the most frequent of the four particles and also the one with the widest variety of correspondences. Apart from the types given in the dictionary, we find verb constructions, independent interrogative clauses, and zero correspondence.

The most frequent type of correspondence of *vel* is adverb, though the proportion is not as high as for *nok* and *sikkert*. The most frequent adverb is *probably*. *Surely* is the only other item in this category that is found more than a few times. The instances that are rendered as *probably* tend to express that the speaker is not or does not want to appear quite certain:

(33) Det er *vel* bare en evangelist som skal ha meg til å tro på det evige liv.
(KA1.2.10.s37)

It's *probably* some evangelist who wants to make me believe in eternal life.

Zero correspondence is the second largest category. It is commonly found in interrogative clauses and in clauses with modal elements. Example (34) with its epistemic modal is a case in point:

(34) Det *må vel* være negeren det. (BV1.3.s180)

It *must* be that nigger.

Not uncommonly, *vel* corresponds to a verb construction in the English translation, usually a modal auxiliary. Note the difference between the zero correspondence in (34) and the insertion of a modal auxiliary in (35):

(35)   Hva som *vel* ligger henslengt der av verdisaker? (KF1.1.1.s53)
       What articles of value *may* be lying around in it.

First-person clauses are another frequent type of correspondence, as in (36):

(36)   Ja, jeg gjør *vel* det, sa han. (SH1.1.8.s336)
       "Yes, *I suppose* I do," he said.

Apart from *I suppose*, which is the most frequent item in this category, we find *I guess*, *I hope* and *I expect*.

Tag questions are found as correspondences of *vel* in about a tenth of the instances, whereas they only occur sporadically with *nok* and *sikkert*, and not at all as a correspondence of *visst*.

(37)   Det er *vel* ikke blindtarmen? spør han. (LSC1.3.s484)
       "It's not appendicitis, *is it?*" he asks.

Less commonly, particularly in translations from English, *vel* corresponds to an independent interrogative clause in English. The category consists of Norwegian declarative sentences containing *vel* corresponding to *wh*-interrogatives or *yes/no*-questions in English.

(38)   "Why don't we all go and look together?" he said. RD1.4.s113
       Vi kan *vel* gå og se etter alle sammen, sa han.

The choice of *vel* in the Norwegian translation follows naturally from the function it has in giving declarative sentences the same illocutionary force as questions (Fretheim 1981: 87). It is also worth noting that a number of declarative sentences containing *vel* do in fact end with a question mark rather than a full stop, as in (37) above. In other words, they are declarative questions.

Comparing the corpus material with the dictionary, we find that two of the translations listed in the dictionary, *presumably* and *I think*, are not instanced in the corpus material, but the correspondences found most frequently in the corpus are given in the dictionary as well. As is the case with the other particles, the zero option which is so frequently chosen by the translators is not given in the dictionary.

3.6. Correspondences of *visst*

The translations given in Kirkeby's dictionary of *visst* when used as a modal particle are: *I think, I believe, I expect* and *I suppose*. All these belong to our category first-person clause but, as appears from Table 1, this is by no means the only category of correspondence found in the corpus material.

The most frequent category is, in fact, verb constructions, which account for about one third of the instances.

(39)   Det er *visst* tynnslitt her på huset om dagen? (EH1.1.7.s18)

   It *must* be nerve wracking around this place these days.

The items in this category are *must, seem*, and *appear*, in that order of frequency.

The next category in terms of frequency is adverbs. As is the case with the other particles (see Section 3.7), adverbs are more important as translations than as sources.

(40)   Men han var *visst* en stri mann. (KAL1.3.s135)

   But he was *apparently* also a stubborn man, reckless and quick-tempered.

The adverbs which occur as correspondences in more than one text are *apparently, sure(ly), perhaps*, and *certainly*. Since the total number of occurrences of *visst* is quite low, none of its correspondences occur more than a few times.

About a fourth of the instances of *visst* are zero correspondences, i.e. a somewhat lower proportion than for *nok* and *vel*. A possible reason may be that the discourse function of *visst* is relatively well-defined. It is used to indicate that the speaker is not willing to guarantee the truth of what is being said, either because it is based on hearsay or because it is inferred on the basis of (more or less reliable) evidence. The instances of zero correspondence thus result in a more categorical statement in the English translation. Compare example (41), where the English version gives the impression that the speaker can read the thoughts of the man referred to.

(41)   Han vil *visst* se på meg først. (LSC1.4.s111)

   He wants to look at me first.

The category that appears to be so important according to the dictionary, i.e. first-person clause, only accounts for about a tenth of the instances.

(42)   Med blikket festet på kortstokken spurte han: "De nevnte *visst* noe om ... narkotika?" (EG2.3.s109)

   His eyes on the pack of cards, he said: "You mentioned something about drugs, *I believe*."

As a source of *visst* this category is more frequent. Here we find the items *I guess, I think*, and *I could tell*.

In the case of *visst*, the match between dictionary and corpus material is not very good. Of the four translations given in Kirkeby's dictionary, only one was found in the corpus material, i.e. *I believe*. Moreover, this correspondence accounts for no more than five per cent of the occurrences. As regards the sources of *visst*, the match between dictionary and corpus material is no better.

3.7. Translations vs. sources

All the Norwegian particles included in the study are far less common in translations than in original texts (see Table 1). It is not surprising that there are differences in linguistic choices in translated texts. These may reflect influence from the source text (cf. Gellerstam 1986) or general features of translation (cf. Baker 1993). The former is the probable reason in our case, as English lacks modal particles comparable with the Norwegian ones.

Modal particles are, however, not infrequent in Norwegian texts translated from English. We find the same categories of correspondences as in going from Norwegian to English, though there are few cases where a category occurs with the same frequency both as source and translation. The most striking difference is that adverbs are consistently more frequent as translations than as sources (see Table 1). The probable reason is that adverbs are a convenient means of filling the gap of this adverb-like category, whereas in translating from English into Norwegian the same category is available (i.e. adverbs in both languages).

Verb constructions and first-person clauses are more common overall as sources than as translations; note especially the higher frequency of verb constructions for *sikkert* and *visst*, and of first-person clauses for *vel* and *visst* (see Table 1). This indicates that modality may be expressed to a greater extent by clauses and verb constructions in English than in Norwegian. The same tendency was observed in Løken's (1996) study of expressions of possibility in the two languages.

The category where perhaps the most interesting differences are found is zero as source vs. translation of *nok* and *vel*. Somewhat surprisingly, zero is considerably more frequent as source than as translation, with 65% vs. 31% for *nok* and 43% vs. 30% for *vel*. This means that a very high percentage of the instances ostensibly appear from nowhere. On closer inspection, this turns out to be less than the whole truth, since many of these sentences contain other elements that function in much the same way (see further Section 4.2 below). Another important point is that most of the instances of particles with zero source are found in direct speech, and the particles may have been inserted in order to give the dialogue more of the characteristics of spoken discourse.

Apart from these tendencies with respect to grammatical form, there is little or no difference between translations and sources. The individual items may vary, but they generally agree in meaning.

4. A comparison of the correspondences of *nok, sikkert, vel*, and *visst*

The account so far has focused on each individual form. The next task is to compare the particles with respect to their correspondences. As in the survey in Section 3, the focus is mainly on English translations of Norwegian original texts.

4.1. Range and grammatical form of correspondences

The four particles are alike in having a large number and a wide range of correspondences (see Appendix 2). The number is largest and the range widest with *nok* and *vel*, and smallest with *sikkert* and *visst*, which probably in part reflects the difference in overall frequency, but may partly also reflect a difference in semantics (see Section 4.3).

The most notable difference with respect to grammatical form (see Table 1) is that the proportion of adverbs is much higher for *sikkert* than for the other particles. The difference is particularly striking in going from English to Norwegian. In a crosslinguistic perspective, *sikkert* is thus treated as more in accordance with English adverbs, and it is no coincidence that it is not normally included among the discourse particles.

4.2. Zero correspondences

The low frequency of zero correspondences, too, sets *sikkert* apart from the other particles (see Table 1), a difference which may have a semantic correspondence (see Section 4.3). The proportion of zero correspondence is highest with *nok* and *vel*, and particularly so in translated texts (see Section 3.7).

As has already been pointed out in passing, zero correspondence does not necessarily mean that the modal meaning is not at all expressed in the English text. A considerable number of the zero correspondences of *vel* are found in connection with independent interrogative clauses or tag questions:

(43) Han visste hva hun hadde sett i øynene hans, men *hva gjorde vel det?* (MN1.1.s289)

He knew what she had seen in his eyes, but *what did that matter?*

(44) Jeg hindret deg ikke i å lese, *gjorde jeg vel?* (EG2.4.s74)

I never stood in your way, *did I?*

More important, a very high proportion of the instances with zero correspondence contain a future-referring expression, a modal auxiliary or a marginal auxiliary construction with a modal meaning:[5] *nok* 64%, *sikkert* 88%, *vel* 50%.

(45) Vi *må nok* finne ut av dette selv. (THA1.26.s10)

We*'ll have to* work this out for ourselves.

---

[5]The percentages apply to Norwegian translations into English. Translations in the other direction show more or less the same picture.

(46)   Da *ville* hun *sikkert* få øye på den mystiske filosofen. (JG1.5.s13)

   If she stood at the window she *would* see the mysterious philosopher.

(47)   Det *må vel* være negeren det. (BV1.3.s180)

   It *must* be that nigger.

Visst is exceptional in that none of the instances with zero correspondence contain a modal verb, probably reflecting a difference in meaning with respect to the other forms (see Section 4.3).

Not infrequently, there are instances of zero correspondence where no modal meaning is expressed at all in the English text, as in:

(48)   Og familien hans *var visst* dau for lenge sia. (LSC2.5.s333)

   And his family*'s been* dead a long time.

(49)   Han *tilhørte vel* det store flertallet. (GS1.5.s56)

   Oh, he *was* one of the silent majority.

(50)   Det så ut som om det rant blod fra munnvikene hennes, men *det skyldtes nok* bare rødbetene. (LSC2.5.s35)

   It looked like blood running from the corners of her mouth, but *it was* just beet juice.

In these cases the English text sounds more categorical than the Norwegian version.

A large proportion of the zero correspondences are found in passages of direct speech or thought. In general, discourse particles are characteristic of spoken rather than written language, as mentioned by Davidsen-Nielsen (1996: 285) in connection with his study of the Danish discourse particles. However, as pointed out above (Section 3.7), the very high frequency of zero correspondences with *nok* and *vel* in going from English to Norwegian may also reflect a tendency on the part of translators to insert particles in order to give the dialogue more of the characteristics of spoken discourse.

4.3. The semantics of the correspondences

The large number and the wide range of the correspondences (see Section 4.1) show that English has no formal equivalents of the particles, but must draw on a variety of other means to express the meaning in the Norwegian text. Moreover, the meanings are such that they need not necessarily be expressed in English, as shown by the large proportion of zero correspondences (see Section 4.2).

To what extent does the crosslinguistic perspective illuminate the differences in meaning and discourse function between the individual particles? The lists in Appendix 2 clearly show that there is a good deal of overlap. As correspondences which only appear sporadically may well be questionable and cannot be properly evaluated without taking the wider context into account, it may be useful to focus on the most frequent correspondences in the material (see Table 2).

Table 2. The most frequent correspondences (Norwegian to English only), broadly ordered according to degree of certainty. To be included in this table, a form must occur at least five times as a translation of one of the particles.

Corresp	*nok*	*sikkert*	*vel*	*visst*
no doubt	6	8	4	0
I'm sure	1	11	2	0
certainly	2	7	1	2
sure(ly)	3	12	13	2
must	7	7	3	9
seem (to)	1	0	1	7
probably	35	12	35	1
I suppose	2	1	16	0
I guess	0	0	5	0
tag question	1	1	20	0

Visst is strikingly different from the other three forms, both with respect to the range and the selection of correspondences. Although there is overlap with the other particles, *visst* has one distinctive correspondence, i.e. *seem*, and this is in fact its most frequent source in going from English to Norwegian (see Appendix 2). Among its correspondences there is just a single instance of *probably*, which is the most frequent correspondence for *nok* and *vel*, and is also a common correspondence for *sikkert*. To use the wording in Section 3.6, *visst* 'indicates that the speaker is not willing to guarantee the truth of what is being said, either because it is based on hearsay or because it is inferred on the basis of (more or less reliable) evidence'. The other particles, on the other hand, express a judgement in terms of probability, based on the belief of the speaker.

Sikkert shares most of its correspondences with *nok* and *vel*, but stands out from these in showing a preference for correspondences with a more categorical basic meaning (*probably* is a notable exception). As *sikkert* also has the largest number of adverb correspondences (see Section 4.1) and the smallest number of zero correspondences (see Section 4.2), it is reasonable to conclude that it is more adverb-like and that its meaning has not been bleached to the same extent as that of the other particles. Moreover, it is frequently stressed, while the other particles are typically unstressed.

Nok and *vel* have many correspondences in common (*probably* being the most striking), but there are notable differences in frequency. In particular, *vel* commonly corresponds to *sure(ly)*, *I guess/suppose*, or a tag question, all of which invite a response from the hearer. Note also the difference in the strength of belief expressed by *must* (more frequent for *nok*) vs. *I guess/suppose* (more frequent for *vel*). Judging by the correspondences, we can then characterize the relationship between the particles in the following way: *nok* expresses a judgement in terms of probability, from the point of view of the speaker; the commitment of the speaker is weaker with *vel*, which at the same time makes an appeal for confirmation from the addressee.

Nok and *vel* are both very frequent and have a high proportion of zero correspondences (see Table 1). The extent to which they are added in translated texts, seemingly without a source, is particularly striking (see Section 3.7). *Vel* is regularly unstressed, and the same is generally true of *nok*. Altogether, this can be taken to mean that these are the particles which have gone furthest in the direction of grammaticalization. A final piece of evidence concerns combinations with modal auxiliaries. In the material examined for this study, *nok* and *vel* were immediately preceded by a modal auxiliary in about a fifth of the cases, as against about ten per cent for *sikkert* and *visst*.[6] When faced with such combinations, the English translator frequently preserves only the auxiliary.

The description above is compatible with Davidsen-Nielsen's (1996) characterization of Danish *nok* as 'assumptive' and *vel* as 'confirmation-seeking'. The description of Danish *vist* as 'putative' seems less appropriate for its Norwegian counterpart *visst*, which is often used as a (weak) marker of connection between cause and effect, or as an indication that there are reasons for the state of affairs that is mentioned.

5. Conclusion

The modal particles *nok, sikkert, vel,* and *visst* all occur far more frequently in original texts than in texts translated from English. This is not surprising. If we examine the frequency of question tags in English, we find higher numbers in original texts than in texts translated from Norwegian. In both cases, we have forms particularly associated with one of the languages. The lower frequency in translated texts is due to the lack of a close formal equivalent in the source language and the tendency of translations to reflect the form of the source text.

How do translators cope with the discrepancy between the source and target language? In the case of the Norwegian modal particles, we find correspondences on different levels: adverb, verb construction, clause. In other words, the translator

---

[6]The combinations found most frequently in the corpus were: *skal nok* and *kan/kunne/skal/skulle/ville vel*. As regards such combinations, see also Løken's (1996) account of expressions of possibility in English and Norwegian.

draws on range of resources in the target language. The range is far wider than suggested in bilingual dictionaries.

The preferred correspondences differ depending upon the direction of comparison, i.e. whether we go from Norwegian into English or from English into Norwegian. In the former case, there is a much higher frequency of adverbs (i.e. the type of correspondence that is closest to the adverb-like Norwegian particles); in the latter, there is a higher frequency of verb constructions. We may infer that the types of meaning expressed by the Norwegian modal particles are more naturally expressed in English by verb constructions, especially modal auxiliaries.

Norwegian and English differ not only in the means of expression, but also in the extent to which the meanings of the modal particles are expressed. For all the particles included, we find zero correspondences, i.e. the lack of an English form that specifically renders the meaning of the Norwegian particle. The number is especially high for *nok* and *vel* (about 30 per cent for original Norwegian texts; 65 and 43 per cent, respectively, for texts translated from English). In other words, these modal particles are very often left untranslated in going from Norwegian to English; to an even higher extent, they are added in translations from English into Norwegian, although there is no obvious source.

The lack of a specific translation or a specific source does not necessarily mean that the modal meaning is totally absent in the English text. In well above half of the cases of zero correspondence, English has a modal verb corresponding to verb plus particle in Norwegian. In the case of *vel*, English may have an independent interrogative clause or a tag question, as against a combination of particle and interrogative structure in Norwegian. From an English point of view, the contribution of the modal particle may be felt to be redundant here.

The contrastive perspective has served to illuminate the relationship between the individual Norwegian particles.[7] There are differences both in the range and types of correspondences. For example, *sikkert* corresponds to English adverbs to a higher degree than *nok*, *vel*, and *visst*. It also has the lowest number of zero correspondences, which indicates that its meaning has not been bleached to the same extent as for the others.

In further contrastive work there is a need to examine the expression of modality in the two languages in greater depth. To what extent do the means of expressing modality correspond? How do the correspondences vary with context? To what extent are modal meanings expressed by a combination of forms? And, perhaps most important, to what extent does the availability of different means affect the degree to which modal meanings are expressed?

---

[7]The usefulness of the contrastive approach is well shown in Aijmer's recent (1996) study of the Swedish modal particles *nog*, *visst*, *väl*, and *ju*. Aijmer stresses the multifunctionality of the particles and the ways in which this is revealed by the contrastive perspective. Unfortunately, Aijmer's paper came to our attention too late to be taken into account in the present paper.

References

Aijmer, K. (1996). Swedish Modal Particles in a Contrastive Perspective. *Language Sciences* 18, 393-427.

Baker, M. (1993). Corpus Linguistics and Translation Studies: Implications and Applications. In M. Baker, G. Francis & Tognini-Bonelli (eds) *Text and Technology. In Honour of John Sinclair*, Amsterdam: John Benjamins, 233-250.

Davidsen-Nielsen, N. (1996). Discourse Particles in Danish. In E. Engberg-Pedersen, M. Fortescue, P. Harder, L. Heltoft & L. Falster Jakobsen (eds) *Content, Expression and Structure: Studies in Danish Functional Grammar*, Amsterdam & Philadelphia: Benjamins, 283-314.

Fretheim, T. (1981). 'Ego'-dempere og 'alter'-dempere, *Maal og Minne* 1-2. Oslo: Det norske samlaget, 86-100.

Gellerstam, M. (1986). Translationese in Swedish Novels Translated from English. In L. Wollin & H. Lindquist (eds) *Translation Studies in Scandinavia*, Lund: CWK Gleerup, 88-95.

Haugen, E. (1984). *Norsk-engelsk ordbok / Norwegian-English Dictionary*. 3rd ed. Oslo: Universitetsforlaget.

Johansson, S. & K. Hofland (1994). Towards an English-Norwegian Parallel Corpus. In U. Fries, G. Tottie & P. Schneider (eds) *Creating and Using English Language Corpora*, Amsterdam & Atlanta, GA: Rodopi, 25-37.

Johansson, S., J. Ebeling & K. Hofland (1996). Coding and Aligning the English-Norwegian Parallel Corpus. In K. Aijmer, B. Altenberg, and M. Johansson (eds) *Languages in Contrast*, Lund Studies in English 88. Lund: Lund University Press, 87-112.

Johansson, S. and J. Ebeling (1996). Exploring the English-Norwegian Parallel Corpus. In C. E. Percy, C. F. Meyer & J. Lancashire (eds) *Synchronic Corpus Linguistics*. Papers from the 16th International Conference on English Language Research on Computerized Corpora (ICAME 16), Amsterdam & Atlanta, GA: Rodopi, 3-15.

Kirkeby, W. (1986). *Norsk-engelsk ordbok*. 2nd ed. Oslo: Kunnskapsforlaget.

Løken, B. (1996). Expressing Possibility in English and Norwegian. Unpubl. *hovedfag* thesis. Department of British and American Studies, University of Oslo.

Appendix 1: Corpus texts

A. English original texts: code, author (translator), title of original text, title of translation

MA1   Atwood, Margaret (Gjelsvik, Inger) *Cat's Eye / Katteøyet*

JB1   Barnes, Julian (Ofstad, Knut) *Talking It Over / En trekanthistorie*

ABR1   Brink, André (Malde, Per) *The Wall of the Plague / Pestens mur*

AB1   Brookner, Anita (Jahr, Mette-Cathrine) *Latecomers / Etternølere*

BC1   Chatwin, Bruce (Greiff, Aud) *Utz / Utz*

JC1   Crace, Jim (Lund, Harald) *Arcadia / Arkadia*

RD1   Dahl, Roald (Dahl, Tor Edvin) *Matilda / Matilda*

RDO1 Doyle, Roddy (Herrman, Bjørn A.) *Paddy Clarke Ha Ha Ha / Paddy Clarke Ha ha ha*

MD1   Drabble, Margaret (Roald, Bodil) *The Middle Ground / Midt på treet*

FF1   Forsyth, Frederick (Hoff, Gerd) *The Fourth Protocol / Den fjerde protokoll*

DF1   Francis, Dick (Kolstad, Henning) *Straight / Dødelig arv*

NG1   Gordimer, Nadine (Bang, Karin) *My Son's Story / Min sønns historie*

SG1   Grafton, Sue (Rogde, Isak) *'D' is for Deadbeat / 'D' for druknet*

TH1   Hayden, Torey (Nergaard, Jan) *The Sunflower Forest / Solsikkeskogen*

JH1   Heller, Joseph (Risvik, Kari & Kjell) *Picture This / Se det*

PDJ3 James, P.D. (Greiff, Aud) *Devices and Desires / Intriger og begjær*

SK1   King, Stephen (Nergaard, Jan) *Cujo / Faresonen*

DL1   Lessing, Doris (Roald, Bodil) *The Fifth Child / Det femte barnet*

DL2   Lessing, Doris (Halling, Kia) *The Good Terrorist / Den gode terroristen*

MM1   Magorian, Michelle (Jakobsen, Ole Skau) *Goodnight Mister Tom / Godnatt Mister Tom*

GN1   Naylor, Gloria (Lange, Mona) *The Women of Brewster Place / Kvinnene på Brewster Place*

BO1   Okri, Ben (Lange, Mona) *The Famished Road / Den sultne veien*

RR1   Rendell, Ruth (Tønnesen, Birgit) *Kissing the Gunner's Daughter / Brent barn*

JSM1 Smiley, Jane (Elligers, Anne) *A Thousand Acres / Fire tusen mål*

ST1   Townsend, Sue (Larsen, Dag Heyerdal) *The Queen and I / Dronninga og Jeg*

AT1   Tyler, Anne (Roald, Bodil) *The Accidental Tourist / Tilfeldig turist*

FW1   Weldon, Fay (Aase, Wivi) *The Heart of the Country / Landets hjerte*

B. Norwegian original texts: code, author (translator) title of original text, title of translation

KAL1 Alnæs, Karsten (Engebretsen, Rune) *Even 1814 / The Boy from Duck River: A Norwegian Adventure Tale*

KA1   Askildsen, Kjell (Lyngstad, Sverre) *En plutselig frigjørende tanke / A Sudden Liberating Thought*

TB1   Brekke, Toril (Born, Anne) *Jakarandablomsten / The Jacaranda Flower*

FC1   Carling, Finn (Muinzer, Louis A.) *Under aftenhimmelen / Under the Evening Sky*

LSC1 Christensen, Lars Saabye (Nordby, Steven Michael) *Herman / Herman*

LSC2   Christensen, Lars Saabye (Nordby, Steven Michael) *Jokeren / The Joker*

KF1   Faldbakken, Knut (Lyngstad, Sverre) *Adams dagbok / Adam's Diary*

KF2   Faldbakken, Knut (Sutcliffe, Hal & Torbjørn Støverud) *Insektsommer / Insect Summer*

KFL1   Fløgstad, Kjartan (Christensen, Nadie) *Dalen Portland / Dollar Road*

EG1   Griffiths, Ella (Cowlishaw, J. Basil) *Mord på side 3 / Murder on Page Three*

EG2   Griffiths, Ella (Cowlishaw, J. Basil) *Vannenken / The Water Widow*

JG1   Gaarder, Jostein (Møller, Paulette) *Sofies verden / Sophie's World*

EHA1   Haslund, Ebba (Wilson, Barbara) *Det hendte ingenting / Nothing Happened*

THA1   Haugen, Tormod (Jacobs, David R.) *Zeppelin / Zeppelin*

TTH1   Hauger, Torill Thorstad (Paulsen, Marlys Wick) *Røvet av vikinger / Captured by the Vikings*

EH1   Hoem, Edvard (Shackelford, Frankie D.) *Kjærleikens ferjereiser / The Ferry Crossing*

SH1   Holmås, Stig (Born, Anne) *Tordensønnen / Son-of-Thunder*

KH1   Holt, Kåre (Tate, Joan) *Kappløpet / The Race*

SL1   Lie, Sissel (Born, Anne) *Løvens hjerte / Lion's Heart*

OEL1   Lønn, Øystein (McDuff, David) *Tom Rebers siste retrett / Tom Reber's Last Retreat*

CL1   Løveid, Cecilie (Christensen, Nadie) *Sug / Sea Swell*

MN1   Newth, Mette (Nunally, Tiina & Steve Murray) *Bortførelsen / The Abduction*

GS1   Staalesen, Gunnar (McDuff, David) *I mørket er alle ulver grå / At Night All Wolves Are Grey*

BV1   Vik, Bjørg (McDuff, David) *En håndfull lengsel / Out of Seasons and Other Stories*

BV2   Vik, Bjørg (Garton, Janet) *Kvinneakvariet / An Aquarium of Women*

HW1   Wassmo, Herbjørg (Simpson, Allen) *Huset med den blinde glassveranda / The House With the Blind Glass Windows*

JW1   Wiese, Jan (Geddes, Tom) *Kvinnen som kledte seg naken for sin elskede / The Naked Madonna*

Appendix 2: Correspondences (excluding zero)

A. Translations (Norwegian to English)

nok

adverb: probably 35, no doubt 6, all right 3, surely 3, enough 2, certainly 2, perhaps 2, undoubtedly 2, indeed, doubtless, of course, always, someday, though, if anything, maybe, beyond dispute, for sure

verb construction:	must 7, bound to 2, inclined to, might, is sure to, could, seemed to, should, agreed
tag question:	1 instance
1st person clause:	I suppose 2, I think 2, I'll say, I expect, I'm sure, I bet
other clause:	don't worry 2, you'll see, you can bet your arse on it
miscellaneous:	emphatic *do*, vil nok -> should, tror nok -> seem

sikkert

adverb:	probably 12, surely 12, no doubt 8, certainly 7, most likely 2, doubtless 2, presumably, possibly, sure, sure as eggs
verb construction:	must 7, bound to, wouldn't hesitate
tag question:	1 instance
1st person clause:	I'm sure 11, I think, I'm pretty sure, I suppose
other clause:	he supposed, there's no doubt

vel

adverb:	probably 35, surely 13, well 4, no doubt 4, of course 3, really 2, perhaps 2, apparently, most likely, certainly, undoubtedly, naturally, right, too, just, as well, anyway
verb construction:	must 3, will, may, can, could, would, seemed, guess, will no doubt
tag question:	20 instances
interrogative clause:	4 instances
1st person clause:	I suppose 16, I guess 5, I hope 3, I expect 3, I'm sure 2, I bet, I know, I should have thought, I shouldn't think
other clause:	he/she supposed 3, she/he thought 2, he reflected, he expected, he assumed, the next thing you know, he's pretty well bound to, don't tell me ... not
miscellaneous:	no reason, so there, but after all

visst

adverb:	apparently 3, sure(ly) 2, perhaps 2, certainly 2, undoubtedly, obviously, evidently, probably, most likely, kind of
verb construction:	must 9, seem 7, appear 2
1st person clause:	I believe 3, I feel, I've heard that
other clause:	it's said that

B. Sources (English to Norwegian)

nok

adverb:	probably 3, surely, well, although, if anything, even though
verb construction:	might 2, would 2, to be sure 2, must, seems
1st person clause:	reckon, I suspect, I reckon, I notice, I think
other clause:	she knew, he supposed, it seemed
miscellaneous:	emphatic *do* 2, fronting, nok ikke <- hardly

sikkert

adverb:	surely 7, probably 6, no doubt 5, certainly 3, undoubtedly
verb construction:	must 5, will 4, would 2, could 2, may, must certainly
1st person clause:	I'm sure 2, I expect 2, I know, reckon
other clause:	it was likely, she was sure of that

vel

adverb:	probably 7, surely 3, at least 2, presumably, maybe, after all, just, anyway, well, like
verb construction:	must 4, would 2, can
tag question:	16 instances
interrogative clause:	8 instances
1st person clause:	I guess 15, I suppose(d) 13, I expect 6, I reckoned 2, I thought, I fear
other clause:	he guessed, he supposed
miscellaneous:	emphatic *do*

visst

adverb:	apparently, certainly, maybe
verb construction:	seem to 10, looks like, always act like
1st person clause:	I guess 2, I think 2, I could tell, I'm thinking
other clause:	it seems, it was supposed to

Modality and Morphology: The Case of *-able*

Alex Klinge

1. Introduction

I was preparing yet another pile of eye-opening handouts for my favourite students in the xerox room in the Department, when one of my colleagues came into the room, clearly intent on doing some xeroxing of her own. Ordinarily, in the busy first few weeks of a new semester the expected exchange would be of the nature "lots to copy?", "well, 20 copies of this and a whole heap of transparencies". Instead, however, she initiated the exchange with a different sort of conversational move. She said "you did some work on modality, didn't you?". This is a type of statement coupled with a there-is-no-denying-it tag question which, in particular when used to initiate conversation, tends to make me apprehensive, because in such circumstances more often than not I find myself confronted with requests for accounts of thoroughly inexplicable data. Colleagues in need of a ready-made explanation for their next language lecture in fifteen minutes do not always appreciate the limitations of the state of the descriptive art.

Unaware of my private concern, she opened a workbook she had brought for xeroxing, and on the inner sleeve of the book was written *PHOTOCOPIABLE*. At least two interesting observations followed, viz. that the utterance on the sleeve was to be interpreted as granting permission to photocopy not merely as stating that it is possible, and that accordingly the semantic input provided was underspecified relative to the pragmatic interpretation that the owner of the book was granted permission to take any number of copies from the book and use them in her teaching as she pleases without facing legal action by the publishers for infringement of copyright. I believe that I mumbled something nebulous to the effect that via metaphorical extension and the principles of indirectness the representational meta-function of language lends itself to directive purposes so that possibility may be transformed into permission. I escaped further interrogation at the time.

I resolved to return to the issue for a more thorough account, and since I subsequently also found that similar forms sometimes present problems for students of legal language and translation, a rather more elaborate explanatory framework appears to me to be called for. Thus is motivated the present investigation of the morpheme *-able*, its semantics and how it enters into higher-level interpretation. Though far from exhaustive, it provides the outline of a framework of description in an underdescribed area of morphology. Primary data have been culled from commercial and legal language.

2. Modality

In the literature on modality in the English language, the modal auxiliaries have spawned the most astute observations, and morphologically realised modality is traditionally part of the standard package only in the form of the subjunctive, which is clearly on the unproductive side in synchronic terms. The morpheme *-able* is hardly mentioned at all in the modality literature, and as far as I know, the permissive function illustrated above has passed practically unnoticed (though see Lyons 1977: 532).

Presumably the modal auxiliaries attract attention partly because their distribution and semantic behaviour may be taken to be a manifestation of an underlying typology of modality, and partly because their distribution and semantic behaviour so abundantly illustrate that modality works in mysterious ways. For purposes of linguistic analysis, two main types of modality are often recognised: (a) *epistemic modality*, which is to do with the extent to which a proposition is presented by the speaker as verified or unverified relative to the situation it represents, ie. p is possibly true, or p is necessarily true, (b) *non-epistemic modality*, which is again sometimes subdivided into *deontic modality*, which is to do with an extrinsically prescribed relation between an individual and an event, ie. permission or obligation to make p true, and *dynamic modality*, which is to do with an intrinsically motivated relation between an individual or an entity and an event, ie. intention, ability or intrinsic potentiality (a phrase coined by Bolinger 1989) to make p true. The modal auxiliaries are distributionally and semantically sensitive to these types of modality. Some writers take this sensitivity to be a semantic property of the modals themselves (eg. Palmer 1990 and Davidsen-Nielsen 1990), other writers take it to be an aspect of contextualisation, which is to be described as interaction between the modals and their contexts of utterance (eg. Perkins 1983, Groefsema 1995 and Klinge 1993 and 1996).

In diachronic terms, the morpheme *-able* has been derived through Middle French and Middle English from Latin *-abilis*, *-ibilis* and *-bilis*, meaning "suitable, fit for a purpose" (Urdang 1982: 140). In present-day English its central, productive function is as a derivational suffix which takes a transitive verb root and turns it into a complex form with the functional properties of an adjective, which is rendered by Lyons (1977: 528) as the formula in (1).

(1)   Vtr + *able* → A

There are other peripheral and incidental derivational patterns which will not be investigated here, such as in *avilalable*, *durable*, *equitable*, *reputable*, and *fashionable*, though at some higer level of analysis they may all be related. The alternative form *-ible*, as in *convertible*, is no longer productive in English and is confined to Latin-derived verbs. It will be assumed that *-ible* formations are to be treated as fully lexicalised. *-ible* will not be separately investigated here. The principles of interpretation outlined in the following are taken in the main to apply also to *-ible*, though idiosyncracies of long-term lexicalisation have perhaps had a more profound effect in the case of *-ible* formations.

Not only has the form of the Latin suffix survived almost intact, but as it appears from (2) and (3), the meaning of the suffix also appears to have been preserved:

(2)   Locally obtainable equipment required for the performance of the contract shall be hired or bought by the Project Manager.

(3)   The genus need not be definable with logical or scientific exactitude ...

In (2) the meaning added by the suffix *-able* to the premodifying adjective phrase of the subject noun phrase, and the meaning assigned by the subject predicate to the subject noun phrase in (3) would be satisfactorily rendered by means of one of the paraphrases *able to be Ved* or *capable of being Ved*, or *can be Ved* (Bauer 1983: 154f and Lyons 1977: 530ff). If we consider the modal element involved in these modalized passive constructions in terms of the above types of modality, it is quite clear that *able*, *capable*, and *can* are to be understood as assigning a modal quality of ability or intrinsic potentiality to the referent of the head noun relative to the event denoted by the transitive verb root of the formula $V_{tr} + able \rightarrow A'$. According to our above typology this qualifies as dynamic modality. But where dynamic modality is ususally conceived of as an active relation between an entity or an individual and the ability or intention to make an event occur, in *-able* we are dealing with a passive relation between an entity or individual and the intrinsic potentiality to be affected by an event. We assume that with the paraphrases offered and the notion of intrinsic potentiality to be a passive participant in the event denoted by the transitive verb root we have accounted for the semantics of the modal element of the suffix. We shall return to the semantics of the whole complex and higher structures in the next sections.

It is readily apparent that the semantics proposed leaves unexplained the *photocopiable* we began with, because in its instance of utterance it communicates a meaning over and above intrinsic potentiality. The utterance on the inner sleeve of the workbook certainly communicates more than "the workbook is capable of being photocopied". Similarly, consider utterance (4) from the articles of a company.

(4)   The Stock is transferable.

The significance of the utterance is that shareholders are entitled to transfer their shares if they so wish without any limitation imposed by the company articles. The point of the utterance is to prescribe a relation of permission between the shares of the company, the shareholders and an event of transfer. In other words, what (4) communicates amounts to deontic modality, rather than the dynamic modality postulated as the semantics of *-able* and found in (2) and (3) above. We shall assume that the sentence uttered in (4) is semantically underspecified relative to its interpretation as an utterance in context.

As an alternative to the underspecification solution, we might choose simply to say that in (4) we have found another, related, semantic meaning alongside intrinsic potentiality, viz. that of permission. And next we can simply record the two related meanings as semantic meanings of -*able*, and that would be the end of this investigation. Such an approach would not be unlike some polysemy and gradience solutions often adopted for similar contrasts of meaning observed in sentences containing the modal auxiliary *can* (see Coates 1983 and Palmer 1990). And indeed, as we shall see below, possibility and permission may be taken to be manifestations of the same basic modality in two different domains of human experience. However, to my mind there are two reasons why we do not wish to say that permission is a meaning of -*able* on a par with intrinsic potentiality. The first, least compelling, reason is that one morpheme would then encode both intrinsic and extrinsic modality. The second reason is that in the corpus used for this investigation -*able* is actually found more often in utterances conveying obligation than in utterances conveying permission. Utterance (5), which is a fragment of a clause from a supply contract, clearly conveys obligation to pay in given way.

(5) All invoices are payable without discount of any kind in pounds sterling within 28 days of the date of the Company's invoice at the Company's premises stated on the invoice ...

We should definitely hesitate to argue that -*able* encodes obligation alongside permission and intrinsic potentiality. In the following we shall pursue the permission and obligation meanings communicated by (4) and (5) as aspects of contextualisation, and we shall seek to explain how -*able* plays a part in the creation of deontic modalities.

3. The syntax and semantics of adjectival qualification

In the previous section I introduced Lyons' derivational formula $V_{tr} + able \rightarrow A$, which states that the derivational morpheme -*able* turns a lexeme of the class of transitive verbs into a member of the class of adjectives. The resulting complex word form owes its semantics to the modality of -*able*, discussed above, the functional properties of an adjective, and the semantics of the verb root. In this section we shall consider the adjectival features assigned by -*able* to the complex form.

I argued above that there are two reasons why the literature on modality in the English language focusses on the modal auxiliaries, viz. the intricate semantic pattern they represent and the assumption that this pattern reflects some underlying typology of modality. But there is an additional reason. The modal auxiliaries, and the subjunctive for that matter, are syntactically realised in the operator position adjecent to the verb, where we find semantic operators with access to the top-most scope positions in the semantic hierarchy of the clause. In the case of epistemically interpreted modal auxiliaries, the modality is assigned scope over the entire propositional nucleus, and in the case of nonepistemically interpreted modal auxiliaries, ie. deontic and dynamic modality, the modality is assigned scope over the relation between the subject and the predicate. In this way the modal auxiliaries may serve directly as the speaker's modification of the propositional content she conveys by means of the sentence she utters. In contradistinction, -*able* formations acquire the functional properties of an adjective and assign their modality to heads of noun phrases at subclausal, constituent level. Fundamentally, we shall be concerned with two syntagmatic relationships: prenominal attributive, ie. NP [AdjP + N], as in (6), or post-copular predicative, ie. CLAUSE [NP + VP [*be* + AdjP]], as in (7).

(6)   The distributable profits of the Company (in so far as they are sufficient) shall be applied first in the payment to the holders of Preference Shares ...

(7)   The Company declares that as and when the security created by this deed becomes enforceable ... the Company shall hold all the property charged upon trust ...

Below I will suggest that -*able* together with the verb root lexeme creates its own sub-propositional event frame which is open to enrichment and expansion by the addressee, and that in predicative relationships the modality of -*able* may be interpreted in the higher operator position.

It is assumed that the possible syntagmatic relationships resulting from the derivational process V_{tr} + *able* → A have identifiable semantic import. Occupying the function of head in an adjective phrase is simply a meaningful occupation. Let us assume with Ferris (1993) that for the purposes of describing this relationship the semantic primitives we need are *entities*, *properties* and a set of possible *relations* between them. Ferris operates with four possible relations, viz. *qualification*, *equation*, *assignment* and *coordination*. The two relations we shall find relevant in connection with the syntagmatic relationships NP [AdjP + N] and CLAUSE [NP + VP [*be* + AdjP]] are *qualification* and *assignment*.

The relation of qualification occurs where an N is expanded with a subordinate preposed AdjP into an NP, so that the property denoted by AdjP narrows down the identification of the N. This is clearly the case in (6), where *distributable* delimits the range of possible entities the addressee can identify for *profits*, ie. not all profits are affected by this article, only those of which *distributable* is an inherent, atemporal feature. The relation of assignment occurs where a CLAUSE is expanded into an NP and a copular VP predicate expanded into a V and an AdjP, so that the property denoted by AdjP qualifies, but does not identify, the entity denoted by the NP. In (7) the property of *enforceable* is assigned to the entity denoted by *the security created by this deed*.

Assignment of qualification differs semantically from simple qualification in two important respects. Firstly, the qualification assigned is subject to the basic illocuationary act performed by the utterance, and accordingly the assignment relation may be asserted or questioned, as in *The security is enforceable* vs. *Is the security enforceable?* Secondly, in the assignment of qualification relation, the qualification is directly governed by any tense or modal auxiliaries of the clause, so the property assigned is accordingly interpreted as applying here and now, there and then, always, merely potentially, etc. The temporal, transient nature of the property assigned is clearly brought out in the subordinating conjunction "as and when" in (7), ie. enforceablility is not a universally inherent quality of the security. This distinction will account for pairs such as *the visible stars*, permanent quality, and *the stars visible*, transient quality, because in *stars visible* the adjective represents a reduced relative clause with assignment, viz. *stars which are/were visible*. Temporalisation or modalisation do not similarly directly affect the prenominal attributive position. The prototypical exponent of assignment is the copular verb *be*, but *become* as in (7) is actually a very frequent alternative in the data investigated. We shall distinguish simple qualification for the purpose of identification, realised as NP [AdjP + N], and qualification for the purpose of assignment, realised as CLAUSE [NP + VP [*be* + AdjP]], where of course the NP is only obligatorily realised in finite clauses.

If we turn now to the question whether the *photocopiable* we started with was intended to be interpreted as simple qualification or as assignment of qualification, we can safely say that it must have been intended as assignment of qualification, ie. as an underlying *this workbook is photocopiable*, rather than an underlying *photocopiable workbook*. First of all, the utterance of *photocopiable* on the inner sleeve of the workbook was hardly intended as narrowing down the identification of an entity, understood here to be the workbook which the reader is already holding in her hand. Moreover, it is crucial to the correct utterance understanding that the quality of *photocopiable* should be seen as being assigned by the speaker in the instance of utterance, and not as a permanent quality of the workbook. We shall come back to the implications of this latter observation in section 5 below.

4. Syntactic and semantic frames

In section 2 above I excluded an unspecified range of forms that are not products of Lyons' derivation formula $V_{tr} + able \rightarrow A$, for instance *actionable, fashionable* and *knowledgeable*, where the root lexeme is a noun. So far I have identified two main utterance functions, the primary one simply relies on the semantics of dynamic modality that *-able* is held to represent, the secondary one is an extension of the dynamic modality into deontic modality via some as yet unexplained context-bound mechanism. But even in formations that satisfy Lyons' formula we find data where neither a clearly dynamic, nor a clearly deontic function seems to be at play.

(8)   The terms of agency are sometimes set out in correspondence between the parties, but where dealings are on a large scale, a formal agreement drafted by a solicitor may be desirable.

Some other possible examples would be *questionable, preferable, regrettable* and *acceptable*. I propose to call this an evaluative function. These complex forms are also in need of an explanation.

The formula $V_{tr} + able \rightarrow A$ states that the input to the derivation is a transitive verb, which is a formulation of a fact of lexically specified syntactic complementation. In other words, the transitive verb root is specified lexically for a syntactic frame with a least one object. A candidate for derivation would then be *pay* as it occurs in (9).

(9)   The Company shall on demand pay to the Lender all money and liabilities now or at any time owing by the Company to the Lender ...

But as it is indicated by the paraphrases proposed for *-able* above, the morpheme seems to be more immediately related with a passive sentence such as (10).

(10)   On each date on which this Agreement requires an amount denominated in sterling to be paid by the Banks to the Agent for account of the Borrower each Bank shall make its portion thereof available to the Agent ...

That the derived complex lexeme is more immediately related with the passive sentence becomes clear when it is realised that it inherits the passive syntactic frame of the transitive verb root.

(11)   Any sums payable by the Warrantors to the Purchaser in respect of the Warranties and under the Deed of Indemnity shall be deemed to constitute a reduction in the Total Consideration.

From data such as (9) and (10) we can deduce the syntactic frames that *pay* requires in the active structure *X pay Y to Z*, and in passive structures *Y be paid by X to Z*, or alternatively *Z be paid Y by X*, where X, Y and Z are all NPs. The complex form *payable* inherits the syntactic frame of the ditransitive lexeme *pay* in the passive structure of (10), but the complements may be reduced to the Y NP, the direct object in functional terms, which becomes the head of the noun phrase modified by the derived adjective. Apparently, the Z NP, the indirect object in functional terms, does not become the head of the noun phrase modified, which rules out *Z be paid Y by X* as a source frame for derivation, cf. (12a) to (12c):

(12a)   She paid the young man the amount. → a payable amount /* a payable young man

(12b)   She read the young man a poem. → a readable poem/* a readable young man

(12c)   She sold the young man a book. → a saleable book/* a saleable youngman

The syntactic frames constitute formal manifestation of a corresponding semantic frame. For our purposes we shall assume that a verb lexeme denotes a type of situation, and that the complements X, Y and Z of the syntactic frame denote entities (including individuals), and properties which may be described in terms of participant roles assigned by the overall pay-situation. The specific participant roles of a pay-situation are the payor = X, the payee = Z and the amount paid = Y. The specific roles are instances of the general participant roles *agent*, *recipient* and *patient*.

A pay-situation is an instance of the more general situation type of *agent-event*. Drawing on Durst-Andersen (1992), I shall recognise *states*, perceived as stability, and *activity*, perceived as instability, as primitive situation types. And modifying Durst-Andersen's terminology, I shall also recognise the complex general situation type of *events* (which corresponds with *actions* in his typology). An event is a complex construct comprising an initial state and a final state which are incompatible and which are causally related by an activity. In semantic interpretation the causal relationship translates into deductive or non-deductive implication between a representation of a final state, an activity and an initial state. An activity may be interpreted as caused either by the world or by a wilful agent, so we can distinguish *world-activity* from *agent-activity*. By extension, since an event is a complex of an activity and two states, an event may also be distinguished as either a *world-event* or an *agent-event*. Agent-activity and agent-events presuppose intentional agent control – the agent could consciously have decided not to produce the activity.

Two points should be made about this scaled-down, modified version of Durst-Andersen's typology. Firstly, in this situation typology time is not the central feature distinguishing states, activities and events, because the crucial distinction lies in incompatability and implication between representations to which time is incidental. Secondly, we need to add the crucial caveat that for English it makes little sense to classify individual verb lexemes as in themselves denoting a state, an activity or an event (Durst-Andersen 1992: 54). Only fully expanded semantic frames may be classified in terms of the type of situation they denote. It is well known that one verb lexeme may enter into different frames and receive different interpretations, such as in *John swims every morning*, an agent-activity, and *John swims ten lanes every morning*, an agent-event. As a rule of thumb, it makes sense to ask about an activity "for how long does/did X V", and it makes sense to ask about an event "how long does/did it take for X toV Y".

Durst-Andersen (1992: 54ff) proposes four situation classifiers, or basic existential modes underlying participants in states, activities and events: *location*, *possession*, *experience*, and *qualification*. So for instance the activity of walking presupposes a location where the activity is taking place, an event of selling presupposes the passing of ownership between the referents of the agent role and the recipient role (though not necessarily of possession in the legal sense), an event of reading presupposes a change of experience in the referent of the agent role or the recipient role (cf. *She read a book*, *She read him a poem*), and an event of repairing presupposes a change of quality in the referent of the patient role.

We can now paraphrase the semantics of an *event frame* as (13).

(13)   Agent X produces an activity with patient Y (for the benefit of recipient Z) and the activity is sufficient to produce a final state with an underlying change of location, possession, experience or quality of X, Y (or recipient Z).

The complex lexeme derived by V_{tr} + *able*→A inherits the semantic event frame of the transitive verb root together with the dynamic modality of *-able* and the complex turns into the paraphrase in (14).

(14)   There is an inherent potential for entity Y to be the patient of an activity produced by X and the activity is sufficient to produce a final state with an underlying change of location, possession, experience or quality of X, Y (or recipient Z).

It should be noted that (14) is no longer only about a quality inherent in some entity, but it also brings out that that quality presupposes that the full pay-event is also a potential event. Some such semantic paraphrase split between the modality and the event frame will have be postulated for the complex lexeme, because we want to be able to say that a negative prefix operates on the modality, not the activity or event denoted by the verb root. So (15) means that there is not an inherent potential for the glass to be the patient in a break-event, and thus there is no potential break-event.

(15)   Some years ago we bought from you a consignment of wrist watches in stainless steel cases with unbreakable glass.

By extension, (16) and (17) can only be intended as not-permission, ie. there is no permitted transfer- or revocation-event, and a permission-not interpretation is not available.

(16)   The shares are non-transferable.

(17)   Any notice given by the Borrower under sub-clause (B) shall be irrevocable.

As a final point in connection with the event frame of the verb root we return to the descriptive problem posed at the beginning of this section: how do formations such as *enviable*, *advisable* and *unthinkable* acquire their evaluative function? Consider the sentence in (18) with the transitive verb *accept*.

(18)   She accepted the payment tendered.

The sentence may be interpreted in two slightly different ways. One interpretation, perhaps the more obvious, is that the referent of *she* received money in settlement, another interpretation is that the referent of *she* took the payment to be satisfactory, but in this latter interpretation she may not have received a penny. The two interpretations rely on the a distinction between a possession-based event and an experience-based event, an ambiguity of reading inherent in *accept*.

The derived complex lexeme *acceptable* seems to prefer the experience interpretation so that *acceptable payment* would be understood in terms of the experience reading as payment that is capable of being held satisfactory, cf. also *unacceptable*, which is clearly reserved for an experience reading. The possession-based reading would probably be ensured by means of *non-acceptable*, though no such form occurred in the data investigated. It is quite plausible that in the process of derivation transitive verbs which denote experience-based events transmit not only the experience interpretation, but that as a result of the adjective features acquired in the derivation, the focus shifts to the subjective evaluative nature of the mental state of experience, rather than on any inherent feature of the thing experienced.

(20)   It has already been submitted that the source of this latter error was an understandable confusion between the provision of consideration on the one hand and its performance on the other.

The subjectivity of the nature of the experience becomes even more pronounced where the verb root is in itself fundamentally negatively evaluative, as in *detestable*, or positively evaluative, as in (21).

(21)   The Licensee shall take out product liability insurance with respectable insurers in respect of the Products manufacture and sold be the Licensee ...

In terms of linguistic description, we are faced with a choice between treating the evaluation element as a result of lexicalisation of a group of adjectives derived from verbs denoting experience-based activities and events, or as a result of extra-lexical interpretation processes. Lyons (1977: 532) also raises this issue. If we say that the evaluation meaning has become lexicalised, we still owe our readers an explanation as to why that particular group should have became lexicalised. Note that if we follow Lyons (1977: 530) suggestion and take the evaluative element of *readable* to be lexicalised, we will find ourselves in trouble with the compound *machine readable* in (22), where there is no evaluative meaning. Since a machine is incapable of experience, (22) can only be understood as possession-based, ie. the machine acquires a representation of the text.

(22)   ... for the purposes only of understanding the contents of such machine readable material ...

The experience-based verbs shift focus from the entity experienced to the experiencer and the quality of the experience. Note here the difference observed by most English speakers between *readable book* and *legible book*, where *legible* is truly a feature of the book and has nothing to do with the experience of the experiencer. In "What Hi-Fi" we find experience-based evaluation in *very listenable sound* (April 1996, p. 21), and I am sure that we would similarly be able to find reviews of *watchable* films, but experience-based *feelable pain* and *seeable paintings* appear distinctly odd, though again of course we have *visible paintings* as a feature of the paintings. The reason is presumable that the experience-based mental states of feeling and seeing are beyond the active intentionality of an agent. However, a possession-based receiving-event is also beyond the intentionality of the agent, and *receivable*, as in (23) from a Power of Attorney, is perfectly acceptable.

(23)   ... and generally to take such steps in respect of the said Rent Act or any other Act affecting my said property or the rent receivable therefor ...

A good deal more work is required in this area since, as we have seen, intricate lexical or derivational constraints seem to operate in the case of experience-based roots.

5. The contextualisation of $V_{tr} + able \rightarrow A$

We have postulated a semantics for the derivational morpheme in terms of its modal element of inherent potentiality, we have captured the semantic consequences of the syntagmatic relationships the derived complex adjective enters into, we have set up a (reduced) situation typology in terms of which we can interpret the transitive verb root and its complements, and finally we have captured how the modal element of inherent potentiality and the semantics of the verb root and its complements combine in a modalised passive event frame. All these are syntactico-semantic resources a speaker can draw on in producing utterances in furtherance of her communicative goals. To make sense of an utterance, the addressee in his turn has to recognise the syntactico-semantic resources invoked, and has to make assumptions about the speaker's communicative goals. He does so by drawing on his linguistic competence and by reference to the context in which the utterance is produced.

For descriptive convenience, we shall assume that it is possible to identify two levels of context available to an addressee. We shall operate with a *metacontext* which shapes rules of interaction and communication and which constitutes the world into which linguistic items are born and have to struggle to survive. The metacontext is relatively stable across members of a speech community, but it also motivates diachronic language change by imposing pressures of functional expediency on linguistic items. We shall also operate with a *communicative context* which is anchored in terms of temporal, spatial and interpersonal coordinates and in which an addressee engages his cognitive powers in on-line processing of specific utterances. In the following we shall investigate how the two aspects of context are brought to bear on $V_{tr} + able \rightarrow A$.

In her well-conceived book on metaphorical and cultural aspects of semantic structure, Sweetser (1990) draws on metaphorical extension between semantic structures to account for diachronic language change. Investigations of the etymology of the English modals strongly suggest that they originated to serve non-epistemic semantic domains, and that they gradually acquired epistemic functions (see Tanaka 1990). Sweetser employs force dynamics with forces and barriers as the point of metaphorical translation between the modal auxiliaries used in the sociophysical non-epistemic domain and the modal auxiliaries used in a domain of internal epistemic reasoning. In this way she provides a very plausible account of how metaphorical mapping takes place between domains of human experience at the metacontextual level. In a somewhat similar vein Perkins (1983) argues that while the modals essentially remain semantically stable and monosemous, they are interpreted quite differently against the background of natural laws, social laws, and rational laws.

On the basis of the framework formulated in the previous sections, we can also trace a possible path of metaphorical mapping, and construct in a plausible manner the functional extension of V_{tr} + *able*→A from the dynamic domain into the deontic domain. As our point of departure, we can revert to example (15) above, repeated here as (24) for convenience.

(24)   Some years ago we bought from you a consignment of wrist watches in stainless steel cases with unbreakable glass.

In (24) we find an entity, *glass*, which is endowed with a physical quality which according to the laws of nature makes it *unbreakable* under normal, non-extreme circumstances. It will be noticed that an event-frame constructed with *unbreakable glass* as input turns out completely unspecified as to whether we are dealing with a world-event or an agent-event. Moreover the distinction is completely irrelevant in this particular context – the laws of nature govern both world and man. In some cases we find complex forms which are clearly interpretable exclusively in terms of an entity which is physically endowed to be a patient in a world-event, such as *perishable goods* and *biodegradable plastic bag*, but which are not derived from transitive verbs. This is dynamic modality in its purest form.

As we saw in the discussion of situation types, we also interpret activities and events as specified for intentional human agency.

(25)   ... and as some of the items in the consignment may prove to be more readily saleable than others, we trust you will do all you can to ensure that the best possible prices are obtained for each separate lot.

Note here that *items* cannot simply happen to be sold by some world-event, and that a sell-event is subject to conscious control by a human agent. We have now moved from merely a quality that an entity is physically endowed with towards what agents can do to entities which have the quality. *items be saleable* can quite clearly only be interpreted in terms of a potential agent-event. We would happily say about a rotten apple that it is *unsaleable* in respect of a greengrocer agent, not because there is a physical, inherent quality of unsaleability in the apple, but simply because sell-situations involving a greengrocer as the agent and a rotten apple as the patient do not occur as part of our normal view of normal situations – so the potential of the event relative to a given agent comes to play a part. We have moved from a purely physical domain into a social domain, where we find types of agent-activities and agent-events which form part of normal social behaviour. This in fact is where we find by far the majority of examples in the data investigated, which is not surprising since the data belongs in the highly conventionalised social domains of law and commerce. Some examples are *excludable, rebuttable, excusable,* and *ascertainable,* which are all prototypically understood in terms of a human agent in control of the underlying events.

The closer we get to the social part of the sociophysical domain, the more likely we are to have assumptions about types of agents relative to types of activitites and events. Assumptions about desirability of activities and events to agents and recipients, and the authority of participants seem to be particularly important. So in some vague sense it is usually undesired to have one's argument rebutted, and it implies intellectual authority on the part of the rebutting agent, it is desired to be excused, and it implies social authority on the part of the excusing agent, but it is neither inherently desired, nor undesired for an entity to be ascertained or for an agent to ascertain.

In (26) we have an utterance where the complex form falls inside the social domain.

(26)   For example, where pension rights are expressed to be non-assignable, it could hardly be suggested that a purported assignment by the pensioner would release the payer of the pension from any obligation to make further payments.

So while we still recognise the semantics of *non-assignable* as assignment of the qualities *not able to be Ved or not capable of being Ved,* this is not the full utterance interpretation in this context. The point is that we interpret the passive event-frame of *non-assignable* in terms of an agent-event with *pension rights* as the patient, and a would-be agent, the assignor. It is a standard assumption that the would-be agent desires the freedom to assign her rights, but in (26) she is expressly blocked from doing so, not by some natural or logical law, but by the operation of some purely social law. Interpreted against such a background, *non-assignable* amounts to non-permission to assign. It is quite clear that, barring information to the contrary, the value we prototypically attach to an assignment-event is that it is desired to the assignor to have the option to assign, and it is this option which is blocked by *non-assignable* in (26). Similarly, the event-frame may represent an agent-event which is clearly desirable and which is made possible relative to the agent who desires it, not by laws of nature, but by social laws. Again barring information to the contrary, the value we prototypically attach to a possession-based claim-event should ensure that *claimable* would be difficult to envisage as meaning anything other than that some agent is permitted or entitled by social laws to claim something.

The metacontext in which metaphorical extension takes place obviously also affects the range of interpretations available to the individual addressee in a communicative context. However, in addition to access to the metacontextual metaphorical connection between natural and social laws, in a communicative context an individual addressee who interprets the complex *-able*-form in terms of an agent-event will rely on assumptions about the illocutionary intent of the speaker, the speaker's authority, and the desirability of the activity or event to the possible referents of the participants of the activity or event, and the likely intentions of those participants. Consider the following clause from a contract of employment:

(27)   Any shortfall of normal hours not worked in the previous 8 weeks must be worked at normal rates before overtime rates are payable.

A reader of this clause is faced with a range of interpretive tasks. Let us say that the reader is well aware that (27) constitutes a clause in a contract of employment, and consequently he also assumes that (27) is governed by the master speech act (Kurzon 1989 and Klinge 1995) THE EMPLOYER AND THE EMPLOYEE HEREBY AGREE, which means that the utterance as a whole is to be assigned the illocutionary force of a contractual provision. If we focus on *payable*, the reader has to identify the underlying passive syntactic frame of *Y be paid by X to Z* of the verb root. *by X* and *to Z* are syntactically unrealised in (27) but are available to the reader through semantic enrichment in his construction of the passive event frame in (28), where the participants are specified for their referents.

(28)   There is an inherent potential for entity Y (overtime rates) to be the patient of an activity (agent-activity) produced by X (the employer) and the activity is sufficient to produce a final state with an underlying change of possession of entity Y (rates) from X (the employer) to the recipient Z (the employee).

Having recognised the pay-event as an agent-event, because prototypically money is only paid if a human agent consciously chooses to produce such an event, the reader has assumptions about normal pay-events, viz. that the agent, the payor, does not desire a pay-event to occur, and conversely the recipient desires a pay-event to occur. Moreover, the desirability parameter is so strong that pay-events are subject to social laws, in particular of course in a contract of employment. The reader recognises a type of agent-event where the laws of society are such that when a pay-event becomes a potential event, the controlling agent becomes responsible for bringing about the event. If we assume that the obligation interpretation of *payable* is lexicalised, we can point to the strong assumptions attached to a pay-event as the motivating factor for lexicalisation. However, as I argued above *claimable* also gives rise to very strong assumptions, but is hardly to be considered lexicalised. Both complex forms may be seen as simply results of the same productive system in metacontext and communicative context.

As a final example, we turn to a type of situation which is much less clear in terms of assumptions, but an example which clearly shows that the case for across-the-board lexicalisation of deontic meanings is highly problematic.

(29)   The wall was to be of the height, thickness and construction specified by the plaintiff in the covenant and when erected was to belong to the defendant and to be maintainable by her.

If we take *Y be maintained by X* to be the underlying syntactic frame, both participants are realised in (29), viz. *the wall* and *by her*. The referent of *the wall* will only become the patient of the activity denoted by *maintainable* if a human agent produces a quality-based maintain-activity. The agent in question is of course the referent of *her*. A maintain-activity in itself carries little in the way of desirability, but an interpretation of (29) in terms of simply "the wall is capable of being maintained" is patently informatively vacuous since this is knowledge we already have of normal walls. We also know about normal walls that as a result of the laws of nature, viz. the forces of erosion, they require the odd job of maintenance. Maintaining a wall costs time and money, but the controlling agent is the referent of *her*, so she is to produce the activity.

The example in (29) also makes plain the important difference between the syntagmatic relationship of attribution for the semantic purpose of identification and the syntagmatic relationship of post-copular attributive for the semantic purpose of assignment. The event-frame of *maintainable* in NP [AdjP + N], as in *maintainable wall*, is not directly affected by the illocutionary force and the tense assignment of the utterance as a whole, and as an identifying, atemporal quality the most immediate interpretation would be in terms of, a capable-of-being-maintained-wall,, ie. the somewhat odd interpretation in terms of purely dynamic modality. In contradistinction, the event-frame of *maintainable* which is assigned in the structure CLAUSE [NP + VP [*be* + AdjP]], as in (29), is directly accessible to, and is merged with, the illocutionary force and the tense assignment of the utterance as a whole. The reason for this merger is that the *be* of CLAUSE [NP + VP [*be* + AdjP]] carries the basic illocutionary force and any tense marking, but it is in itself semantically vague and unspecified as to the situation type denoted by the clause. Semantically, the illocutionary force and the tense marking require a situation type to operate on, so they pick the situation type of the verb root of the complex lexeme in the predicate position. So in a very fundamental sense (30) is an utterance about a maintain-activity.

(30)   The wall is maintainable by the defendant.

This semantic trait of assignment, where the higher-level semantic information carried by *be* is transferred to the situation denoted by the following verb root, actually recurs in other constructions. *She was maintaining the wall* and *Was she maintaining the wall?* denote a quality-based maintain-activity, *The wall was maintained* and *Was the wall maintained* denote the final state of a maintain-event.

6. Conclusion

In this investigation I have taken a first step towards formulating a framework that can handle the semantics and pragmatics of the derivational process and product of V_{tr} + *able* → A. However, since this is an underdescribed and overlooked area in the literature on modality in English, much still remains to be done. In particular, more work is required to capture how the agent-event denoting potential of V_{tr} + *able* → A is used for deontic purposes. Part of the explanation may well run parallel with an explanation of the modal auxiliary *can* and be based on the principles of metaphorical extension in metacontext. A much more crucial shortcoming of this investigation is that the focus on reception has left unaddressed the problem of constraints on the morpho-syntactic derivation process, cf. ? *givable*, and constraints on the availability of deontic interpretation. But then of course we must appreciate the limitations of the state of the descriptive art.

References

Bauer, L. (1983). *English word formation*. Cambridge: Cambridge University Press.

Bolinger, D.L. (1989). Extrinsic possibility and intrinsic potentiality: 7 on MAY and CAN+1. *Journal of Pragmatics* 13, 1-23.

Coates, J. (1983). *The semantics of the modal auxiliaries*. London and Canberra: Croom Helm.

Davidsen-Nielsen, N. (1990). *Tense and Mood in English: a comparison with Danish*. Berlin & New York: Mouton de Gruyter.

Durst-Andersen, P. (1992). *Mental grammar: Russian aspect and related issues*. Columbus Ohio: Slavica Publishers.

Ferris, C. (1993). *The meaning of syntax: a study in the adjectives of English*. London & New York: Longman.

Groefsema, M. (1995). *Can, may, must* and *should:* a relevance theoretic account. *Journal of Linguistics* 31, 53-79.

Klinge, A. (1993). The English modal auxiliaries: from lexical semantics to utterance interpretation. *Journal of Linguistics* 29, 315-357.

Klinge, A. (1995). On the linguistic interpretation of contractual modalities. *Journal of Pragmatics* 23, 649-675.

Klinge, A. (1996). The impact of context on modal meaning in English and Danish. *Nordic Journal of Linguistics* 19, 35-54.

Kurzon, D. (1989). *It is hereby performed: explorations in legal speech acts*. Amsterdam & Philadelphia: Benjamins.

Lyons, J. (1977). *Semantics*. Vol. 2. Cambridge: Cambridge University Press.

Palmer, F. R. (1990). *Modality and the English modals*. 2nd ed. London & New York: Longman.

Perkins, M. R. (1983). *Modal expressions in English*. London: Frances Pinter.

Sweetser, E. E. (1990). *From etymology to pragmatics: metaphorical and cultural aspects of semantic structure*. Cambridge: Cambridge University Press.

Tanaka, T. (1990). Semantic changes of CAN and MAY: differentiation and implication. *Linguistics* 28, 89-123.

Urdang, L., A. Humez & H. G. Zettler (1982). *Suffixes and other word-final elements of English*. Detroit: Gale Research Company.

The Danish and English Sound Systems: Complications of a Contrastive Analysis

Fritz Larsen

In 1970 Niels Davidsen-Nielsen published a phonetics textbook for Danish students of English, *Engelsk fonetik*. In various guises it has been the faithful companion of students of English in this country (and Norway) ever since. A revised version, in which I was involved, appeared in English in 1994 under the title *An Outline of English Pronunciation*.

The revision was far from radical. Any description of contemporary pronunciation will inevitably be in need of intermittent updating, but we did not want to change fundamentally a description that had proved pedagogically useful over a quarter of a century. The strength of the book lies in its systematic comparison of Danish and English. The remarks that follow will be concerned with some difficulties inherent in a contrastive analysis; they will not question the value of the undertaking as such.

1. Differences and difficulties

The basis of contrastive analysis is the observation that differences between two languages give rise to difficulties in going from one to the other. A comparison of the two systems will have pedagogical implications in that it points to those problems that a native speaker of a particular L1 will encounter when attempting to learn a particular L2. The observation seems innocent enough; in a less systematic form, a comparison of the target language with the mother tongue of the pupils has been the stock-in-trade of all language teachers. There has, nevertheless, been a long and occasionally acrimonious debate about the merits of contrastive analysis. As the discipline was developed in the 1950s and 1960s, it laid itself open to attack by an unfortunate association with the dominant behaviouristic learning theory of the day.[1] The debate need not concern us here. There are certainly difficulties of learning that a contrastive analysis will not predict, and that which is most different between two languages is not necessarily most difficult. The criticism of the excessive claims made by some proponents of contrastive analysis has not, however, shaken the basic

---

[1] After writing this I was reminded of the long shadows cast by this battle of extremes when I read an article (Sheen 1996) which reveals how even today, in North America at least, advocates of contrastive analysis feel that they are up against a hostile establishment.

assumptions: properly applied, a contrastive analysis of L1 and L2 is a powerful pedagogical tool, not least in phonology.

But it is not a straightforward undertaking. One problem immediately presents itself. A contrastive analysis assumes that there exist two sound systems that we can proceed to compare. But what is the sound system of Danish or of English? A language is a collection of varieties. It varies geographically and socially, and even if we can agree on the choice of one sociolinguistic variety as a standard, that variety will not be stable over time.

These two aspects, synchronic and diachronic variation, are well-known problems for any contrastive analysis, and I will comment on them only briefly below. The main purpose of the article is to introduce yet another complicating aspect.

Not only does a contrastive analysis assume the existence of two fairly well-defined and stable systems for comparison, it also implicitly assumes that these two systems are independent of each other and are two equal 'opponents' that come up against each other, as if under laboratory conditions. In the real world, of course, the relationship between two languages such as Danish and English is very different. A speaker of Danish about to learn English is not in the same situation as a speaker of English about to learn Danish. The target language is not an unknown system to be approached armed only with the L1 system. What is more, Danish is under influence from English. Some of the variation in the L1 is due to the dominance of the very language that is our L2.

In this complex situation, some difficulties that a contrastive analysis predicts turn out not to be real difficulties. That has to be taken into account if a contrastive analysis is to be turned into pedagogical advice. The teacher will obviously need to focus on the real problems, not the problems that might have been if the two languages had existed in a vacuum.

I will come back to the influence of English on Danish and the status of English as a dominant language. First a few remarks about the two traditionally recognized problems for a contrastive analysis.

2. The choice of a standard

The choice of target accent can be debated and has been debated. For British English there is in reality not much of a choice. It may seem odd to set up RP, with its upper-class connotations, as the accent to be emulated by every lowly Dane. But it is no viable alternative to substitute a regional accent, however comparable sociolinguistically to the L1 of the learners. Try to imagine a situation where people from, say, Aalborg in Northern Jutland, were to be taught a Manchester or Aberdeen accent, sociolinguistically graded to accord with the status of their L1 variety.

In any case, the problem is more theoretical than real. Very few Danes acquire an accent that identifies them with the upper classes of Britain. What they develop is an accent that is clearly foreign, hence outside the British social hierarchy altogether. The danger that they may be mistaken for members of the Royal Family is pretty slight.

It is the choice of standard for the L1 that is the real problem. For a contrastive analysis to make sense, the L1 that is described must be the learner's mother tongue. Only with that as the starting-point can the analysis make valid predictions about the learner's difficulties in the acquisition of the L2. But learners do not of course share one accent.

For a textbook that aims widely at students from all backgrounds, there is no perfect solution. Not surprisingly, Davidsen-Nielsen has chosen the Copenhagen standard of Danish. In the chapter on intonation, it is said explicitly (1983: 125, 1994: 127) that the description is of 'East Danish'. Again there is no obvious alternative, but it is important to point out that half the population is not East Danish, and even among those who are East Danes there is not one standard.

Unlike the debate about the L2 norm, this turns up a genuine pedagogical problem: for many groups of learners our predictions will simply be wrong. The results of a contrastive analysis must be handled with care. The practical application needs to be undertaken by teachers who are able to modify the description so that the point of departure becomes the actual L1 of the learners.

3. The variability of variation over time

Contrastive analysis ultimately exists for the benefit of learners, and they are typically young. Among the age-related varieties we would thus be best advised to select for our standard a younger variety of the L1, younger than our own. This would seem indisputable, but I am afraid I have to enter yet another caveat here. We may well run into a conflict between this consideration and the wish for geographical coverage. Pronunciation changes emanate from the capital and spread, rapidly or slowly, westwards. Choosing the most recent type of Copenhagen speech for our description may make it less useful in the rest of the country, at least until the pronunciation there catches up.

I can illustrate this trade-off situation with the changing relationship of the vowels of English *hat* /hæt/ and Danish *hat* /had/.[2] In Davidsen-Nielsen's original 1970 edition, English /æ/ was described as lying between Cardinal Vowels 3 and 4, coinciding with Danish long /a:/ as in *bade*, whereas the short Danish /a/ was described as more open and retracted. That description and the consequent advice to learners is now outdated, as Livbjerg & Mees rightly point out (1995: 437).

The standard pronunciation has changed in both languages. As for English, no one can help noticing the opening of the /æ/ that has taken place even in the most

---

[2]Unless otherwise noted, I transcribe Danish with the IPA-based symbols used by Davidsen-Nielsen. There is no generally accepted system of transcription for Danish.

conservative type of RP since Prime Minister Chamberlain declared war in 1939 from what he called the *Kebinet* Office (example from Honey 1989). An investigation by Laurie Bauer (1985, also summarized in 1994: 115ff) of recordings of RP speakers over a long time-span showed some marked vowel developments that had been slow to find their way into textbook descriptions. One such development was a retraction of /æ/. The standard pronunciation today is far from the Cardinal 3 value that you may hear in old recordings, and the opening and retraction of /æ/ is progressing further among young speakers of RP.

In Danish the development has been in the opposite direction. In their description of the (then) youngest Copenhagen vowel system, Brink & Lund (1975: 701) have long /a:/ at C3, whereas short /a/ occupies a half-open to open somewhat retracted position, i.e. overlapping with the short vowel in RP. We have thus reached the fortunate situation where the Danish *hat* and the English *hat* have identical vowels.

Or do they? Some Danish accents have a closer short vowel; according to Brink & Lund the 'Low Copenhagen' short /a/ is as close as the long /a:/. We could well be heading for a situation where the short English /æ/ becomes problematic for Danes again, but now because the corresponding short vowel in Danish is not open enough.

The question is what our pedagogical advice should be in the present situation. Livbjerg & Mees conclude that Danish learners should aim at a more open quality. That is certainly good advice if the learners in question actually have a pronunciation that is markedly different from modern RP. But many learners do not. One needs to take account of the variation that exists in both languages, and for many young Danes there is still a fair degree of overlap between the two short vowels in Danish and English. For the moment at least, a conservative statement along these lines seems to strike a reasonable balance. The 1994 edition of Davidsen-Nielsen was revised accordingly.

4. Substitution in loanwords: how to say oh

The influence of English on Danish has come under close scrutiny in recent years, as a linguistic and more widely as a cultural phenomenon (see e.g. Hansen & Lund 1994, Jarvad 1995, Sørensen 1995, Larsen 1994, 1995, 1997). The focus is on vocabulary, the importation of several thousand loanwords and the indirect borrowing that comes out in translated compounds and collocations as well as semantic extensions copied from English. This is as it should be: it is primarily in vocabulary change that the dominant cultural and linguistic status of English reveals itself.

Pronunciation has received much less attention, and when it is treated (the only treatment of any length is in Sørensen 1973, but see also Hansen & Lund 1994: 95ff), the question that is posed is not whether the pronunciation of Danish changes under English influence but how and to what extent loanwords are adapted to fit the existing phonology of Danish. This is also where I will begin.

For most English sounds there is a similar Danish sound that acts as an automatic substitute: the second /l/ of *volleyball* becomes 'clear' like the first, the /dʒ/ of *badge* becomes voiceless as in *batch*, and so on. In other cases the adaptation is less straightforward. Perceptions of what is a suitable corresponding sound may change, due to changes in Danish itself or to increasing familiarity with English pronunciation. In a situation where everybody learns English and hears English practically every day, the latter aspect becomes important.

I will take as my first example loanwords with /əʊ/ in English. I have classified about 85 of this type. (Needless to say, nobody can determine how many loanwords there are; my figures represent a minimum count.) As with all the other examples that follow, I have checked the two Danish dictionaries of pronunciation (Hansen 1990, Brink et al. 1991) but have had to rely heavily on my own impressions, not only when it comes to words that are not listed but also because the two dictionaries often disagree. The procedure will not meet ordinary reliability criteria, but it will suffice for the purposes of this article where I am aiming only at establishing some general trends.

The standard substitution for /əʊ/ is the diphthong found in *sproglig* (the dictionaries transcribe /åw/ and /ɑ̊w/ respectively) or /œʊ/ as in *støvle* (in the dictionaries /öw/). The majority, about 50 words, follow this pattern, e.g. *slow-motion*. A group of about 20 have exclusively, or almost exclusively, some further adaptation, typically a spelling pronunciation with the long monophthong /o:/ (*totem*) or the short /ɔ/ (*pony*). Most of these are old loans, but not all, cf. *coca-cola* with /o-o:/ – though *coke* has a diphthong.

The remaining 15 are highly variable; older more adapted pronunciations compete with the modern standard substitution. Examples are *bulldoze(r)* (earlier only /o:/), *poker* (earlier only /o'/). Older pronunciations with /o'/ or /ɔ/ are still found in *joker* – though not in *joke*. Some fully integrated loans may be taking the first steps back in the direction of English: *folklore*, *globetrotter*, *smoking* ('dinner-jacket'). The pattern here is what we can observe with several other sounds, too: with improving knowledge of English, the modern standard substitution spreads to older more adapted loans.

Although it is easy to understand what is going on here, there is an important point to be made. Some of the literature has a simplistic conception of what happens when a language borrows words from another. A loanword is assumed to become formally adapted to fit the structure of the recipient language, and the older the loan the more assimilated it will become. If a word from another language appears in an unadapted form, it is not a loanword but a case of code-switching.

There are several reasons why this description will not hold water. For one thing, there is always some degree of adaptation even if the foreign word is clearly making a nonce appearance. Most people are simply not capable of more than an approximation to the original pronunciation, and even perfect bilinguals tend to avoid a pronunciation that makes the word sound like a demonstration piece in a language class.

Secondly, although it is a good working assumption that assimilation occurs over time, the process need not in fact take time. Many loanwords happen to be of such a form type that they immediately become as assimilated as they will ever be. The verb *linke* in Danish may serve as a recent example: I have registered a couple of occurrences, but it cannot be said to be an established loanword, yet formally there is nothing foreign about it, and I wonder if people who hear or read it for the first time will even notice that it is new. There simply is no reliable formal distinction between code-switching and borrowing, only a vague frequency criterion: a loanword is an instance of code-switching that has caught on.[3]

Thirdly, *must* total assimilation occur? Certainly thousands of old loans have been adapted to the point where nobody recognizes their foreign provenance. But is there necessarily such a development? This is where our /əʊ/ example comes in. The status of English in Denmark (or in the heads of the Danes, if you like) hampers what in other circumstances would be a natural assimilation process. As we saw, the process may even be reversed: younger pronunciations being closer to English. We will see that again with some other examples where it becomes clearer that this faithfulness to the donor language may be doing something to the sound system of Danish.

First the /əʊ/ example must be rounded off. As we heard, there are two standard substitutions in this case. Brink & Lund (1975: 221ff, 587) state that the diphthong with a rounded back first element (/åw/ in their transcription) has been partly supplanted, especially among young people, by a diphthong whose first element is rounded front (/öw/ in their transcription). The entries in their pronouncing dictionary reflect this. Now, I am not sure that /öw/ is in fact as widespread as this, but the interesting thing is the assumption behind the statement, and behind the development that may or may not be under way: that /öw/ is more English than /åw/. This also comes out explicitly in Molbæk Hansen's introduction to his dictionary (1990: 20) where he explains that the transcription /åw/ has been left out in loanword entries because /öw/ is closer to British English pronunciation. (Not, incidentally, a relevant argument in a dictionary of *Danish* pronunciation.)

But the Danish diphthong in *sproglig* is in fact quite close to well-known English variants with a rounded back first element, old-fashioned in RP but certainly English. That is not true of /öw/ (=/œʊ/) whose rounded front vowel is clearly un-English. If young Danes insist on saying /öw/ (=/œʊ/) in loanwords like *go* or *show*, so be it, but one cannot argue for it on the grounds that it is especially English.

---

[3] The same point is made by, among others, Penelope Gardner-Chloros (1995: 73f). Discussions of borrowing, code-switching and code-mixing tend to become bogged down in terminological confusion. It is characteristic of code-switching research that the editors of the volume in which her article appeared had to give up an attempt to standardize the terminology across contributions (Milroy & Muysken 1995: 12).

There is a general remark to be made in this connection. Standard substitutions are practical means to adapt loanwords. What is the best substitution in Danish is the privileged decision of the Danes. If their preferred solution diverges markedly from English, it is not for others to tell them that their Danish is wrong.[4] But they would be wrong to think that the same pronunciation is wonderful when speaking English. It is a consequence of loanword adaptation that Danes may have to master two pronunciations of the same word, one for the loanword in Danish, another when speaking English.

What this example has shown is the vacillation that may arise in the adaptation of loanwords. But it still shows adaptation to the existing system, not Danish changing under the impact of English.

5. Reversing the process of adaptation: the status of /w/

The accepted wisdom is that there is no /w/ in standard Danish. Or rather: there is no initial /w/. The sound is found medially and finally, although the phonemic status is not absolutely clear. One should not be too impressed by the appearance of /-w/ in transcriptions of Danish diphthongs. That simply reflects a particular branch of phonological analysis, a tradition that happens to be also common among American linguists.

But is it still true to say that there is no (initial) /w/ in Danish? I have looked at 60 loanwords with /w/ in English. (Some of the items are from Jacobsen 1994: 6 and Jarvad 1995: 68). It is only true of about 10 of them that the standard substitution /v/ is mandatory. Not surprisingly, the list comprises old loans like *watt* and *quilt* (also with the assimilated spelling *kvilt*), but there are a few newer ones like *quiz(ze)* – as well as the oddity *wrangler* with a spelling pronunciation. On the other hand, about 20 nearly always have /w/; (it would be too categorical to say 'only'.) These are mostly recent loans, e.g. *hardware, wok, workout*.

This leaves about half the items in an unstable middle group. They are not equally unstable, though: in a handful /v/ predominates (*whist, wing*), in more of them /w/ is typical (*goodwill, speedway*). When there is vacillation, the characteristic situation is that younger people have /w/. Once again, the development is clearly *back* in the direction of the donor language. Of the 60 items under consideration, an estimated 45 either already have, or will have among the next generation, /w/ as the standard pronunciation. That would seem to justify an analysis of /w/ as an established phoneme of Danish.

There is an alternative analysis which has been applied to Dutch by J. Posthumus

---

[4] It follows that I will have to distance myself from Brink & Lund who (1975: 590) call the use of /w/ and front /r/ in English loanwords an improvement. Adaptation to the existing Danish system is a perfectly respectable process.

(1986: 35ff, 1995). In addition to the old-established set of 'primary' phonemes, a language may have a number of 'secondary' phonemes that are used in the integration of loanwords. One of his examples is /g/ which does not appear in indigenous Dutch words. Despite their limited function, the secondary phonemes are readily available to all native speakers.

This analysis is psychologically appealing. All phonemes need not have the same status for the speaker. Instead of debating whether a phoneme /w/ exists in Danish, we could say that /w/ is at present well on its way to becoming a secondary phoneme, i.e. employed by all but for restricted purposes. Such a special status, it seems, may persist for a long time. According to David Crystal (1995: 69), /ʒ/ in English, after more than 300 years, may still be felt to have 'French overtones'.

Whichever description we prefer, a contrastive analysis that predicts problems for Danish learners in the acquisition of /w/ will be wide of the mark. That is not to say that all problems have disappeared, alas. There are enough to keep English teachers busy (and employed). First, /w/ words have to be kept separate from /v/ words. Confusion is very common; the form *wolleyball* has even found its way into the Brink et al. dictionary.[5] Secondly, final /v/ as in English *have* no longer exists in the Danish of young speakers, and medial /v/ as in English *over* rarely appears. What a contrastive analysis must focus on is the distribution of /v/ not a putatively missing /w/.

6. /eɪ/: as Danish as bacon

A similar story can be told, only more convincingly, about the new diphthong /eɪ/, or /ɛj/ in Danish transcription.[6]

Of the 120 items I have tried to classify, about half are found with a monophthong in at least one of the dictionaries. But only in a small minority is the monophthong mandatory or dominates over a preserved diphthong, in fact only in 14 or 15 items. These are old loans like *es* (<- *ace*) and *kvæker* (<- *quaker*), with assimilated spellings, or spelling pronunciations like *radar* /ɑ:/ and *steak* if pronounced with a pseudo-English /i:/.

In about 40 items the monophthong /ɛ:/ is characteristic of older people while young people have a diphthong (*baby, bacon*, etc.). I have included many examples

---

[5]*wolfram* with /w/ in Molbæk Hansen's dictionary must be a slip!
[6]Strictly speaking, it may not be correct to say that there was no /ɛj/ in Danish until the influx of loanwords from English. In a handful of words of the type *lægen* ('the doctor'), the development of a former velar fricative into /j/ does produce a sequence of /ɛ(:)j/. It is hard to tell what status this combination has in the minds of speakers. Or had, because among young speakers of standard Copenhagen the /j/ has gone too, leaving /lɛ:n/ (Brink & Lund 1975: 298f). Still, they do not monophthongize English loanwords.

in this category in accordance with the Brink et al. dictionary although I find it difficult myself to imagine monophthongs in them, e.g. *cocktailshaker, crazy, spray*. It is not so important what exact share is allocated to the vacillating middle group at this particular point in time; what is clear is, once again, that the development is contrary to the expected process of adaptation.

The remaining 65 items I think can only have a diphthong, e.g. *aids, case, layout*. When Davidsen-Nielsen, in his advice to Danish leaners of English (1982: 14), says that /eɪ/ is among the four vowels most unfamiliar to Danes, I humbly beg to differ. It is certainly not the case now.

7. Splitting the /a/

I now turn to a slightly more complex case. We looked at the opposite developments of English /æ/ and Danish /a/, resulting in a (temporary?) overlap of English *hat* and Danish *hat*, a straightforward case of change within each of the two languages. When it comes to the integration of English loanwords in Danish, we need to pay attention to a couple of complicating differences between the two languages.

First there is the existence of length allophones in English. The vowel of *cat* is drastically shortened by the following fortis consonant as compared with *cad*; where there is no fortis/lenis opposition, as in *can*, the length is intermediate (see Davidsen-Nielsen 1994, Ch. 6.5). This distinction cannot immediately be imitated by Danes as Danish has no fortis/lenis opposition, so the /æ/ in the loanword *badge* may be no longer than that of *batch* – in fact the two loanwords will mostly be indistinguishable. Before nasals, however, a lengthened vowel predominates, as in *band, handle* (verb), *hamburger, spanking*.

Secondly, and of more interest for the purposes of this article, there is the different status of front versus back vowel in the two languages; the integration process is different for words like *cat* and *band* on the one hand and *hamburger* and *spanking* on the other. Put in the simplest terms, front /æ/ and back /ɑː/ are contrasting phonemes in English, whereas front versus back in Danish is allophonic variation, a function of the environment. The short front [a] in Danish, whose happy coincidence with English /æ/ we have noted, is only found before alveolar consonants; followed by labial and velar consonants, and also in combination with r, the allophone is a central to back [ɑ].[7] The result is that whereas the *cat* type is easily integrated, problems arise with the types *kidnap(pe), camp(ing)* (+labial), *back, tank* (+velar) and *rap, brandy* (/r/+).

---

[7]The divide actually steers an uncertain course right through combinations with /n/ and /l/, *Anders* (name) having a back [ɑ] but *and* ('duck') a front [a], *aldrig* ('never') having a back [ɑ] but *alder* ('age') predominantly a front [a].

There are many of these. I have tabulated no less than 160 loanwords with /æ/ in English, and that is after leaving out of consideration a further 25 or so which have a front vowel in American English (and several other accents) but an /ɑ:/ in RP. It is a striking demonstration of the strength of the traditional British orientation of English teaching in Denmark that even items with an American association such as *basketball, breakdance, fastfood* and *ghettoblaster* are normally integrated as loanwords with an RP /ɑ:/.

Of the 160 items only 65 fall in the +alveolar category, and half of those are of the *band* type where the lengthening is a complication even though the front vowel as such is not, compare a loanword like *handling* ('managing') with the short vowel of the existing Danish noun *handling* ('action').

In close to 100 words the English front vowel is foreign to the Danish system. As with my earlier examples, we find various degrees of adaptation. A handful of old loans like *sjækkel* (<- *shackle*) are completely detached from modern loans and can be disregarded here. What we are concerned with is the difference between *back* with [ɑ], *comeback* with [a], and *backgammon* with either. The recent loan *fax* has an adapted pronunciation with [ɑ], but that is an exceptional type. By far the majority keep the English front vowel, with the result that new minimal pairs have come into existence: *hacke* with a front vowel (only about computers) / *hakke* with a back vowel ('hack' in general), *slacks / slags* ('sort'), *snack / snak* ('chat'), as well as near-minimal pairs like *gang /gang* ('walk', 'corridor'), *tank* (armoured vehicle) / *tank* (general word, itself from English originally), *rap* (music) / *rap* ('smack' or 'quack'), *crack* (drug) / *krak* ('crash').

The development of an allophonic distinction into a phonemic contrast is not a rare occurrence in language history. How common it has been for such a split to be brought about by contact with another language is hard to know, but cases can be found. Old English had no phonemic contrast between voiced and voiceless fricatives, although both series existed as conditioned allophones. A word like *heofon* had the same medial [-v-] as in modern *heaven*, but in initial and final position the written *f* was indeed pronounced [f]. It is generally assumed (see e.g. Gimson 1994: 166, McMahon 1994: 210, Nielsen 1994) that it was the influx of Norman French loans, in this case words like *virtue, visit* and *very* with initial /v-/, that led to the split into contrasting phonemes. We may be witnessing a similar process at work in modern Danish, the establishment of an extra phoneme, at least a 'secondary' one.[8]

---

[8]In my simplified presentation, I have assumed that there has hitherto been only one /a/ phoneme in Danish. But as Davidsen-Nielsen points out (D-N et al. 1982: 13), you do in fact have a minimal pair *ka'* /a/ versus *kar* /ɑ/, and similarly for the long vowel *Ane* /a:/ versus *Arne* /ɑ:/. Consequently, it may not be strictly correct to say that the English loanwords are establishing a phoneme contrast out of something that has only been an allophonic difference, rather what is happening is that an existing contrast with a limited distribution is being extended to all environments.

8. Is one /r/ enough?

With items like *rap* and *crack* we have already approached what will be my last example of the possible influence of English on the Danish sound system, and left till last because I am uncertain about what is happening.

Both languages have an /r/ phoneme, but the difference in articulation is of course manifest, English having an alveolar liquid and Danish a uvular-pharyngeal fricative – let us call them 'front' and 'back' for short. In the integration of loanwords, Danish can either substitute a back /r/ or keep the English sound. If unadapted takeover is common, we may see the acquisition of an additional (secondary) phoneme. Is this happening? Let us first survey the evidence.

Out of 180 (!) items, 60 (or one third) have a Danish /r/, and another 25 typically have it, although an English pronunciation may be heard among young people, e.g. in *crawl(e), rally, trust*.[9] Another 40 also vacillate, but with a front /r/ dominating, e.g. *all right, dry, roastbeef, spray*. In the remaining 55 or so, e.g. *break, ranking, strike* (as opposed to *strejke*), a front /r/ is standard – which does not mean that it is universal, though.

The items are distributed fairly evenly across a continuum. Moreover, cases where an earlier fully integrated loan appears to be reacquiring an English pronunciation are comparatively rare (although instances do exist, e.g. *brandy, evergreen*). For once, the traditional hypothesis of a gradual formal integration of loanwords might seem a tempting explanation. But it does not fit the data in one important respect. The words that have a Danish /r/ are not exclusively old loans like *crosse(d), drible, revolver, rollmops, rommy, sherif*; many are quite new and yet are instantly assimilated by old and young alike: *printe(r), producer*. (Further items may be found in Jarvad 1995: 69f). The process seems almost haphazard: in the pronunciation of young people, *rock and roll* has front /r/ (twice), but *rock* and *rocker* do not.

There seems to be something special about the status of English front /r/ in Danish. Although it can be acquired by Danes and is used in many loanwords, it seems to retain its foreign stamp. Although we do find some age-grading, it is far from clear that the drift is back in the direction of English.

The best analysis may still be in terms of a 'secondary phoneme' for this sound too, but the front /r/ appears to be meeting with more resistance than, for instance, /eɪ/. Note how in cases like *grapefrugt, behaviorisme, interrail*, the substitution of a Danish back /r/ may go together with retention of the diphthong, but not the other way round. The /eɪ/ is obviously felt to be less foreign. Apparently the use of an English /r/ is such a strong signal of unintegrated status that it blocks a number of

---

[9]In some cases I have had to disregard Molbæk Hansen's dictionary which tends to give an English pronunciation first where a Danish back /r/, to my ear, is clearly more common, e.g. in *jury, kricket, rockwool, trawler*.

standard substitutions. Thus the recent loan *rap* with a front /r/ will also retain a front /a/ before the labial, whereas the older *scrapbog* with a back /r/ has also changed the vowel to a Danish back /ɑ/; a word like *rally* has two pronunciations, the vowel depending on the choice of an English or Danish /r/. Similarly, you may find adaptation in the form of loss of /d/ and addition of glottal stop in *trend* but not unless the ordinary Danish /r/ has also been substituted.

Is the English /r/ too peculiar for export? Is there a natural resistance to having more than one /r/ phoneme? Whatever the motivation, the outcome looks uncertain.

9. More hutducks than ogly docklings

After these demonstrations of English influence on Danish, the reader may well have drawn the conclusion that there is precious little left to worry about for Danish learners of English and for their teachers. Not only are Danish learners exposed to English from an early age, their Danish L1 has incorporated a large number of English loanwords, and in so doing appears to be establishing a helpful set of extra phonemes. Psychologically, these units may only have secondary status, but if they are available for the integration of loanwords, they are also available for the acquisition of English as an L2.

Certainly much has become easier, but the conclusion would still be wrong. My examples have been selected to highlight points where the status relation between donor and recipient languages is promoting new developments. There are more areas where nothing has happened, where the structure of Danish remains an almost insurmountable barrier to the acquisition of a near-native pronunciation of English. Or, to put it in a different perspective: there are a number of points of contrast that together account for a characteristic Danish accent of English. These characteristics can be expected to persist even if it comes to a situation where a large part of the Danish population has become bilingual with English as their second language.[10]

A prominent characteristic of that type of English is (along with intonation) the lack of distinction between fortis and lenis consonants outside initial position and between the vowels /ʌ/ and /ɒ/. As a result, *duck, dock, dug, dog* are typically pronounced the same.[11] I will now look briefly at the vexed /ʌ/ versus /ɒ/ contrast. I apologize for the compressed treatment of a topic that really deserves an article of its own.

First on the integration of loanwords. My list runs to no less than 240 items with one of these two vowels in English. The vast majority have the common standard

---

[10]It is legitimate to ask the question "What is wrong with an accent? Aren't there enough native speakers of English already?" But a consideration of the possible inclusion of non-native varieties of English under the umbrella of 'World Englishes' lies outside the confines of this article.

[11]During the preparation of this article, a mock-up was constructed of a proposed extension of the Royal Theatre in Copenhagen. Yes, it did appear in print as a *muck-up*.

substitution that will be our concern here. The exceptions are mostly spelling pronunciations of words with *u*, mandatory in about 15 items, possible in another 15. The vowel may be an /u/, as in *klub*, or, more commonly, the mid vowel that Brink et al. transcribe /ǻ/, as in *jungle*. Although most of these exceptional items are old, spelling pronunciations are also possible in a few later loans, e.g. *puck* with /u/ and *tumbler* with /ǻ/. Among the words with /ɒ/ in English there are fewer special cases. I have noted 24, but almost half of these are due to the possibility of long vowels in *off* and *soft* and compounds with these, probably in imitation of the competing English pronunciation with /ɔː/.

In approximately 200 items, then, we have the standard substitution which gives English *cup* the same vowel as Danish *kop* and collapses the two loanwords *pop* and *pub*. What exactly is this vowel? And why do Danes find it almost impossible to acquire the English contrast? A tour of the literature leaves one confused. It is not without reason that Davidsen-Nielsen sounds almost despondent:

> There is no simple answer to the question of why the English opposition /ʌ/ ≠ /ɒ/ should be so difficult for Danes, and this problem certainly cannot be read off from a contrastive analysis of English and Danish. (D-N et al. 1982: 17)

I agree that the answer is not simple, but I think that a contrastive analysis does help if we take a second look at the structure of the two systems we want to compare. The main thing to keep in mind is that vowel qualities are not dots on a diagram but more vaguely delimited combinations of features. It is practical to indicate focal points of articulation in a vowel diagram, but the range of variation between speakers and between different articulations by the same speaker is striking. The variation is such that many tabulations of the formant frequencies of vowels have had to be based on averages of a number of measurements. Some vowels vary more than others, because of sociolinguistic and age-related differences but maybe also because certain types of vowel are inherently unstable – there may, for example, be a reason why unrounded back vowels are so rare among the world's languages.

The place of articulation of the English /ɒ/ of *cop* is fairly stable at an open and back position. The /ʌ/ of *cup*, however, varies within RP between centralized back and centralized front with a height quality between half-open and open.

In their description of the youngest Copenhagen system, Brink & Lund (1975: 701) plot the vowel of *kop*, commonly transcribed /ɔ/, as open central. As their /ɑ/ is also defined as central, it looks as if all that keeps the two vowels apart is lip-rounding. It is clear from their description elsewhere, though, as well as from descriptions by other phoneticians (see e.g. Basbøll & Wagner 1985: 35), that /ɔ/ varies widely between open central and half-open back, i.e. over an area that is very different from that of /ɑ/.

The similarity as to range of place of articulation between Danish /ɔ/ and English /ʌ/ is noticeable, and it is surprising that /ʌ/ has so consistently been proclaimed a problem for Danes. A contributing reason is probably that the classification of

Danish /ɔ/ as rounded leads easily to an identification with English /ɒ/ which is similarly classified (and was earlier often transcribed with /ɔ/ too, as it happens). But for the sounds under consideration here, rounding is not much of a distinctive feature in either language. It is primarily place of articulation that keeps /ʌ/ and /ɒ/ apart in English; lip-rounding for /ɒ/ is slight (Ladefoged 1993: 82, 219).[12] The impression of roundedness is probably due more to the strong retraction; note that the quality can be achieved without the help of lip-rounding.

In Danish the /ɔ/ may be more or less rounded, the main thing is that even among people who have a rounded back variety (primarily but not exclusively speakers of 'Low Copenhagen') it is rarely the case that the articulation is open enough to allow identification with /ɒ/. Anything that is not both retracted and open enough will be heard as /ʌ/. I agree with Livbjerg & Mees whose practical experience with Danish students of English leads them to conclude (1995: 442) that the problem for most Danes is not the /ʌ/ but the retraction of /ɒ/. Hence my subheading.

As I said, traditions of transcription, although they cannot bear responsibility for the complex nature of the problem, have no doubt contributed to the confusion in the analysis. For Danish learners of English, Molbæk Hansen's transcription of *kop* as /kʌb/ may be more instructive; it is not the /ʌ/ of *cup* but the /ɒ/ of *cop* that is the big stumbling-block for Danes.

10. Concluding remarks

Davidsen-Nielsen's phonetics books have had a long life, but they may not after all last another 25 years. The textbooks that take their place, however, will have to build on similar principles of contrastive analysis. It goes without saying that the description will have to be updated as the two standard languages change, but I hope to have shown that there is more involved.

What is at play in the mental process of acquiring another language is not of course a description of language structures but what people have in their heads. The learners we are concerned with here, young Danes at the beginning of the 21st century, do not have one sound system pure and simple. The second language they are acquiring is a language they are exposed to before teaching starts and the language that currently influences their first language most, with the result that they possess mechanisms for the integration of loans from English, including a set of secondary phonemes.

They do not, however, have two native sound systems in their heads, and very few Danes will ever achieve that. Teaching may help the learner to go some of the way, especially if the pedagogical advice is based on a description that takes a fair

---

[12]Note that in General American pronunciation, where *cop* is /kɑp/, the distinction is solely one of place of articulation – and works all the same.

number of the complicating factors into account. An important complication is the variation that is found in the L1 of learners. No textbook, however, can predict everything; successful exploitation of contrastive analysis depends on teachers who do not go uncritically by the book.

References

Basbøll, H. & J. Wagner (1985). *Kontrastive Phonologie des Deutschen und Dänischen. Segmentale Wortphonologie und -phonetik*. Tübingen: Niemeyer.

Bauer, L. (1985). Tracing phonetic change in the received pronunciation of British English. *Journal of Phonetics* 13, 61-81.

Bauer, L. (1994). *Watching English Change*. London: Longman.

Brink, L. & J. Lund (1975). *Dansk rigsmål. Lydudviklingen siden 1840 med særligt henblik på sociolekterne i København*. 2 vols. Copenhagen: Gyldendal.

Brink, L., J. Lund, S. Heger & J. N. Jørgensen (1991). *Den Store Danske Udtaleordbog*. Copenhagen: Munksgaard.

Crystal, D. (1995). *The Cambridge Encyclopedia of the English Language*. Cambridge: Cambridge University Press.

Davidsen-Nielsen, N. (1970). *Engelsk fonetik*. Copenhagen: Gyldendal.

Davidsen-Nielsen, N. (1977). *English Phonetics*. Translated and adapted for use in Norway by B. Bird and P. Moen. Oslo: Gyldendal Norsk Forlag.

Davidsen-Nielsen, N. (1983). *Engelsk udtale i hovedtræk,* 2nd edition. Copenhagen: Gyldendal. Reprinted 1991 by Odense Universitetsforlag.

Davidsen-Nielsen, N. (1994). *An Outline of English Pronunciation*. Translated and revised by F. Larsen and H. F. Nielsen. Odense: Odense University Press.

Davidsen-Nielsen, N., C. Færch & P. Harder (1982). *The Danish Learner*. Tunbridge Wells: Anthony Taylor.

Gardner-Chloros, P. (1995). Code-switching in community, regional and national repertoires: the myth of the discreteness of linguistic systems. In Milroy & Muysken 1995, 68-89.

Gimson, A. C. (1994). *Gimson's Pronunciation of English,* 5th edition, revised by A. Cruttenden. London: Edward Arnold.

Hansen, E. & J. Lund (1994). *Kulturens gesandter. Fremmedordene i dansk*. Copenhagen: Munksgaard.

Hansen, P. M. (1990). *Dansk udtale*. Copenhagen: Gyldendal.

Honey, J. (1989). *Does Accent Matter: The Pygmalion Factor*. London: Faber & Faber.

Jacobsen, H. G. (1994). Sprogændringer og sprogvurdering. Om nogle aktuelle engelskinspirerede ændringer i dansk og vurderingen af dem. *Danske Studier* 1994, 5-28.

Jarvad, P. (1995). *Nye ord – hvorfor og hvordan?* Copenhagen: Gyldendal.

Ladefoged, P. (1993). *A Course in Phonetics*, 3rd edition. New York: Harcourt Brace.

Larsen, F. (1994). More than loan-words: English influence on Danish. *RASK* 1, 21-46.

Larsen, F. (1995). Review of Jarvad 1995. *RASK* 3, 145-152.

Larsen, F. (1997). Review of Sørensen 1995. *RASK* 5/6, 187-198.

Lewis, J. W. (ed) (1995). *Studies in General and English Phonetics: Essays in honour of Professor J. D. O'Connor*. London: Routledge.

Livbjerg, I. & I. M. Mees (1995). Segmental errors in the pronunciation of Danish speakers of English: some pedagogic strategies. In Lewis 1995, 432-444.

McMahon, A. M. S. (1994). *Understanding Language Change*. Cambridge: Cambridge University Press.

Milroy, L. & P. Muysken (eds) (1995). *One Speaker, Two Languages: Cross-disciplinary perspectives on code-switching*. Cambridge: Cambridge University Press.

Nielsen, H. F. (1994). On the origin and spread of initial voiced fricatives and the phonemic split of fricatives in English and Dutch. In M. Laing & K. Williamson (eds) *Speaking in Our Tongues*. Cambridge: D. S. Brewer, 19-30.

Posthumus, J. (1986). *A Description of a Corpus of Anglicisms*. Groningen: Anglistisch Instituut.

Posthumus, J. (1995). Describing the pronunciation of loanwords from English. In Lewis 1995, 445-453.

Sheen, R. (1996). The advantage of exploiting contrastive analysis in teaching and learning a foreign language. *IRAL* 34/3, 183-197.

Sørensen, K. (1973). *Engelske lån i dansk*. Dansk Sprognævns Skrifter 8. Copenhagen: Gyldendal.

Sørensen, K. (1995). *Engelsk i dansk. Er det et must?* Copenhagen: Munksgaard.

The Appeal of Otto Jespersen's
Growth and Structure of the English Language

Hans F. Nielsen

Among the many books written by Otto Jespersen none became more popular than his *Growth and Structure of the English Language*, which was first published in Germany in 1905, and which by his death in 1943 had appeared in nine editions. In his autobiography from 1938 Jespersen observes that

> 33 years after its first appearance, it is still being used at many universities in several countries, including England and America, as an introduction to the history of the English language. (Juul et al. 1995: 137)

A few months ago, I came across a tenth edition of *Growth and Structure*. In his 'Foreword' to this edition from 1982, Randolph Quirk ponders over the appeal that the book has been able to retain over the years, concluding that it is due neither to Jespersen's constant revision and updating of the book nor to its modern outlook. Instead Quirk offers this explanation:

> Jespersen's continuing appeal lies in the sheer scholarly quality of the man: our awareness in reading him that we are engaged with a supremely learned and cultivated mind. He is indeed the most distinguished scholar of the English language who has ever lived, in my view. ... A further and related reason is this. While being a deeply serious theoretical linguist to whom such daunting labels as phonetician and grammarian pre-eminently apply, Jespersen was above all a *philologist* in the older senses of the word, a lover of language and of the arts that are realised in language. (Quirk 1982)

The second reason given by Quirk comes close to an explanation of the success of the book referred to by Jespersen himself in his autobiography:

> Those who mention it nearly always stress the way in which cultural history and language have been used to shed light on each other. (Juul et al. 1995: 137f)

It would be hard to disagree with these viewpoints, but perhaps there is more to it than what has been advanced here. Could there be other reasons why a book written by a Danish scholar and published in Germany should achieve such popularity in England and America? Let us go through Jespersen's presentation of English language history chapter by chapter with a view to finding clues that might enable us to come up with additional answers.

In his background chapter (II), entitled 'The Beginnings', Jespersen assigns

English to the Germanic branch of Aryan (i.e. Indo-European). Jespersen describes Aryan as a grammatically and lexically extremely complicated language with numerous inflexional endings and full of irregularities (1938: 18).[1] The most important change in setting Germanic off from Aryan was, according to Jespersen, the fixation of the Aryan movable stress on the first syllable, i.e. the root syllable, which had the advantage that the most important syllable had also the strongest stress. Jespersen (1938: 22ff) explains the stress shift in Germanic as the result of a psychological process of value-stressing that was tied up with the national character of the Germanic peoples. Although the French, with their specific system of accentuation, may express themselves more elegantly and artistically, the English, Scandinavians and Germans prefer a system where the most significant element receives the strongest phonetic expression in accordance with their desire to say things bluntly and to emphasize what is essential.

English eventually established itself as a separate language after Germanic tribes had settled in Britain in the fifth century as described in Ch. III, 'Old English'. Prior to this settlement the colonizers must have lived 'as the neighbours and relatives' of the Frisians on the Continent owing to the great similarity between English and Frisian (1938: 32f). Jespersen even operates with the concept of an English-Frisian group of Germanic intermediate between, but separate from both, German and Scandinavian (1938: 18), cf. above. The topic with which Jespersen is most concerned in this chapter, is the linguistic effects of the christianization of England at the beginning of the seventh century (1938: 37ff). A number of the ideas and items associated with Christianity were expressed in Old English by means of Latin and Greek borrowings, but to Jespersen it is significant that most of these loans were short words which were treated grammatically just like native words, cf. OE *ancor* 'hermit', *biscop* 'bishop', *decan* 'dean', *mæsse* 'mass', *preost* 'priest', *scrin* 'shrine' etc. And what to Jespersen is even more significant, is the considerable extent to which Old English used its own native resources to render Christian concepts, e.g. (a) by adding native suffixes to loan-words as in OE *biscopscir* 'diocese', and *preosthad* 'priesthood'; (b) by changing the meaning of native words as in the originally pagan terms OE *eastron* 'Easter' and *god* 'God'; and (c) by forming new Christian words on the basis of native language material as in *heahfæder* 'patriarch' and *þrines* 'trinity', literally 'three-ness'. Jespersen regards the Old English principle 'of adopting only such words as were easily assimilated with the native vocabulary ... and of turning to the greatest possible account native words and roots ... as a symptom of a healthful condition of a language and a nation' (1938: 44f).

The following three chapters (IV-VI) deal with, respectively, the Scandinavian, French and Latin (and Greek) elements in English, foreign influences that between

---

[1] The references to *Growth and Structure* are, with one exception, all to the ninth edition from 1938, reprinted 1962.

them were to alter the Old English system of utilizing native lexical resources for new concepts. The most striking thing about the Scandinavian borrowings was their everyday character, e.g. *gate, husband, root, skill, skin, sky; ill, low, meek, scant, ugly; call, die, drown, scowl, scream*, words that denoted no new ideas, but which represented only fresh labels for semantic ground already covered by the English lexicon. Jespersen can see no other reason for such borrowing than that after the Viking settlement in England in the late ninth century, the Scandinavians and their descendants had a social status comparable to that of the English; this eventually led to 'a more intimate fusion of the two nations than is seen anywhere else'. The following memorable phrase epitomizes the situation, 'They fought like brothers and afterwards settled down peacefully, like brothers, side by side' (1938: 71). Jespersen points out that the Scandinavian borrowings are felt very much like native lexical elements, not just because they were non-specialised but 'because their shortness too agrees with the monosyllabic character of the native stock of words' (1938: 74). As far as grammar is concerned, Jespersen observes that the processes of reduction and levelling of suffixes were accelerated in the areas in which the Vikings had settled (1938: 76).

In comparison with the 'democratic' nature of the Scandinavian element in English the French loan-words are described by Jespersen as 'aristocratic' (1938: 74, 79). French became the language of the ruling classes after the Norman Conquest in 1066, and not surprisingly a number of administrative, feudal, military, legal and religious terms entered English. However, a great many non-technical expressions were borrowed from French as well, and especially the late thirteenth and the fourteenth centuries saw a substantial French lexical influx (1938: 87). Jespersen suggests that it became *fashionable* for the English to imitate their French-speaking betters, but points out that whenever two synonyms have survived, one English and the other French,

> The former is always nearer the nation's heart than the latter, it has the strongest associations with everything primitive, fundamental, popular, while the French word is often more formal, more polite, more refined and has a less strong hold on the emotional side of life.

Cases in point are *clothe* vs. *dress*, *folk* vs. *people*, *help* vs. *aid*, and *hut* vs. *cottage* (1938: 91f). It should finally be mentioned that numerous French loan-words had their accent shifted from the last to the first syllable, according to Jespersen (1938: 96f) because 'the first syllable was felt as psychologically the most important one', cf. what was said above concerning 'value-stressing' in Germanic.

With the Renaissance a vast number of – sometimes very learned – borrowings from Latin (and Greek) were introduced into English. The French loan-words had paved the way, and in some cases French words were latinized, cf. *describe* and *adventure* which first entered English as *descrive* and *aventure*. Jespersen grants that the Latin borrowings entailed an enrichment of the English language in that its stock of synonyms and international words increased, but a major drawback was that much useless lexical material was introduced, and not just that: many of the Latin words were so difficult as to require a classical education for a person to construe and employ them properly.[2] The Latin loan-words were therefore seen by Jespersen, the Social-Democrat,[3] as 'undemocratic', contributing towards accentuating class divisions and hindering the spread of education (1938: 133f). From a language historical viewpoint the increasing use of borrowed expressions had the negative effect of stunting the growth of native formations, as Jespersen puts it (1938: 139). Speakers of English failed to utilize the potential of their own language for forming new words, preferring instead – out of mental laziness – the Latin terms available (1938: 122). Thereby the language was thrown into an 'unnatural state' (1938: 130ff), manifesting itself in, e.g., the adoption of irregular Latin and Greek plurals (*nuclei, indices, phenomena,* etc.), awkward sets of words belonging to the same semantic spheres (*father, paternal, parricide*) or stress-shifting (as in *solid, solidity*), 'which is so contrary to the Germanic tongues'.

As described in Ch. VII, 'Various Sources', English later borrowed words and expressions from numerous other languages, but Jespersen attributes 'this linguistic omnivorousness' as he calls it (1938: 145), to the linguistic laziness 'fostered especially by the preference for words from the classical languages'. However, Jespersen stresses that it is not the English language itself that is inherently deficient, a point which is borne out in Ch. VIII, where the 'native resources' of English are seen as much more important for the enrichment of the language than foreign loan-words. Jespersen focuses especially on the ease with which in Modern English nouns can be made into verbs and verbs into nouns (1938: 152ff). The historical basis for this is the Old English nouns and verbs which went back to the same etymological roots, but which inflexionally were clearly differentiated, e.g. OE *lufu* 'love' (n.) which exhibited specific endings indicating case, number and gender: *lufu* itself was a nominative singular feminine form as indicated by the suffix *-u*, whereas, e.g., *lufum* was a dative plural form. The corresponding verb, *lufian* (inf.), had suffixes denoting person, number, tense (present, past) and mood (indicative, subjunctive, imperative); *lufast*, e.g., was the 2nd person singular present indicative form as signified by the ending *-ast*. In the course of time the endings were reduced and/or lost, so that very many nouns and verbs became formally identical. Something similar happened to words of French origin. So after *love* and many other words had come to function as both nouns and verbs, there was no reason why, e.g., the nouns *cook* and *time* should not also be used as verbs (*cooked, timed*) or, conversely, why the verbs *laugh* and *move* should not acquire

---

[2]As a point of interest, it might be mentioned that around the turn of the century Jespersen had himself worked hard at – and succeeded in – reducing the role assigned to Latin in the Danish educational system. For the details, see Juul & Nielsen 1992: 100f.
[3]Cf. Juul et al. 1995: 270.

nominal functions (*a laugh, a move*) as well. According to Jespersen (1938: 161), English has a great advantage 'in its power of making words serve in new functions': he sees no problem in the loss of grammatical endings and no ambiguity in a sentence like *Her eyes like angels watch them still*, in which *eyes, like, watch* and *still* might all belong to more than one words class and *her* might be both an object form and a possessive. In this connection it should be noted that except for the Christian loan-word *angel* all the words in his sentence are monosyllabic. The morphological developments discussed here along with other morphological processes have contributed to the monosyllabism of Modern English, but additional factors have been at work as well: some words have simply 'been shortened by regular phonetic development' like the nouns *ant* (< OE *æmette*) and *lord* (< OE *hlaford*); new, frequently occurring monosyllabic words have emerged such as *bad, big, fun* and *job*; and long foreign words have been clipped, cf. *bus* 'omnibus', *phone* 'telephone', *prep* 'preparation', etc. (1938: 165ff).

In addition to English word-formation, Jespersen, in Ch. IX 'Grammar', sees the historical development of English grammar as a gradual movement 'from chaos to cosmos' (1938: 168), from Old English with its 'difficult' formative elements, its numerous inflexional endings, irregularities and anomalies to Modern English, where grammatical simplicity and regularity have come to prevail. Cases in point are the strong verbs, which have both been reduced in number and simplified in their use of distinct vowels,[4] and especially the adjectives, where in Modern English one form has replaced no fewer than eleven different inflexional forms in Old English. Jespersen ascribes this development in English to linguistic 'progress' (1938: 169). Among several causes bringing about this effect, Jespersen regards as the most important one the disruption of the Old English inflexional system, which in his view was brought about by the failure of each of the unaccented flexional vowels *a, e, i, u* to be associated unequivocally with the same meaning. The lack of semantic clarity led to the blurring and subsequent loss of such vowels.[5] A further consequence of this 'progressive tendency' was, according to Jespersen (1938: 169ff), the analogical extension of particularly distinct suffixes such as the *s*-endings in the genitive and in the plural. In Old English there were several genitive endings in the singular and plural of nouns, the genitive case had a variety of

---

[4] An extreme example given by Jespersen (1938: 169) of the simplification of distinct vowels is *burst, burst, burst* as compared with OE *berstan* inf., *bærst* pt.sg., *burston* pt.pl., *borsten* pp. The conjugation of this and the other 23 irregular verbs in Modern English with unchanged preterite and past participle forms is discussed in Nielsen 1989: 74f, where such verbs are seen as somewhat awkward, irregular minority forms stemming from normal phonetic attrition, and not from any 'progressive' drift, cf. below.

[5] This reflects a 'functional' view of language change in line with the Horn-Lehnert school, cf. Horn 1921 and Lehnert 1957 with further references; see also Nielsen 1989: 72. It goes counter to the concept of blind inflexional loss through 'sound-law' as assumed by the Neogrammarians. It should be noted that Jespersen's 'functional' views go all the way back to his doctoral dissertation from 1891, cf. 1891: 100ff.

functions, and the word order was not fixed in relation to the governing word. Eventually the genitive suffix -(e)s, which in Old English was restricted to the singular of the most common types of masculine and neuter nouns, was extended to all nouns and not just in the singular, but in the plural as well. Today the s-genitive is used primarily in connection with persons, and it is always placed in front of the governing word (1938: 170f). The extension of the substantival plural marker -(e)s, which historically goes back to the most common type of nominative/accusative masculine plural suffix in Old English, -as, also led to 'a greater regularity and simplicity' in accidence. Of all the OE plural suffixes -as was the most distinct and therefore gradually selected for general use (1938: 174f).

Similarly, Jespersen stresses the 'clearness and simplicity', which the English language has gained by giving up the word-gender system of Old English, which had three gender-classes. According to Jespersen, the advantage achieved by English in this respect will be especially felt by 'Anyone acquainted with the intricacies of the same system (or want of system) in German' (1938: 180). English also compares favourably with languages such as German, French and Italian in being the only one to have got rid of the 'useless distinction', as Jespersen puts it (1938: 223) in the eleventh and final chapter of the book, between the familiar and polite pronominal terms of address: the old 2nd person singular form *thou* was ousted by the 2nd plural form *you* (*ye*), which had thereby become the only term of address. Jespersen speaks of 'democratic levelling'[6] and concludes that English has 'attained the only manner of address worthy of a nation that respects the elementary rights of each individual' (1938: 223f).

On the background of such simplificatory 'progressive' measures it is not immediately comprehensible[7] why Jespersen should praise Modern English for having built up a 'rich' system of tenses (e.g. with perfect and pluperfect auxiliary constructions) in comparison with the Old English two-tense system (present – preterite) or for having developed a distinction between the simple and expanded tenses, 'a wonderful means of expressing temporal and emotional nuances', as he puts it (1938: 192f).

By way of summing up his theoretical views on language change, Jespersen (1938: 198) stresses that he sees in the evolution of human speech

> a wise natural selection, through which while nearly all innovations of questionable value disappear pretty soon, the fittest survive and make human speech ever more varied and flexible, and yet ever more easy and convenient to the speakers.

In other words, 'advance in usefulness' is the principle by which Jespersen evaluates language evolution. But where does that place English among the languages of the

---

[6] I am not quite at ease with this label seeing that it was the polite plural form that gained the upper hand. 'Aristocratic levelling' might be a more appropriate designation!
[7] Or perhaps it is even contradictory.

world? Jespersen faces this question in the very first chapter of the book, 'Preliminary Sketch', clearly basing his statements on much of the material presented in the subsequent chapters of the book and frequently discussed by us in our search for possible explanations of the popularity of *Growth and Structure* in England and America in addition to those offered by Quirk.

Jespersen describes Modern English as more masculine than any other modern European languages including its Germanic next of kin, German and Danish. The virility of English grammar emerges clearly from a comparison of English *all the wild animals that live there* with German *alle diejenigen wilden Tiere, die dort leben*: English has reduced or lost endings while German has retained a superfluity of plural markers. The retention of *-e, -en* gives German sentences a 'drawling' ring, while the English forms are 'the shortest possible', the sense being 'expressed with the greatest clearness imaginable' (1938: 5). The terseness of the English language is also seen in its syntax, where words 'do not play at hide-and-seek, as they often do .... in German, where ideas that by right belong together are widely sundered in obedience to caprice, or more often to some rigorous grammatical rule' (1938: 10). To Jespersen, the masculinity of the English sound system is evident from its voiced and voiceless consonants that are symmetrically patterned, and which are clearly pronounced unlike 'the indistinct or half-slurred consonants that abound in Danish', cf. *ha_de, hage, li_vlig*, and unlike the palatalized consonants that give, e.g., Russian such an 'insinuating grace' (1938: 2). In phonetic structure, English differs from such European languages as Italian and Spanish where words end much more frequently in vowels than they do in English, cf. *feasts, helped, hence, months, tempts*. The final consonants or, rather, consonant groups make English sound energetic and harsh, whereas word-final vowels tend to give a 'childlike and effeminate' impression (1938: 3). Childishness is also the impression rendered by an excessive use of diminutives as, e.g., in Italian and Russian and even in the Germanic languages, German and Dutch (1938: 9). Obviously, vigorous and no-nonsense Englishmen rarely resort to such devices. Finally, in very general terms, French is said to be a language 'where everything is condemned that does not conform to a definite set of rules laid down by grammarians'. No such 'rigorous regulations' were enforced in English, which is described as a language spoken by 'great respecters of the liberties of each individual', who were 'free to strike out new paths' for themselves (1938: 14).

If we are to believe Jespersen, only one language in the world has qualities that surpass those found in English, namely Chinese. In accordance with his 'progress' theory, successful language evolution was, to Jespersen, synonymous with reaching a high degree of communicative effectiveness with the fewest and simplest means, as he pointed out as early as in his doctoral dissertion (1891: 9, cf. also 1894: 13). He praised Chinese for its monosyllabism, fixed word-order and logical precision, calling it 'the highest, finest, and accordingly latest developed expedient of speech to which man has attained' (1894: 90). Although in *Growth and Structure* Jespersen does see clear masculine aspects about 'the enormous richness of the English vocabulary' (1938: 16), 'the great number of long foreign, especially Latin, words' have prevented English from acquiring a degree of monosyllabism comparable to that found in Chinese (1938: 5f) and consequently from attaining a regularity of word-order and linguistic logic similar to that language (1938: 10ff).

As we have seen, the 'progress in language' theory as summarized here was conceived in Jespersen's early days, it pervaded the theoretical foundations of the first edition of *Growth and Structure* from 1905 and all subsequent editions, and it raised its head again in his later published work, including *Efficiency in Linguistic Change* that appeared only two years before his death in 1943. Davidsen-Nielsen (1990: 38) has, in my view correctly, classified Jespersen's belief in 'progress in language' as one of the possibly two heroic failures of his life.[8] Since I have discussed Jespersen's theory elsewhere, I shall not go into detail here with its shortcomings.[9] But we can return now to the question asked at the beginning of the article. Ironically, I think that the success of Jespersen's *Growth and Structure* as an introduction to the history of the English language was very much tied up with his 'progress' theory. Jespersen sums up Ch. I, 'Preliminary Sketch', in the following way (1938: 16):

> The English language is a methodical, energetic, business-like and sober language, that does not care much for finery and elegance, but does care for logical consistency and is opposed to any attempt to narrow-in life by police regulations and strict rules either of grammar or of lexicon.

The 'progressive' tendencies of English clearly underlie this description, and Jespersen goes on:

> As the language is, so also is the nation,
>
> > For words, like Nature, half reveal
> > And half conceal the Soul within.
> >
> > > Tennyson

As if this were not enough, Jespersen writes in the very last paragraph of the book (1905: 249):

> Whatever a remote future may have in store, one need not be a great prophet to predict that in the near future the number of English-speaking people will increase considerably. The curse of Babel is beginning to lose its sting, and it must be a source of gratification to mankind that the tongue spoken by two of the greatest powers of the world is so noble, so rich, so pliant, so expressive, and so interesting as the language whose growth and structure I have been here endeavouring to characterize.

---

[8]The other was Jespersen's absorption in constructing a well-functioning international auxiliary language, which can be seen, however, as 'a revealing application of his linguistic thought' (Larsen 1989: 120, cf. also Davidsen-Nielsen 1990: 43f).
[9]See Nielsen 1989.

I have no wish to detract from the scholarly qualities of Jespersen in general nor of *Growth and Structure* in particular, far from it. But who would not like to have the history of one's language presented in the way that Jespersen describes the evolution of English, the intrinsic merits of the present-day language and of those who speak it? No wonder that the book was loved in England and America, indeed by all Anglophiles round the globe.[10]

References

Davidsen-Nielsen, N. (1990). Essentials of Jespersen's Growth and Stature. Remarks on "Otto Jespersen: Facets of his Life and Work". *Sprint* 1990/1, 37-45.

Horn, W. (1921). *Sprachkörper und Sprachfunktion* [= *Palaestra* 135]. Leipzig.

Jespersen, O. (1891). *Studier over engelske kasus*. Copenhagen: Klein.

Jespersen, O. (1894). *Progress in Language with Special Reference to English*. London: Sonnenschein.

Jespersen, O. (1905). *Growth and Structure of the English Language*. Leipzig: Teubner; 9th edition 1938, reprinted 1962 (Oxford: Blackwell); 10th edition 1982 (Chicago: University Press, Oxford: Blackwell), 'Foreword' by Randolph Quirk.

Jespersen, O. (1941). *Efficiency in Linguistic Change*. (Det Kgl. Danske Videnskabernes Selskab. Historisk-filologiske Meddelelser. 47, 4.) Copenhagen: Munksgaard.

Juul, A. & H. F. Nielsen (1989). *Otto Jespersen: Facets of his Life and Work*. Amsterdam & Philadelphia: Benjamins.

Juul, A. & H. F. Nielsen (1992). Otto Jespersen and the introduction of new language-teaching methods in Denmark. In A. Giroud (ed) *Aspects de l'histoire de l'enseignement des langues: 1880-1914* [= *Bulletin CILA* 56]. Neuchâtel. 91-105.

Juul, A., H. F. Nielsen & J. E. Nielsen (eds) (1995). *A Linguist's Life. An English Translation of Otto Jespersen's Autobiography with Notes, Photos and a Bibliography*. Odense: University Press.

Larsen, F. (1989). Jespersen's New International Auxiliary Language. In Juul & Nielsen 1989, 101-122.

Lehnert, M. (1957). The Interrelation between Form and Function in the Development of the English Language. *Zeitschrift für Anglistik und Amerikanistik* 5, 43-56.

Nielsen, H. F. (1989). On Otto Jespersen's View of Language Evolution. In Juul & Nielsen 1989, 61-78.

Quirk (1982). See Jespersen 1905 (10th edition 1982).

---

[10] I would like to thank Arne Juul and Fritz Larsen for their comments to an earlier version of this paper.

Tendencies in the Syntax of the Verb in American and British English[1]

Bent Preisler

In a world of many 'World Englishes', is a description of American English (AE) by means of comparison with British English (BE) becoming an irrelevancy? The answer, in my opinion, is negative: the major varieties of English are so similar that a non-contrastive description of each would be uneconomical. Only BE has a strong tradition of being described as a language in its own right, and so the obvious norm for comparison is BE.

It is generally agreed that grammatical differences between BE and AE are fewer, and less likely to affect mutual comprehensibility, than lexical differences (see e.g. Strevens 1972: 47). While this point cannot be argued, it is the aim of this article to show that the extent of grammatical differences between BE and AE has been underestimated, due to a limited (historically determined) conception of what constitutes 'standard AE.'

It is clear from historical treatments of standardization in AE (e.g. Baron 1982; Gallardo 1984) that the grammar of the written language as it is taught in American schools and universities has, in the main, remained faithful to the norm of literary BE. The spoken language, to the extent that it differs from this norm, has made sporadic imprints on the, largely prescriptive, American grammatical tradition, but has never been systematically codified (cp. Preisler 1995). As a result, references to 'Standard American English' tend to be references to *written* AE, and Švejcer (1978), for example, equates it with 'belles-lettres' usage (p. 75).

In other words, although it is true that, even with regard to the grammar of written AE, 'It's generally quite easy ... to distinguish between UK and USA produced texts, as long as they are not too short' (Peter Trudgill)[2] – there are many more AE-BE differences in the spoken language, whose manifestations make their way into writing only whenever realistic colloquial language happens to be an aspect of the author's style.

However, even if we look only at the spoken language, AE and BE are not two distinct and easily recognizable grammatical varieties. Many, probably most, grammatical differences are frequency differences, AE tending to use one variant,

---

[1] I'm greatly indebted to Tim Caudery, John Dienhart and Knud Sørensen for their invaluable comments on an earlier version of this article. These kind colleagues are not, of course, responsible for any errors that remain.
[2] Personal communication.

BE the other. In fact, it is such tendencies in the pattern of linguistic choices which cause us, particularly when we are reading an American author whose style is influenced by speech, to intuitively recognize the variety as American English. Functional variation, too, such as register variation, is characterized by a preponderance of relative over absolute differences. This does not, of course, mean that we regard functional variation as irrelevant in linguistic terms, nor should it cause us to regard geographically and culturally based variation as irrelevant.

The traditional identification of standard AE with written AE has made it easy to write off many distinctly American patterns of grammatical usage, in writing influenced by speech, as 'local coloring' intended for 'characterizing through speech characters who speak local dialects' (Švejcer 1978: 75). This is obviously well justified in many cases, including some of those Švejcer mentions. But for many such grammatical usages, some of which I will point out below, automatic relegation to 'local coloring' – to the extent this implies 'nonstandard English' – would clearly be unreasonable. The main reason for this is that it would class a large proportion of the American educated middle class as speakers of nonstandard English. Peter Trudgill points out that it is a 'basic error ... [to assume] ... that Standard English speakers sometimes use nonstandard forms. They don't.'[3] Forms that are used regularly (i.e. forms that are not performance phenomena or humorous usages in imitation of dialect speakers, etc.) in the speech of educated Americans should be considered Standard English, regardless of whether or not they conform to the norms of the written language.

A case in point is constructions such as *want in/out* etc. (an AE alternative to *want to come in/out* etc.), which Švejcer characterizes as having a 'clearly expressed local coloring,' being 'widely distributed in the Midwest and partially in the Middle Atlantic region.' They are, furthermore, 'deviations from the norms of the standard language ... found only in the speech of informants with little education' (Švejcer 1978: 75). To this one could argue, first, that it seems strange to designate the expression 'local coloring' to constructions that are widely distributed in such large parts of the US; and that it is precisely the Western US which since the Second World War has had the greatest influence on spoken middle class AE, most conspicuously in the area of pronunciation. Secondly, on *either* side of the Atlantic, 'there is regional variation, even in Standard English' (Trudgill and Hannah 1982: 43). Thirdly, and most importantly, although constructions like *he wants in* may once have been confined to the speech of people with little education, this is certainly not true any more – as recognized by the LDELC, which characterizes them as 'AmE infml.'

Three more factors make it difficult to pinpoint the grammatical differences between standard AE and BE. One concerns a general problem in language

---

[3]Personal communication.

description – that of differentiating grammatical differences from lexical differences. I am not here offering any hard and fast criteria: the expressions discussed below have been chosen because they represent structural or functional options which seem relevant to grammatical description. The second problem is the fact that the two varieties influence each other, and that the influence of AE on BE, in particular, means that there is a steady influx of AE forms and expressions into BE, where they often become integrated in a very short time (for manifestations of this process, see comments on examples (51) and (89) below). To keep up with this development, any comparative grammar of American English would have to be revised continually. This, however, is made difficult by the third (and biggest) problem: the lack of a comprehensive computer-based corpus of Spoken American English, comparable to those now available with regard to the written language.

The area I have chosen for the following discussion is the syntax of the verb. Several characteristics of AE, as compared with BE, are generally recognized in this area (see e.g. Algeo 1988; Benson et al. 1986: 20ff; Strevens 1972: 44ff; Švejcer 1978: 75ff; Trudgill and Hannah 1982: 43ff). They include a greater tendency to use nouns as verbs and vice versa; some distinctive irregular-verb patterns (cp. Preisler 1995: 352ff); auxiliary *do* in connection with *have* in certain cases (AE *do you have* – BE *have you got*); the past tense vs. the present perfect (AE *did you see him this morning* – BE *have you seen* ...); AE *have to* corresponding to some meanings of BE *must* (AE *that has to be lemonade* – BE *that must be* ...); and, finally, some lexical verbs whose complementation varies in AE and BE. However, even as an account of the *types* of differences to be found (cp. Strevens 1972: 53), this list is inadequate. Algeo (1988), Benson et al. (1986) and Trudgill and Hannah (1982) include several more types, involving e.g. verbal derivation (cp. AE forms like *citify, burglarize*), modal-verb usage generally (e.g. differential use of *shall/should, need* and *dare*), the subjunctive (previously dealt with by Preisler (1977)), verb-phrase substitution with/without *do* (AE and BE *she hasn't bought one yet, but she may* – BE (optional) ... *but she may do*), as well as a more comprehensive typification of complementation differences (Algeo 1988: 22ff).

Still, the primary aim of these accounts is to enable students of English to recognize (some of) the *types* of differences between the two major varieties. They do not represent exhaustive treatments of the grammar of the American English verb, even in contrastive terms. This is obviously also true of the present article, the aim of which is simply to demonstrate that research has so far only scratched the surface, and to indicate some of the directions that the further exploration of Standard American English may take.

Most of the verbal phenomena dealt with here, some of which are well-known whereas others may not be, have been selected for discussion in a context in which they appear to represent general tendencies or principles that have not hitherto, as such, received much attention. They are: (1) the greater tendency to observe tense and aspect distinctions in BE, and the (often converse) tendency to observe distinctions related to modality, in AE; and (2) the tendency for AE and BE to choose differential patterns of complementation, particularly in connection with lexical verbs of potentially modal meaning.

My empirical material, for want of a corpus of Spoken American English, consists of a variety of written sources. I am thus not confining myself to a discussion of the spoken language, though many of my examples represent – or seem clearly influenced by – the spoken language, as confirmed by their content. My sources are a combination of novels that employ colloquial AE to a greater or lesser extent, other primary sources, and (for some areas of complementation) Gustav Kirchner's *Die syntaktischen Eigentümlichkeiten des amerikanischen English* (Kirchner 1970). Kirchner's huge material, which includes examples from both before and after 1950, has to be used with a good deal of caution, particularly as it does not systematically distinguish non-prestigious forms, and because a large number of examples are no longer specifically AE. The examples selected for this article represent Standard-English contexts, and the rarity in BE of the exemplified constructions has been verified through BE manuals and, especially, the CobuildDirect/Bank-of-English corpus of written and spoken English. This corpus consists of 11 subcorpora, amounting to 50,000,000 words, including three of US texts (see the list of Abbreviations). Comparison between AE and BE has been done by asking (in the query language) the same 'question' of the US corpora (npr, usbooks, usephem: 9,000,000 words) and the three corresponding UK corpora (bbc, ukbooks, ukephem: 11,000,000 words). Confirmation of BE low frequency of a particular form has occasionally been sought in the remaining UK corpora, as well. Relevant syntactic environments are generally too infrequent in a corpus of 9,000,000 words for particular AE-BE differences to show statistical significance, and the informal procedures employed can best be described as those of a pilot investigation.

1. The first diverse AE/BE verbal differences to be discussed here in terms of a general principle concern features which in themselves have often been commented on, cp. the works referred to above. The principle guiding their priority in AE and BE, consisting of three points, may be tentatively stated as follows:

(1.1) Verbal distinctions of tense and aspect, time and time relation, often seem less important in AE than in BE.

(1.2) This is the case especially where such distinctions compete with indications of the *pragmatic* (interpersonal) potential of the clause.

(1.3) The pragmatic potential of the clause tends to be more important in AE than in BE, as indicated in particular through distinctions of modality.

1.1. Verbal distinctions of tense and aspect, time and time relation, often seem less important in AE than in BE

1.1.1. The classic example of principle 1.1 concerns the past-tense/present perfect distinction. My own favorite example of the clash between AE and BE usage in this respect is the following piece of dialog from an American talk show, which I recorded some years ago, in which Dick Cavett, the host, interviewed the actress Katharine Hepburn, a speaker of the once aristocratic New-England variety (influenced by British English), which was favored by Hollywood up till around 1950:

(1)   Cavett: Are you sorry you never acted with Olivier?
      Hepburn: Well, neither of us is dead yet.

In Hepburn's language, Cavett's utterance had to be interpreted as distinct from ... *you have never acted* ... (hence her reply). Cavett, however – in accordance with present-day Standard AE – may well have intended the latter meaning.

1.1.2. The past-tense/perfect difference is usually represented as if it concerned only present-time contexts, as in (1), where BE would have had the present perfect, cp. Trudgill and Hannah 1982: 57, Preisler 1992: 100. Actually, however, the difference applies to past-time contexts as well, to the extent that, in reported speech, AE tends to generalize the past tense:

(2)   [The Reverend] Koukla ... said briskly, ... 'I'm having some people in this evening ... Could you possibly join us ...?' I figured Dr. Thorndecker had put the Reverend up to it, and sometime during the evening I'd get a casual explanation of what happened [cp. *had happened*] to Chester K. Petersen (LSS 159).

BE – to place an event in the past before the reported event (represented by *figured*, in this case) – would more frequently than AE use the past perfect, though the choice would not necessarily depend on meaning in terms of absolute vs. relational time (see e.g. Preisler 1992: 101; cp. also my comments on example (13) below, and cp. Algeo 1988: 19. Thus it is a three-way, not a two-way, distinction that AE fails to observe, in generalizing the use of the past tense in environments where BE is more likely to use the perfect.

1.2. Verbal distinctions of tense and aspect seem less important in AE than in BE especially where such distinctions compete with indications of the pragmatic (interpersonal) potential of the clause.

1.2.1. In AE it is often (different) aspects of the pragmatic potential of a clause which determine matters of tense cohesion. Thus the *present* subjunctive governed by deontic[4] lexical forms and conjunctions, which is less frequent in BE, remains unchanged in *past*-tense contexts:

---

[4]Deontic meaning represents speaker attitude – the proposition is more or less *desirable* – as opposed to epistemic meaning, which is speaker assessment of the truth value, or *probability*, of the proposition.

(3)   It seemed fair to her that before she accepted Edith's suggestion, Edith know her [sic] truth (WG 5).

(4)   Victor and Dolores ... tried not to look at each other lest they break out in laughter (MF 90).

BE more frequently uses a construction with *should*, though the present subjunctive is often possible in formal language. Interestingly enough, there is another (reported speech) construction in which a past-tense verb of reporting tends to attract past-tense forms in the indirect quotation in BE,[5] but where in AE it is more likely to be followed by present-tense forms 'if the indirect quotation is a statement of timeless truth or of current events' (Algeo 1988: 19). Algeo's BE example is from the *Times*: 'She said that there *was* nothing in the bible that *had* anything to do with ordination as we *knew* it today'). I suggest that the present tense in past-tense reported-speech types of context (whether indicative or subjunctive) may carry connotations of greater relevance and urgency, and that its more frequent use in AE is thus a question of the pragmatic potential of the clause.

Deontic use of the present subjunctive, in fact, seems increasingly to be determined by pragmatic *as distinct from* lexico-grammatical context in AE. In (3) the subjunctive is separated from the form that governs it by a finite subordinate clause, even though the deontic force of the governing form, *fair*, in semantic terms is not very strong (cp. e.g. *important*). However, deontic meaning may rest solely in the subjunctive; thus – while it is possible to argue that the occurrence of deontic *be* as governed by *idea* in (5) is facilitated by the presence of *urged* in the nonfinite clause – the subjunctives of (6) and (7) are not governed by forms of inherent deontic content:

(5)   A third idea – urged by flight insurance companies – was that passengers' baggage be opened for examination (AH 196).

(6)   the notion that a linguistic description be based exclusively upon the phonemic shape of expressions is a modern development (RL 207).

(7)   Pitt ... indicated with his hand that Admiral Bass be the first to enter the aircraft (CC 197).

In other words, the present subjunctive does not here reproduce a deontic component of meaning already residing in, respectively, the forms *idea*, *notion* and *indicated* (cp. Preisler (1977)). On the contrary, the deontic interpretation of these forms derives from the context as represented by the subjunctive (and, in (5), by the form *urged*).

---

[5] 'Although British English also permits the present tense in such cases, reportage in quality newspapers favors an attraction into the past, perhaps as a device for distancing the reporter from the opinions reported' (Algeo 1988: 19f).

Conversely, the presence of a potentially deontic lexical form does not guarantee that the present subjunctive will follow, which is further evidence that the context is decisive:

(8)   I would have preferred they swung outward, in case I had to bust through in a hasty exit. But you can't have everything (LSS 288).

The speaker's 'preference,' in a contrary-to-fact context, is irrelevant in terms of influencing future action. Hence *would have preferred* – and *swung*, not *swing*.

1.2.2. The auxiliaries, not least the modal auxiliaries, offer many differences between AE and BE in details of syntax as well as semantics, see e.g. Trudgill and Hannah 1982: 46ff. However, in regard to the topic concerning us here – the AE tendency to disregard tense and/or time relations in contexts of modality – one particular feature which has as yet escaped notice deserves a mention. It concerns the expression of non-reality in the past, which, both in AE and BE, is regularly expressed by adding perfect *have* to the past-tense form of the modal auxiliary, the meaning ranging from 'remoteness' (contrary-to-fact or hypothesis) to possibility. An example:

(9)   ... people on the street might have assumed he was English or French ... but he was in fact ... American (DI 38).

However, recently it seems that the form *may (have)* can be used, in the same past-time context, to signal possibility *as distinct from* remoteness. In this way a modal distinction is gained at the expense of a (redundant) formal indication of past-time context:

(10)   What sins had he committed before ...? For one thing, he may have shot an old man's dog eight years ago (PCA 239) [cp. '*might* have ... eight years *before*'].

(11)   Thus Morgan had not adjusted Mrs. McGuane's testimony. Morgan may have just missed the facts. After all, the man had other things to worry about (CH 61).

(12)   Again she smiled ... Kwani may have stolen Kokopelli – after he had chosen her, Tiopi, not once but twice for mating! – but Kwani would learn she could not steal the necklace, too (LS 283).

(13)   No fingerprints had been discovered from them, and if anything, their purpose may be to make us think what the person who had left them wanted us to think (PCA 238).

In (13), a potential contrary-to-fact perspective is actually discarded by the introduction of *may* rather than the expected *might have*, while the time perspective is blurred by *may* and by the simple past-tense form *wanted* (instead of *had wanted*, cp. 1.1.2 above).

Semantically, this replacement of *might* by *may* in examples such as (10) - (13) marks the obliteration of a distinction between a past- and a present-time reference point (on the time line, see e.g. Preisler 1992: 98): *May* as a modality is regularly used to express the current speaker's assessment of probability, in AE as well as BE, in terms of which the reference point coincides with the point of speaker utterance, even if the 'event' is in the past, as in,

(14)   She may have been emotionally turbulent, but she also had a lucid, organized mind (CBD usbooks B9000001237).

Replacing *may* by *might*, in (14), would only make the speaker's assessment more tentative. However, in (10) - (13) above, *may* substitutes for *might* as a means of reporting some character's assessment (of something) in the past. The tendency for *may* to do this in AE is confirmed by the CobuildDirect corpus, though the relevant context did not occur frequently enough for the findings to be statistically significant: 5 examples were found in the US material (out of 33 relevant contexts), whereas comparable UK material yielded none. An example from the US material:

(15)   Arch slipped away from the table to deal with a situation which may have reached crisis proportions: Cleavon had not shown up with the coffee (CBD usbooks B9000000463).

1.2.3. In some contexts, contrary-to-fact meaning – occupying the negative pole on the scale of epistemic modality (the opposite pole being 'fact') – does not represent any significant degree of *pragmatic* tentativeness. The fact that AE seems – more often than BE – to avoid contrary-to-fact use of the perfect in favor of more 'open' expressions of hypothesis might therefore also be seen as a manifestation of principle 1.3:

(16)   It might even be ... that if you gave me half a chance, I would have apologized (ST 54).

In the context of *I would have apologized* (contrary-to-fact) we might have expected *if you had given me* ..., but that would close the matter (indicating it was decided in the past). On the other hand, *if you gave me* ..., by expressing a hypothesis, leaves the possibility open that 'you' might still give 'me' a chance.[6]

In connection with *would*, too – in contrary-to-fact contexts – the perfect is often left out (as in (17) and (18)); or – in environments where this is not possible in standard BE – *would* cooccurs with the perfect (19), or replaces the simple past tense (20):

(17)   ... it doesn't appear that her wounds bled out much, if at all, otherwise I would expect more predator activity (PCB 15) [cp. *would have expected*].

---

[6]The modality *it might (even) be (that)* – cp. *maybe* – is hardly variable to the extent of making *it might (even) have been (that)* a likely option.

(18)   I wonder what these couples would be doing now, if they'd still be with each other, what difference that might have made (PCA 256) [i.e. 'if they *would* still *be* ...'; but in BE, in a contrary-to-fact context, a more likely construction would have been, 'if they *had* still *been* ...'].

(19)   ... if you'd have seen her afterwards – she was just *drained* [author's italics] (JK 42) [cp. *if you had seen* ...].[7]

(20)   Charles knew that if it would happen, it would happen immediately (RC 127) [cp. *if it happened* ...].

In (20) the context is not actually contrary-to-fact, but still *would* is used in a conditional clause where BE (and often AE) would have had the simple past tense.

Were, as a past-tense subjunctive, is used mostly for the expression of contrary-to-fact meaning both in AE and BE (e.g. in conditional, concessive and comparative clauses), which may be why – contrary to what has sometimes been suggested (cp. Benson 1986: 24) – subjunctive *were* is not generally more frequent in AE than in BE. For the explicit expression of hypothesis, e.g. in interrogative clauses, we might have expected *were* (instead of indicative *was*) to be more frequent in AE than BE, as in

(21)   ... as it got dark, he sighed to himself, not knowing if he were relieved that he was free, or if he were more miserable than he had ever been (NM 293).

but a comparison of occurrences of *were* after pronominal subjects in the singular, in the CobuildDirect corpus, shows no noticeable differences between US and corresponding UK materials for this or any other clause type. As *were* is the only common, though fairly formal, epistemic subjunctive in English (the epistemic present subjunctive being confined to highly formal contexts), this means that the epistemic subjunctive – contrary to the deontic subjunctive – is *not* more frequent in AE than in BE, though descriptions often lump together deontic and epistemic subjunctives in characterizing the subjunctive generally as being formal and more frequent in AE than in BE (e.g. Trudgill and Hannah 1982: 56f).

1.3. In general, however, AE does tend to emphasize the pragmatic potential of the clause particularly through distinctions of modality. Thus the greater inclination to use the deontic subjunctive may even result in AE choosing a finite construction where BE would tend to choose a nonfinite one: after some deontic verbs which in BE would more likely govern an infinitive clause (e.g. *I recommend you to* ...), AE often chooses a finite object clause (*I recommend that you* ...); in other words, even

---

[7]Trudgill and Hannah, too, characterize this construction as 'USEng only' (1982: 47), but according to Tim Caudery it is in fact quite common in (nonstandard) BE speech.

where both constructions are possible, AE more often than BE chooses the finite one. The finite construction allows AE to employ the deontic present subjunctive, which may explain why AE tends to prefer the finite construction (cp. Algeo 1988: 22):

(22)   '... the documents we've subpoenaed. They're due today.'

   'Well I'm afraid we shall be a bit late providing them. You are basically asking that Mr. Hartnell ... stop running his business and look for records for weeks' (ST 55) [cp. *You are asking Mr. Hartnell ... to stop ...*].

(23)   I'd prefer you direct that question to Dr. Thorndecker (LSS 97) [cp. *I'd prefer you to direct ...*].

(24)   Fortunately, no one required that he like becoming a German agent again (FF 197) [cp. *... no one required him to ...*].

Again, we seem to have a case of AE preferring a construction in which pragmatic potential can be explicitly (and even redundantly) indicated.

2. As we have just seen in 1.3, differences involving categories of modality extend into the area of complementation, which area I shall now focus on.

As with auxiliary usage, it is not possible here to give an exhaustive account of all the differences in complementation, whether absolute or statistical, between AE and BE. Some of them are well-known, involving e.g. some copula constructions, the order of direct and indirect object, and infinitive constructions with or without *to* after the verbs *come, go* and *help* (cp. Trudgill and Hannah 1982: 53ff; Preisler 1992: 28n., 39n.). Further differences have been pointed out by Trudgill and Hannah, as well as by Benson et al. (1986: 25), Strevens (1972: 52), Švejcer (1978: 84ff) and – in particular – by Algeo (1988: 22ff).

Still it seems to me that the area of complementation offers numerous usage differences which have not yet been described – especially as pertaining to the spoken language – or which have only received random treatment. Many of these involve verbs of epistemic or deontic meaning, i.e. modal lexical verbs (as in 1.3 above). In the following, I will discuss some examples.

2.1. Some constructions that are usually mentioned in connection with particular verbs are really constructional types, of which each can be found with a larger group of verbs.

2.1.1. The group *come, go* and *help* mentioned in section 2 above should possibly be expanded by at least one other member, *beg*, which appears sometimes to be followed by an infinitive without *to* in informal AE. Kirchner cites a few examples, e.g. (25). My own example (26) might be a case in point; alternatively, it represents the finite construction discussed in 1.3, cp. *I must beg (that) you help me out of here.*

The CobuildDirect corpus yields very few examples of *beg,* and none in environments relevant for verification.

(25) He begs him go over to Cursitor Street and see what can be done (GK 595).

(26) I must beg you help me out of here (BF 198).

2.1.2. Several accounts mention that the verb *order* may be constructed with a past-participle object clause in AE, where BE has a passive infinitive clause; cp. Strevens' example (Strevens 1972: 52):

(27) The President ordered controls clamped on wages, prices and rents [AE].

(28) The President ordered controls to be clamped on wages, prices and rents [BE].

However, this construction may be generally more frequent in AE than in BE, with other modal lexical verbs; cp.

Cognitive verbs of epistemic meaning (states):

(29) One well-known novelist conceives his work done when he hands over ... (GK 563).

(30) Imagine Versailles decorated by Dr. Dolittle, and you have some idea of Kersner's pink-tinged palace (CBD npr S2000921207).[8]

(31) She knows her life-purpose well-accomplished (GK 563).

Epistemic verbs, including performatives (acts):

(32) As soon as his ballot was announced voted H. left the shop hurriedly (GK 563).

(33) Some are rumored parachuted into Poland (GK 563).

Cognitive verbs of deontic meaning (states):

(34) Will the party desire commissars introduced ...? (GK 561).

Performative verbs of deontic meaning (acts):

(35) He refused to permit his name entered (GK 562).

The CobuildDirect corpus suggests a slight confirmative tendency, but comparison is made difficult by the fact that the relevant syntactic environment is rare: no examples of the alternative construction with *to be* after these verbs were found for AE *or* BE in the relevant US and UK material.

---

[8]Tim Caudery has called my attention to the fact that BE would not normally use a passive infinitive clause here, as it would have a different meaning.

2.1.3. Another object clause construction, which as an AE feature is usually associated with the verb *like* (e.g. Trudgill and Hannah (1982: 54)), is the *for ... to ...* infinitive where BE would leave out *for*:

(36)   I'd like for you to sit around for a week (CBD usbooks B9000000492).

However, the *for ... to ...* infinitive is found with many other verbs in AE which do not normally combine with this construction in BE:

Deontic verbs referring to a cognitive state:

(37)   I would adore for you to give it a little publicity (CBD usbooks B9000000463).

(38)   He aims for me to lie, he thought (CBD usbooks B9000001423).

(39)   How can you expect for me to drink the whiskey with him or what (CBD npr S2000930519).

(40)   I hated for Ben to hear the squabbling (GK 614).

(41)   I didn't mean for you to give a lecture (CBD usbooks B9000000418).

Deontic verbs referring to an act, including performatives:

(42)   I gave you a party flat on its back and grown men crying for you to get in (CBD npr S2000911116).

(43)   With me it was living with a drunken uncle ... and every year pleading for him to let me go back to school (CBD usbooks B9000000447).

(44)   ... it's been ... five years since she started pushing for me to go for help (CBD usbooks B9000001282).

(45)   He said for us to stay here (CBD usbooks B9000000492).

Most of these were quite common in the CobuildDirect US material, whereas they were practically non-existent in the corresponding UK material (including (42) - (44), which appear to be possible[9] in BE). Another group of verbs with a *for ... to ...* infinitive, all of them meaning approximately 'to signal to somebody to do something' – though not uncommon in the relevant UK material – also seemed to be more frequent in the US material:

(46)   McKee motioned for Miss Leon to start the motor (CBD usbooks B9000000447).

(47)   ... here she was, signaling for Lydia to join her (CBD usbooks B9000001399).

(48)   Suzie Keller yelled for him to take it out (CBD usbooks B9000001059).

---

[9]According to Tim Caudery (personal communication). Caudery suspects, though, that BE would have 'pleading *with* him' in (43).

An exception was the verb *gesture*, which is quite common with a *for ... to ...* infinitive in the UK material (cp. AE *motion* in (46)).

Furthermore, after the same (deontic) types of verb in AE, the *for ... to ...* infinitive may be used to syntactically simplify the second of two parallel clauses, of which the first one is a finite or a different nonfinite type:

(49)   I'd rather you didn't give me a birthday present at all than for you to stop at one of those awful places (GK 615).

(50)   He said that didn't matter and for me to come up here (GK 616).

Of two UK examples of this from the CobuildDirect corpus, one is likely to be a loan from an American news source (cp. *help us show*, see 2.1.1):

(51)   The background changes now going on in the whole region because of the Gulf crisis are bound to help us show Iran, and for Iran to show us, that we really have a crucial interest between us in improving relations (CBD bbc S1000900903).

2.1.4. Finally, by way of finishing this section on differences relating to modal lexical verbs, I would like to point out that the cognitive verb *figure* offers several interesting features of complementation, in spoken AE – over and above those commonly recognized, which are the following (from LDELC, marked as 'esp. AmE'):

(52)   I figured (that) you'd want to see me about it [epistemic *figure* + finite clause].

(53)   I figured on him leaving [deontic *figure on* + *-ing* clause].

These additional features include, first, other nonfinite constructions besides the *-ing* clause:

(54)   ... the men assigned to the case figured it for a murder by a prostitute (LST 214) [epistemic *figure* + verbless clause, with subject *it* linked by *for* to subject complement *a murder* ...].

(55)   I figured her to faint (GK 610) ['thought she would ...': epistemic *figure* + infinitive clause].

(56)   '... you've lived here a long time, haven't you?' 'Thirty years ... And I figure to live out the rest of it right here' (LSS 171) ['intend ...': deontic *figure* + infinitive clause].

Secondly, an intransitive construction – reflected in the idiom *that figures* (which is not marked as 'AmE' in LDELC) – is actually productive in AE but not in BE:

(57)   It could still figure as a female, but the cops were going by probabilities (LST 215) [cp. 'they figured it could still be a female': epistemic].

(58)   Moses, a young black man, was a crackerjack lawyer – he figured for great things (ST 250) [cp. 'they figured he would accomplish great things': epistemic].

(59) 'But we wanted to go [to Mexico], and it seemed worth the risk.' 'Worth another stretch in Lansing?' 'That didn't figure. See, we never intended coming Stateside again' (TC 251) [cp. 'we didn't figure that was a possibility': epistemic].

The CobuildDirect corpus yielded no UK examples of any of the types in (54) - (59).

2.2. Finally I intend to focus on features of complementation concerning other lexical verbs that have not been (sufficiently) dealt with elsewhere.

2.2.1. The complementation of the verbs *come* and *go* offer several interesting differences between AE and BE (cp. section 2 above). For example, the use of *go* with an object expressing a high value, to signify 'accomplishment,' seems particularly common in AE, apparently influenced by the language of American sports commentaries:

(60) If the play-offs go seven games, Minnesota will have played 13 of its last 17 games against Toronto (CBD npr S2000911005).

(61) There was the 1924 convention for the Democrats in New York which went 104 ballots (CBD npr 2000920713).

(62) ... he's burning the calories off at twice the pace of ... Yard Stevens.' ... Yard Stevens ... went maybe three hundred pounds (SK 59).

(63) If I could have a twenty-six-year-old, Britt would go me two years younger. She was that competitive (EJ 230).

As seen in (63), *go* may even take an indirect object when used in this way. The CobuildDirect material only yielded 2 BE examples in the relevant UK corpora, both in expressions with *better*: *go (sb.) one/two better*. The corresponding, though smaller, US material showed 7, more varied, examples (cp. (60) and (61) above). These findings may be suggestive of a tendency.

2.2.2. The question of transitive or intransitive construction is involved in many differences of complementation between AE and BE. Some of them (concerning e.g. *battle* and *protest*, which tend to combine with an object in AE but a prepositional phrase in BE) have been pointed out before, e.g. by Benson et al. (1986: 21ff) and Trudgill and Hannah (1982: 56). Many others remain to be included, a few of which will be pointed out here, cp. the following AE examples of, first, transitive constructions which in BE would more likely be intransitive:

(64) She wants you to sit Tommy (Am. TV film 'The dark end of the street') [cp. *babysit*, LDELC: intransitive *(for)*].

(65) It might be Marie, calling to ask if he was still working and should she wait dinner (TC 225).

(66) ... why don't you come give me a hand at the café. Cook a little. Wait counter (TC 134).

Note that the two transitive occurrences of *wait* in (65) - (66) have very different meanings. The second one in fact represents a highly productive construction used in AE to express what a person does for a living (cp. also Preisler (1992: 91)), except that the verbs of this construction are *typically* transitive, as opposed to *wait*: [10]

(67)   Kate herself taught school (ST 22) [cp. *school teacher*].

(68)   I hop bells and hump bags and get you room service (LSS 28) [cp. AE *bellhop* (n.)].

The complex verb *tune in*, which is followed by the preposition *to* in BE (LDELC: *tune in*, intransitive, *to*), is often transitive in AE:

(69)   ... when you tune in a station on a radio (CBD usbooks B9000000397).[11]

(70)   Ali Hassan ... kept trying to tune in the news on his car radio (CBD npr S2000910226).

(71)   She flicked on the little TV by my dresser and tuned in The Today Show (CBD usbooks B9000001088).

Secondly, AE may use an intransitive construction where BE would prefer a transitive one, well-known examples being *meet* and *visit*, which in AE tend to become *meet with* and *visit with (somebody)*, see e.g. Trudgill and Hannah (1982: 56).

In fact, the tendency for the object of a transitive verb to become the subject of the same verb used intransitively – though found also in BE – seems to be particularly strong in AE; cp.

(72)   He had conquered his impulse to anger now (CBD usbooks B9000000447) [i.e. to get angry, cp. 'something angered him'].[12]

(73)   I still hurt thinking of it (TC 162) [cp. 'it still hurts me to think of it'].

(74)   I don't impress easily (LSS 63) [cp. transitive (passive) 'I'm not easily impressed,' corresponding to an active (less idiomatic) sentence like 'people don't impress me ...'].

(75)   ... the trucking concerns which had located here originally ... (ST 159) [cp. 'which located themselves here originally ...'].

(76)   'Have you talked to Pat Harvey?' 'Since the articles ran in the *Post*?' (PCA 315) [cp. 'since they ran the articles ...'].

(77)   Dick and Perry ... had been living ... in a double room renting for eighteen dollars weekly (TC 227) [cp. 'which they rented for ...'].

---

[10]This was pointed out to me by John Dienhart.
[11]The CobuildDirect text providing this example is *The Harper Dictionary of Science in Everyday Language* (!).
[12]In the CobuildDirect UK material, the intransitive use of the verb *anger* is attested only in the expression *quick/slow to anger*.

Thirdly, in AE, some transitive verbs allow an indirect object where such a construction would be much less usual in BE. Cp.

(78) Knock out a preliminary version tonight ... and you can phone me in the final touches from Heathbury (DF 146).

(79) Her grandparents had traded her parents the mansion for the cabin (LA 80).

Inserting a pronominal indirect object, which is coreferential with the subject, between *have (got)* and its direct object is often used in depicting AE characters as speakers of rural varieties, which is why it is often accompanied by indisputable manifestations of nonstandard English like *ain't* and double negatives. The feature is a common colloquialism, however, which should not be considered nonstandard in AE; thus the speakers in the following examples – though portrayed in terms of local origin in various ways – are both highly educated middle class characters whose grammar is standard English:

(80) ... sometimes I think he oughta have himself a peckerectomy (ST 125).

(81) 'I'll bet you a box of cigars ... you can't get that stuck airplane clear ...' 'Keep her moving, son. Now I got me an incentive' (AH 245).

BE examples of this seem mostly confined to speakers of nonstandard BE, as in

(82) I had me a man once ... I loved that man something awful (CBD ukbooks B0000000115).

The last AE-BE difference of verbal grammar that I will discuss in this article concerns the occasional use of *be* before a past participle, in AE, where in BE (and often AE) one might have expected perfect *have*. I have chosen to deal with this as a question of complementation, seeing it as a greater tendency in AE to produce copula constructions on a par with e.g. *(when she came home, she noticed that) one of the windows was broken*. In other words, rather than declaring *be* an alternative perfect auxiliary in AE, I prefer to regard *be* in such examples as a copula, with a subject complement consisting of a past-participle (clause) describing a state.[13]

(83) And underneath the pocket, chilly flesh that was stiffened into rigor mortis (SK 262).

(84) We're borrowed up to the hilt (NW 30).

(85) I was already packed (EJ 179).

(86) It was become so routine (NM 149).

(87) Clear liquors are become more popular at the expense of ... grain colored whiskeys (CBD npr S2000920413).

---

[13]The inherent transitional meaning of *become* in (86) and (87) is not as easily reconciled with that interpretation as the meanings of the other participles.

I found one example (with *become*, besides a few doubtful or spurious ones) in the CobuildDirect UK material (all UK corpora included). Similar forms to (83) and (84) were all passive constructions in the UK material, e.g.

(88)   ... will continue ... until the rules are stiffened (CBD ukmags N0000000547).

Interestingly enough, the only UK example with *packed* comparable to (85)[14] was one in which *pack* means 'to carry a gun regularly,' which usage, according to LDCE, is 'AmE infml.'(!):

(89)   The chicks are packed! (CBD ukmags N0000000493) [*chicks* in the sense of 'girls'!]

In conclusion, I have tried to show – for just one grammatical area (the verb) – that grammatial differences between AE and BE tend to be more numerous than they are often claimed to be, especially in (language reflecting) the spoken language. Many of them are relative rather than absolute differences, which is why the use of informants is practically impossible. To paraphrase Hymes 1971: 281, an informant may accept a construction as possible, feasible and even appropriate in his/her variety, but this is still no guarantee that it is actually used (much) in that variety. Comparative descriptions of AE and BE, therefore, require the use of huge text corpora for statistical analysis.

Some AE-BE differences may be trivial in terms of mutual understanding. A good example not dealt with in this article is *that* used as an optional conjunction, which in informal usage is more often absent in AE, to the extent that the relative absence of *that*-conjunctions in many AE texts is in itself enough to give them an American 'flavor.' However, as I have pointed out, adjectives like 'relative' and 'trivial' could also be used to describe *functional* variation; if we recognize that the study of language in its social functions is important, then surely the study of geographically, hence *culturally*, determined variation is equally important.

The grammatical differences between AE and BE – though the manifestations of each of them may be infrequent – together make up variety-specific, identifiable patterns whose particulars can often be subsumed under general headings at a higher level of linguistic description. It is true that their variables concern us as *geo*linguistic, not sociolinguistic variables, as the focus is on their geographically specific, *standard* variants only. Still, just as I have previously suggested that the concept of Inherent Variability (e.g. Trudgill 1974: 45f) could be applied to the description of Standard English in functional terms (cp. Preisler 1995: 349f), I suggest that this concept might also prove extremely useful in the geolinguistic delimitation of Standard AE as opposed to Standard BE.

---

[14] Tim Caudery has pointed out to me that the *Shorter Oxford Dictionary* gives an example quoting from J. Cannan.

Abbreviations – Primary Sources

AH   Arthur Hailey, *Airport*, New York: Bantam, 1981 (first published 1968).

BF   Bruce Fraser, Hedged performatives. In P. Cole and J. L. Morgan (eds.) *Syntax and Semantics 3: Speech Acts*. New York: Academic Press, 1975, pp. 187-210.

CBD CobuildDirect, 50 million word corpus consisting of 11 subcorpora, of which the following have been used for this article:

bbc	3m	BBC World Service radio
ukbooks	5m	Books: miscellaneous (UK)
ukephem	3m	UK ephemera
ukmags	5m	Popular magazines (UK)
times	5m	Times newspaper (UK)
today	5m	Today newspaper (UK)
ukspok	10m	Informal speech (UK)
npr	3m	National Public Radio (US)
usbooks	5m	Books: miscellaneous (US)
usephem	1m	US ephemera

CC   Clive Cussler, *Vixen 03*, New York: Bantam, 1979.

CH   Colin Harrison, *Break and Enter.* Toronto etc.: Bantam, 1991.

DF   Dick Francis, *Forfeit*, London: Pan, 1970.

DI   David Ignatius, *SIRO*, New York: Avon, 1991.

EJ   Erica Jong, *How to Save Your Own Life*, New York: Signet, 1977.

FF   Frederick Forsyth, *The Odessa File*, London: Corgi, 1973.

GK   Gustav Kirchner, [AE examples from] *Die syntaktischen Eigentümlichkeiten des amerikanischen English*, see Kirchner (1970).

JK   Jonathan Kellerman, *Devil's Waltz*, New York: Bantam, 1993.

LA   Lisa Alther, *Kinflicks*, Harmondsworth: Penguin, 1983.

LDCE *The Longman Dictionary of Contemporary English.*

LDELC *The Longman Dictionary of English Language and Culture.*

LS   Linda L. Schuler, *Voice of the Eagle*, New York: Signet, 1993.

LSS Lawrence Sanders, *The Sixth Commandment*, New York: Berkley, 1979.

LST Lawrence Sanders, *The Third Deadly Sin*, London: Granada, 1981.

MF   Marilyn French, *The Bleeding Heart*, London: Sphere, 1980.

NM   Norman Mailer, *The Deer Park*, London: Granada, 1978.

NW   *Newsweek* 1986-12-08.

PCA   Patricia Cornwell, *All that Remains*, New York: Avon, 1993.

PCB   Patricia Cornwell, *The Body Farm*, New York: Berkley, 1994.

RC   Robin Cook, *Fever*, New York: Signet, 1982.

RL   R. B. Lees, A multiply ambiguous adjectival construction. In *Language*, Vol. 36, No. 2 (1960) 207-221.

SK   Stephen King, *Thinner*, New York: Penguin, 1984.

ST   Scott Turow, *The Burden of Proof*, New York: Warner Books, 1990.

TC   Truman Capote, *In Cold Blood*, New York: Signet, 1965.

WG   William Goldman, *Control*, New York: Dell, 1982.

References

Algeo, J. (1988). British and American Grammatical Differences. In *International Journal of Lexicography* Vol. 1, No. 1, 1-31.

Baron, Dennis E. (1982). *Grammar and Good Taste: Reforming the American Language*. New Haven: Yale University Press.

Benson, M., E. Benson & R. Ilson (1986). *Lexicographic Description of English*. Amsterdam: John Benjamins.

Gallardo, A. (1984). *The Standardization of American English*. Universidad de Concepción, Chile.

Hymes, D. H. (1971). On Communicative Competence. In J. B. Pride & J. Holmes (eds) *Sociolinguistics*. Harmondsworth: Penguin (1974), 269-293.

Kirchner, G. (1970). *Die syntaktischen Eigentümlichkeiten des amerikanischen English*. München: Max Hueber.

Preisler, B. (1977). The place of the Subjunctive in the System of Modality in English. In Working Papers in Language and Linguistics (Tasmanian Coll. of Advanced Ed., Launceston) 5, 16-40.

Preisler, B. (1992). *A Handbook of English Grammar on Functional Principles*. Aarhus: Aarhus Univ. Press.

Preisler, B. (1995). Standard English in the World. In *Multilingua* 14-4, 341-362.

Strevens, P. (1972). *British and American English*. London: Collier-Macmillan.

Švejcer, A. D. (1978). *Standard English in the United States and England*. The Hague: Mouton.

Trudgill, P. (1974). *Sociolinguistics*. Harmondsworth: Penguin.

Trudgill, P. & J. Hannah (1982). *International English*. London: Arnold.

Understanding Semantics

Torben Thrane

1. Language understanding[1]

Language understanding is considered the preserve of psycholinguistics, and has been for a long time. Yet it is far too important to be left to the devices of experimental psychologists. To show why, I shall sketch a manifesto about the policies of linguistics. Then I shall show how the new linguistic policy in conjunction with information theory affects two well-defined topics in English linguistics: article usage and the lexical semantics of nouns.

I shall begin with a small anecdote. Two priests are discussing if it's permissible to smoke and pray at the same time. They disagree, so they write to the Pope for guidance. One writes: "Is it permissible to smoke while you pray?". He receives the reply: "Of course not. *Nothing* should interfere with the solemnity of prayer". The other writes: "Is it permissible to pray while you smoke?" and receives the reply: "Of course it is. It is *always* permissible to pray, no matter what you are doing."

The point is this: *The quality of the answer is embedded in the shape of the question.*

Now, what is the shape of the questions you usually ask of linguistics? According to Chomsky 1986: 3 there are only three questions worth asking, or (1995: 17f) only three of the potentially interesting questions available for precise answers at present:

(1)   What constitutes knowledge of a language?
(2)   How does such knowledge develop?
(3)   How is such knowledge put to use?

I think there are other questions worth asking about language and linguistics, and I think that they may be available for precise answers. I think, for example, that it would be interesting to know

---

[1] This paper is a slightly revised version of a lecture given at the Aarhus School of Business in 1995. Since then, many people have been kind enough to ask me to publish it, but I have felt that both its content, style and presentation called for a rather less austere form of publication than that provided by the standard learned journal. Such an occasion is being offered by the publication of this *Festschrift* – and it is the more apposite since its recipient was much involved in the circumstances around the original lecture.
    The context of the paper is the long-term project *COmputational Dynamic tEXt UnderStanding*, which has occupied me on and off over the last half dozen years. Previous articles in the project are Thrane (1992a, 1992b, 1993, 1994a, 1994b). The functional view of meaning behind the project goes back to Thrane (1980, 1983).

(4)   What constitutes understanding of a language?

Chomsky would probably say that this is a less general question than his number (3) and therefore included in it. The reason would be that in order to understand a language, you have to know it. *When* you know it, understanding it is one of the ways in which you may put your knowledge to use.

Given the Innateness Hypothesis this is a sound argument. Yet I prefer one that does not crucially presuppose, but rather sustains, its validity:

Knowing and understanding are both cognitive capacities. But whereas knowing is a cognitive *state,* understanding is a cognitive *process*. Both are *information-based* capacities for imposing internal order on the chaos of external things. But whereas knowing is the state of having such order, understanding is the process of creating it. Knowing and understanding are the static and dynamic counterparts of each other.

I would argue, therefore, that questions (1) and (4) are two versions of the same *underlying* question, and that the answers you get for each of them may be qualitatively different, much in the way of the two versions of the question about smoking and praying. For the quality of the answer is embedded in the shape of the question.

It is time to comment on the ambiguity of the title. If your concern is language understanding, then you'll start looking for properties of sentences that make them *interpretable*. This is reflected in reading (5a) of the title:

(5a)   under`standing se$_1$mantics = the semantics used in understanding (something)

If there is truth to my claim that the quality of the answer is embedded in the shape of the question, then the answers to questions (1) and (4) are likely to lead to different conceptions of the very nature and practice of semantics. This is reflected in reading (5b):

(5b)   under$_1$standing se`mantics = understanding the subject matter of semantics

There is another way to explain the ambiguity of the title. One of the leading questions in semantics has always been 'what *is* meaning?'. This is connected to reading (5b). In order to understand *semantics*, you should at the very least know what *meaning* is. Even so, it has proved a remarkably tough question to answer.

I have therefore followed my usual tactics of replacing it with another: 'what does meaning *do?*' This is related to reading (5a). If you understand a sentence, then it's because the semantics of the sentence has *let* you. It is also a more linguistic than a philosophical question, for it assumes a functionality of meaning that can be addressed by general linguistic methods, developed to account for the functionality of language.

And yet it also matters to philosophers, or at least to Frederick Dretske:

> I have become increasingly preoccupied with the question, not of what meaning (or content) *is* but what meaning (content) *does*. It is no good having a theory of meaning if the meaning in question doesn't *do* something, something that both needs to be done and will, without the help of meaning, not be done. Does the mind do something the brain can't do? Is there something that meaning does that a material bearer-of-meaning can't do? Is there, for that matter, something that information (understood as a semantic commodity) does that a signal or event *carrying* that information can't do? If not, why are philosophers (some of us anyway) so interested in getting a theory of meaning or semantic information? People stopped talking about the soul when they realized that there was nothing for the soul to do. Information and meaning deserve the same fate. (Dretske, 1990: 6)

So, what I set out to do in these somewhat lofty terms is no less than trying to salvage information and meaning from the tragic fate of the soul.

What I am setting out to do *here*, in more specific terms, is to answer the question:

(6) Given that language understanding is a cognitive, information-driven process, what is the role of linguistic meaning in the provision of the information needed for understanding natural language sentences?

2. Meaning as instructions for cognitive activity

The view of meaning behind this paper is that conventional, linguistic meaning is not representational but *instructional*. Linguistic meaning somehow makes explicit the information that the cognitive processes involved in language understanding need in order to run. This view involves a number of additional notions that have to be clarified: *concept, semantic content, model* and *mental model*.

I shall give proper explanations of 'concept' and 'semantic content' in due course. For reasons of space, however, I shall give no comprehensive explanation of models and mental models, but simply assume that a model is a scheme for the representation of knowledge, and that a *mental* model is a special *dynamical* kind of model for what is assumed to be involved in human knowledge manipulation.[2] Whenever I just talk of 'models' in the following, it should be understood that I think of 'mental models'. Since the main character in this paper is *meaning*, however, I shall begin by stating the relevant propositions for that:

(7) Natural language expressions have semantic *effects* on models in virtue of carrying conventional meaning.

Proposition (7) is the basic principle of semantic effect. It first says that meaning *does* something. Then it says what meaning *does*. The notion of semantic *effect* must

---

[2]The main sources of inspiration for (mental) models in this connection are Kamp 1981, Johnson-Laird 1983; 1993, Fauconnier 1985, Dinsmore 1991, Kamp & Reyle 1993.

be seen in relation to models. The semantic effect of a linguistic item is the contribution made by that item towards the construction, maintenance, or handling of models.

(8) The semantic effect of a complex expression is a function of the semantic effects of its parts, plus the semantic effects of the structural rules by which it is composed.

This may look familiar. It is the dynamic counterpart of the semantic principle of compositionality. It says, in effect, that a model is not one big, unstructured affair, but is composed of partial representations, interrelated in various ways. In particular, a model may be recursively embedded in a larger model, which is ultimately embedded in a Top Model. This is not what you may think it is. The Top Model contains the background knowledge – including lexical knowledge – available to the model as a whole.

(9) The semantic effects that a linguistic item has in virtue of being a carrier of meaning is always the same. This I call the principle of *uniformity of semantic effect*.

This proposition is no doubt the most controversial and least obvious of the three. What it *says* is that whichever semantic effect an item may have on a model, it will have the *same* effect on any other model.

Since it is far from obvious how this could be true, the rest of the paper is designed to show that it not only *can* be true, but indeed *must* be, if we are to give a principled account of interpretation and understanding at all. The topic I shall use for illustration is one of the most well-studied topics in English grammar: the articles, and in particular the definite article. But we cannot discuss the articles independently of nouns. Therefore we must make a detour into the jungle of informational and semantical properties of lexical nouns. The reader may well find this a strenuous tour, for we may have to take some unfamiliar pathways, and even cut some new ones.

3. The articles in English

Descriptive grammars of English offer detailed instructions for the *use* of the articles, which is quite as it should be. They do not usually say anything about what the articles mean *in themselves*, which is also quite understandable. To say that the meaning of the definite article is "definiteness" isn't very helpful. Therefore, descriptions of article usage are always given in terms of the types of noun they can appear with, and in terms of the kind of reference such combinations can be used to express. The picture is often generalized in schematic form, something like this:

The reference types are referential in the sense that they are supposed to pick out something in the physical world. Cutting across this extensional kind of reference, there is another, textual one, which deals with the correlations between NP's in a

NOUN TYPE	FORM	REFERENCE TYPE		
		Generic	Specific	
			Indefinite	Definite
Count	Sg	*the lion* *a lion*	*a lion*	*the lion*
	Pl	*lions*	*(sm) lions*	*the lions*
Noncount	Sg Pl	*whisky* *(the) measles*	*(sm) whisky* **(sm) measles*	*the whisky* **the measles*

sentence or text. A definite NP *refers anaphorically* to an indefinite NP in the textual context. An indefinite NP introduces a new object into the universe of discourse. This, at least, is the standard assumption.

All this indicates that article usage cannot be adequately described without appeal to various *presupposed* kinds of reference, situational or textual. I am certainly not argueing that this is wrong for a descriptive account. But I *am* going to argue that this will not do for an account of article interpretation. It is in clear violation of the principle of uniformity of semantic effect, for it leads to the awkward conclusion – as appears from the table – that there are in fact *two* sets of definite and indefinite articles in English, one pair concerned with generic, the other with specific reference. And the picture would be even messier if we introduced the opposition *specific-nonspecific* for the indefinite, and the opposition *referential-attributive* for the definite article.

It might be objected that this is just theory-dependent criticism, for who says that the principle of uniformity of semantic effect is true? But then try this. It cannot, in principle, be right to base a theory of language understanding on its ability to predict the referential intentions of the speaker. For there is no accounting for speakers' intentions. We must base our theory on the assumption that a NP carries the information needed for its interpretation. In other words, it must be the various types of reference that should be predictable from an account of NP interpretation.

I will quote a few examples to sustain my account of the descriptive approach to article usage. At the same time, they appeal to some kind of mental activity, the first by the speaker, the second by the listener:

> In discussing the use of the articles, it is essential to make a distinction between specific and generic reference. If we say

>   a lion and two tigers are sleeping in a cage
> the reference is specific, since *we have in mind* specific specimens of the class 'tiger'.
>
> (Quirk et al. 1972: 147; my italics)
>
> (46) Before I go to bed I always turn down the heating
>
> In example (46) there is no point in asking 'Which heating?': **we assume on the basis of our familiarity with the situation** that there is *one* heating system in **the room** or in **the house** and that it is this particular heating system that is turned down.
>
> (Ek & Robat 1984: 120; my emphasis)

Here is clear indication that 'what we have in mind' and 'what we assume' plays a role in descriptive explanations. Such expressions suggest the involvement of a mental model.

But how is the reader of the last passage supposed to be able to understand it? The writers use phrases like *the room* and *the house*, but neither rooms nor houses have been introduced into the text before. So it is not anaphoric reference. And it cannot be *this* room I am in *here and now* which is referred to. Indeed, is anything specific referred to? If there is we should know which room and which house it is, otherwise the use of *the* would be wrong. Is the reference perhaps generic? No, for then they would be talking about houses and rooms in general, and example (46) indicates that talk is about the house belonging to whoever *'I'* refers to. And who is that? Ek or Robat? Anyone? The point clearly is that instead of asking what the definite article *means*, we should ask: What does the definite article tell us to *do*?

There are, in fact, *two* things that the definite article tells us to do. One of them can be inferred from an insight about article usage by Schibsbye (1956), who says that the definite article basically has something to do with *identification*. So the definite article tells us to *identify* something.

The second relates to an insight by Hawkins (1978). It says that the definite article has something to do, not with *uniqueness*, but with *inclusiveness*. If I say *the children are in bed*, my listener may assume that I mean *all* the relevant children, and not just some of them. So the second thing the definite article tells us to do is to identify *all* instances of something.

Now, in order to *identify* anything, we must *look* for it – and we must look for it *somewhere*. Unfortunately, the definite article does not tell us *where* to look, nor what to look *for*. As for *where* to look, it has always been assumed that it should be somewhere *near*, like the situational or textual context, but at the *very* least, somewhere outside our *heads*. Hence the various reference types. When *this* did not quite work, new reference types were invented – like the generic, the associative and the attributive. These two are exemplified by sentences like

(10)   I was *driving* along merrily when *the car* broke down (association from *driving*)

(11)   *The winner* must have been fast (whoever he is – since Linford Christie was in the race)

The *where-to-look* question has also led to all sorts of philosophical controversies over examples like

(12)   The Golden Mountain does not exist

– for there was supposed to be an existential presupposition on the definite article, and if you could not find a referent in the *real* world, you must invent a *possible* one, with Golden Mountains in it. All this, just to avoid looking inside the head.

I think *now* – but I did not use to – that the place to look is precisely into our heads, and not directly into the real or some possible world. In fact, I do not think we can give an account of *understanding* without looking inside people's heads, for after all – that is where it *happens*. And that is what mental models are for.

What still needs explaining is what the *something* is that we are supposed to identify, and *how*. This point concerns the *noun* in the NP. This is where we leave the beaten track to veer off into an information-theoretic account of lexical semantics.

4. Information and concepts

I have already introduced the notions of *concept* and *semantic content*, but without explanation. It follows here. Concepts are *not* the same as words. The *concept* "lion" is not the same as the *word* 'lion'. Concepts are private, words – so far at least – are public. *My* concept of "lion" may differ from your concept of "lion". I can use the word 'lion' to communicate to you the fact that I *have* the concept "lion", but it will not be *my* concept of "lion" that you receive. It will be your own, which is *evoked* by my use of the word 'lion'. So, although words and concepts are not the same, they are related in some way. This section explains how.

Words – and for now, words are lexical nouns – are structures carrying lexical meaning, as I think everyone agrees. Concepts, I shall argue, are also structures carrying meaning. But whereas words, as public creatures, carry their meaning on their sleeve, openly, socially, concepts carry their meaning privately, inaccessibly to others. They carry *cognitive* meaning. But what is that, and where does it come from?

The short answer is: from *information*. Let me explain by example. Imagine that someone asked you: *what's this?* – handing you a tumbler with amber liquid in it. You look at it, smell it, taste it, and decide that it is *whisky*. So this is what you say: 'whisky'. Now, you *could* have said instead: '*information*'. That would have been true as well, but only in a derivative sense. When people ask you what something *is*, then they want you to tell them *what* it is, not *how you came to know* what it is.

And that would be what you did by replying 'information'. For it was by interpreting the *information* carried by the liquid that you came to decide what it was.

The information processing that led to the decision consisted in comparing the pattern of incoming information against patterns of information that you already had. Let us say, for example, that you immediately, just by looking at the colour, discarded the possibilities of milk, wine, fruitjuice, coffee, water, and a great many others. Then, by smell, you discarded cold tea, white port, stale beer, and many others. Finally, let us say, the choice was between brandy, calvados and whisky. These possibilities you eventually reduced by taste to one: *whisky*. During this process the incoming pattern of information has been generalized, transformed and greatly reduced. These comparisons were attempts to decide if the incoming pattern of information was a token of an already existing type of information pattern. The decision that the incoming pattern was a token of a preexisting type amounted to an instantiation of the type in some mental model.

The patterns of information that you already had are *concepts*. It is important to note that you *have* them whether or not you have *words* for them. It would not be inconsistent for you to say: *I don't know what it's called, but I've tasted it before.* You can also have a *private* word for it, for it would not be inconsistent for you to say: *I don't know what* you *call it, but I call it 'uisgebeah'*. But the *public* word for it, in English, is *whisky*. You could also have a mistaken word for it, for it would not have been inconsistent for you to have said *brandy* instead of *whisky*. It would just have been wrong.

Let us now say that you are somewhat of a whisky connoisseur. You are not in doubt, then, that it is *whisky* in the tumbler, but *which?* Is it a Lagavulin 10 years old or a Laphroaig 16 years old? They are both Islay malts, they are both quite peaty, and if you could be sure they were the same age you wouldn't be in doubt, for although Laphroaig is usually *more* peaty than Lagavulin, it tends to loose a little of its peatyness with age.

Now, these are quite conscious deliberations, and you are down to a very finegrained analysis of information. Not many could do it – *not* because they would not have access to the same *information* that you do, but because they do not have the *conceptual discrimination* that you have. In addition, many people would not have 'Lagavulin' and 'Laphroaig' in their vocabulary.

So what is going on here? A straightforward answer seems to be that you – the expert – have *more* concepts, and concepts with *more* information packed into them, than the non-expert. The bundle or cluster of information packed into a concept is its *semantic content*. Your concept of "Lagavulin" – a concept the layman does not even *have* – contains far more bits of information than the layman's concept of "whisky" – indeed, your concept of "whisky" is sure to contain more bits of information than the layman's concept of "whisky" – bits that reflect your knowledge of how it is made, what its history is, and so on.

Once a concept is 'packed', as it were, it has aquired *cognitive meaning*. To you, the concept "whisky" now *means* whatever information is packed into it. So the cognitive meaning of concepts arises in virtue of information. It is, in a sense, *distilled* information. But this is not the information the layman is getting when you use the word 'whisky' in a sentence which he hears. As already mentioned, he gets at most whatever information is packed into his concept of "whisky". So how can we understand each other? Well, the truth is that quite often we do not – at least not *precisely*.

That we do at all is due to the role of lexical meaning in the flow of information.

5. Lexical meaning and information

Once again, let us replace the question of what lexical meaning *is* by the question of what it *does*. For once, this is a question that semantics has dealt with. The reply usually is: it conveys *information*. Or, to be more precise, language is said to *convey* information in virtue of the fact that it *carries* meaning, where 'meaning' at least *includes* lexical meaning. But how does it do that? This is the question we will pursue.

Now if you, the connoisseur, show me, the layman *without* the concept "Lagavulin", a tumbler with something in it and say: *This is Lagavulin,* has your utterance *conveyed* any information to me? Yes, lots: that you speak English, that you are an adult, that you don't have a cold, and a great many other things besides. This information is *source-oriented*.[3] It contributes to the creation in me of a mental model in terms of which I interpret the utterance situation as a *physical* occurrence. But has it informed me *what is in the glass?* No – except in the trivial sense that you are prepared to call it 'Lagavulin'. But that, presumably, was precisely what you *wanted* your utterance to convey. You did not specifically want it to convey the fact that you speak English, nor any of the other things it *did* convey (though you may have, of course – for there is, as I said, no accounting for speakers' intentions).

Nonetheless, 'Lagavulin' carries *meaning*. But if it carries meaning, and if it conveys information *in virtue of* its meaning, how can it have failed to inform me? Well, obviously because I do not *know* the meaning of the word. But what is it to know the meaning of a word, or simply to be able to *understand* it? It is the ability to create a mental model with inclination of fit, not towards the signal, or source, but towards something else, a target which is *different* from the signal and the source. The difference between mental models with inclination of fit towards the source of the signal and those with inclination of fit away from it corresponds to the difference between non-symbolic and symbolic representation.

---

[3]Cf. Thrane (1992a,b; and especially 1993) for detailed discussion of the notions of inclination of fit, source and target in this connection.

I hope we agreed that we could have a concept without having a *word* for it. But this is the opposite question: Can we *have* a word, in the sense of knowing its *meaning* and being able to *understand* it, *without* having a concept joined with it? The answer, I am sure, is *no,* and I will try to explain why.

Think of a jigsaw puzzle. The joint between a word and a concept within the same mental model is just like the joint between two pieces of a jigsaw puzzle, like this:

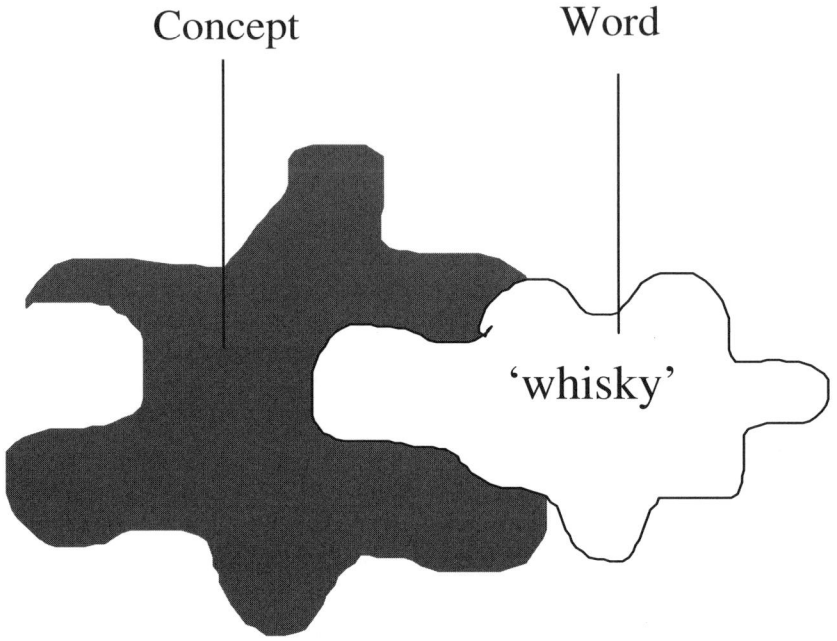

This is supposed to represent a revival of the Saussurean, biplane sign in new clothing: the piece representing the word 'whisky' bears the inscription 'whisky'. This is the *signifiant*, or expression. The *shape* of the piece is the *signifié*, or the content, which defines its place in lexical structure. They are inseparable, but neither is immutable.

As I said, the concept linked to the word 'whisky' differs in cognitive meaning from expert to layman. I shall represent this difference like this:

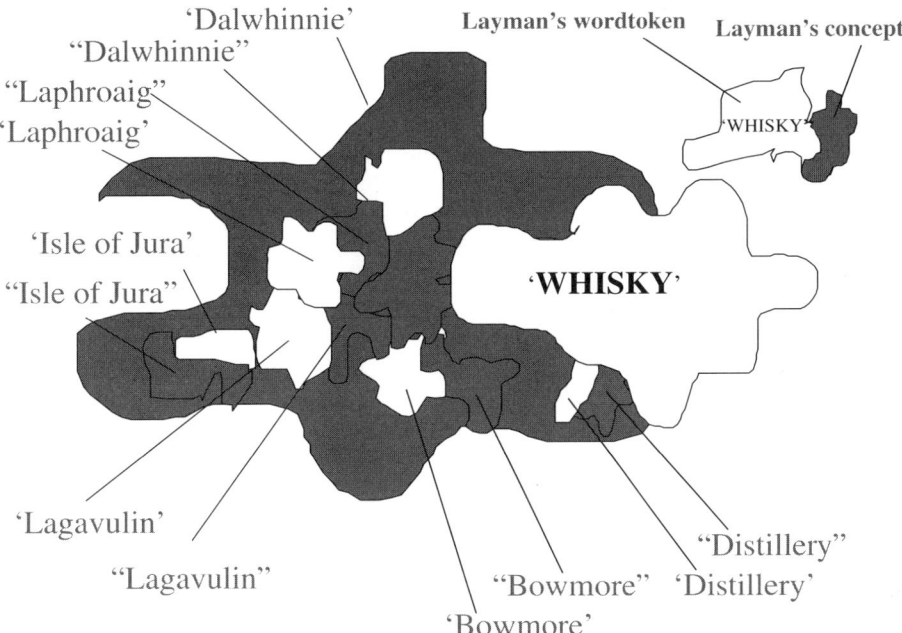

Puzzle 2: Connoisseur's concept and word token 'whisky'

What has happened, graphically speaking, is that the piece representing the expert's concept "whisky" has been cut into a whole jigsaw puzzle of its own, with two adjoining pieces representing, respectively, the concept "Lagavulin" and the word 'Lagavulin'. Other two-piece combinations represent other concept-word pairs. The piece representing the layman's concept, on the other hand, is still undivided: to the layman, we assume, whisky is whisky, and there's an end to't.

The type-token distinction now shows itself again. Obviously, the expert and the layman each has his own private *token* of the public word *type* 'whisky'. The expert's word-token 'whisky' looms larger in *his* vocabulary than the layman's does in *his*. But since the two tokens are tokens of the same *type*, they share the same *meaning*. The larger amount of information that the expert gets access to for dealing with utterances containing the word 'whisky' stems from the semantic content of the concept linked to his private word 'whisky', not from the meaning of the public word.

The picture that emerges from this you may find very strange. It can be drawn like this:

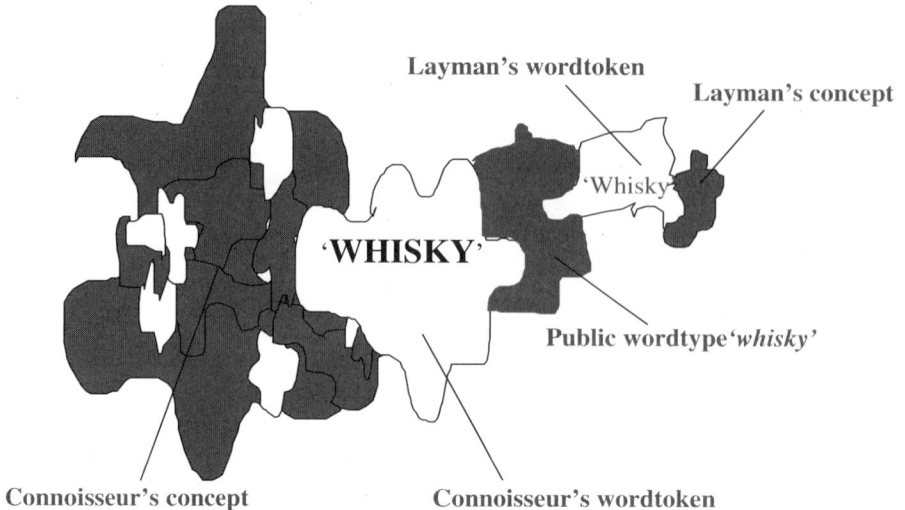

The idea behind it, however, is quite simple in an information-theoretic context. It is the idea that *the uniform semantic effect of lexical items is to establish communication channels between concepts in different mental models.* Public wordtypes trigger corresponding private word tokens, which in turn trigger private concepts linked to them. But where does that leave lexical *meaning*?

I said before that it was the *transformation* and *reduction* of incoming information that resulted in the distillation of semantic content into cognitive meaning. But this was on the *personal, individual* level, for cognitive meaning is covert. Now we are looking for an account of meaning on the *public, social* level, for lexical meaning is *overt*.

Presented in these terms, the problem points to its own solution. The lexical meaning of a noun must be the meaning of the public noun *type*. It is therefore an *abstraction,* obtained from the generalized, transformed and reduced information carried by all the *tokens* of that type. In other words, the semantic content of a lexical noun-*type* is the *average amount of information that has ever been transmitted through its tokens* from a transmitting concept to a receiving concept on every occasion of use. *Although* it is an abstraction, this entity is stable enough to count as the *lexical meaning* of a noun and to account for the possibility of compiling dictionaries. At the same time it is flexible enough to allow for explanations of semantic change, metaphorical usage, and many other phenomena.

Matters of lexical meaning are not *quite* as simple as this account has made them out to be (they never are, are they). But even this simplified account has done what we set out to do in this section.

It has made sense of the claim that language *conveys* information *in virtue of carrying* meaning. It does so by taking lexical meaning as a sort of *transmission channel* through which *one* concept may transmit information to another. The information actually passing *through* the channel is about *which* concept has been transmitting, and so acts as an instruction for, which concept should be the receiver. But the actual *meaning* of what we hear and read, stems from the cognitive meaning of our *own* conceptual structures.

Along the way it has been argued that words are public word types with private word tokens. We can now see why both are needed. If I can have a private or a wrong word for a concept which in other mental models would be linked to a private token of the public word 'whisky', then it is because there is no causal – but only an informational[4] – relation linking concepts to private words to public words. And if I can utter a token of a public word (say 'sesquipedalian') without the slightest idea of what it means, then it is because there is no concept linked to my (private) token of it. This is just another way of saying that we cannot have a public word – in the sense of knowing its meaning – without having a concept linked to a private token of it. Taken together, these two points constitute the grounds of the claim that both public and private words are needed.

This ends our rough ride through lexical semantics. I shall now turn to the last point: to present a recipe for the interpretation of an NP consisting of the definite article followed by a single noun, like *the lion*. It will respect the principle of uniformity of semantic effect, and it will show how the various types of reference in fact may be deduced from it.

6. Recipe for the interpretation of simple *the* + *N*

To remind you, I have mentioned four points that an account must satisfy in order to respect the principle of uniformity of semantic effect:

(1)   It cannot appeal to the *prior* existence of reference types as the basis of explanation. Different reference types must be different *consequences* of essentially the same procedure. Therefore it is necessary to operate with mental models, rather than with extensional models.

(2)   It must make it clear what *identification* is

(3)   It must make it clear what *inclusiveness* is

(4)   It must respect the *semantic effect* of lexical nouns

These four points lead to the suggestion that a NP like *the lion* carries information that will activate an interpretive procedure, which could be described like this in semiformal terms:

---

[4] I am here once more following Dretske (1980: 26ff) in his distinction between causal and informational relations.

- look in the *current mental model* for *every instantiation* of the concept "lion"
- if *one and only one instance* is found then EXIT with *SUCCESS*

    (1) look at *the lion*. Isn't it magnificent? → singular, definite reference

    (2) there was a lion .... *The lion* ..... → anaphoric reference

- if *NOT SUCCESS* then look for any *instantiation* of a concept with a semantic content that *includes* a concept with the semantic content of "lion"
- if *one and only one* such inclusive concept is found, then *instantiate* the concept "lion" in the current mental model and EXIT with *SUCCESS*

    (3) (On returning from the ZOO). *The lion* was old → associative, situational

    (4) There were many animals. *The lion* was the biggest → associative, anaphoric

- if more than one *instance* of the concept "lion" is found then *FAIL* and EXIT

    (5) (You are both looking at a pride of lion). 'Look at the lion' → ID failure

    (6) 'There were five lions in the cage. The lion ...' → ID failure

- if *no instance* is found in the current model then *shift* to the mental model including the current model and *repeat* process *until* you reach Top Model

    (Yesterday there was a TV-news report of a lion which had escaped from the circus. You watched it with your children. Now, today, you are reading in the paper that it has been caught, and you say:)

    (7) *The lion* has been caught → singular, definite reference, larger situation use

- if *NOT SUCCESS*, but if you have a concept attached to the word 'lion' as a type, then revise its semantic content and EXIT with *SUCCESS*

    (8) the lion is the king of the animals

- if not *SUCCESS*, then *create* new concept type with semantic content "king of the animals" and attach it to the word 'lion' in Top Model; EXIT with *SUCCESS*

    (9) Now I know what 'lion' means → concept formation

- if *NOT SUCCESS*, then EXIT with *FAIL*

    (10) I'm not sure I understand what you mean by 'lion' → request for further information

Input to the procedure is the current mental model and the NP *the lion*. What the procedure now does, in plain language, is this:

If there is one and only one lion represented in the current model then this is the one you are looking for. Therefore, you can stop looking. These are the steps leading to simple cases of singular, definite and anaphoric reference, as exemplified in (1) and (2).

If you could not find a lion directly, look for representations of something with which lions can be associated. If there is one and only one of these, then make a representation of a lion and stop looking. This leads to associative types of reference, situational and anaphoric, as exemplified by (3) and (4).

If there are more than one representation of a lion in the current model, then you do not know which one is to be identified. Therefore stop. This is exemplified by the referentially deviant examples (5) and (6).

If there are no representations of lions in the current model, then shift into the embedding model and look for one there. Keep doing this until you have found one or reached the Top Model. Picking up a conversation from the day before would be an example of this, as that sketched in connection with (7).

If you *still* have not found any representations of lions, but you have the concept of "lion" in your Top Model, then this is what you want. This leads to generic types of reference, exemplified in (8).

If you do not have the concept, you can now either *create* it or abandon the search, asking for further information. Both are strategies involved in concept formation, as exemplified in (9) and (10).

Identification is explained in terms of the *instantiation* of a *concept* in a *mental model*. Inclusiveness is explained as a search for *all* instantiations of the relevant concept in the same model. If there are more than one (when the noun is singular), identification *fails.*

The distinction between specific and generic reference is explained in terms of the distinction between concept *instantiation* and concept *type*, whereas no principled distinction between situational and anaphoric reference can be deduced.

So, to conclude, it has been my aim to substantiate a claim that meaning *does* something – in fact that it provides the information in terms of which mental models are constructed, manipulated and searched. And if you feel that what I've said has done something to you, I may have succeeded!

References

Chomsky, N. (1986). *Knowledge of Language. Its Nature, Origin, and Use.* New York: Praeger.

Chomsky, N. (1995). *The Minimalist Program.* Cambridge Massachusetts: MIT.

Dinsmore, J. (1991). *Partitioned Representations. A Study of Mental Representation, Language Understanding and Linguistic Structure.* Dordrecht: Kluwer.

Dretske, F. (1981). *Knowledge and the Flow of Information.* Oxford: Blackwell.

Dretske, F. (1990) Does Meaning Matter? In Enrique Villanueva (ed) *Information, Semantics, & Epistemology.* Oxford: Blackwell.

Ek, J. A. van & N. J. Robat (1984). *The Student's Grammar of English*. Oxford: Blackwell.

Fauconnier, G. (1985). *Mental Spaces. Aspects of meaning constructions in natural language.* Cambridge: CUP, 1994.

Hawkins, J. A. (1978). *Definiteness and indefiniteness: a study in reference and grammaticality prediction.* London: Croom & Helm.

Johnson-Laird, P. N. (1983). *Mental Models.* Cambridge, Massachusetts: Harvard UP.

Johnson-Laird, P. N. (1993). *Human and Machine Thinking.* London: Lawrence Erlbaum.

Kamp, H. (1981). A theory of truth and semantic representation. In J. Groenendijk, T. M. V. Janssen & M. Stokhof (eds) *Formal Methods in the Study of Language.* (MC-Tracts 135). Mathematical Centre, Amsterdam, pp. 277-322.

Kamp, H. & U. Reyle (1993). *From Discourse to Logic.* Vols. 1-2. Dordrecht: Kluwer.

Quirk, R. et al. (1972). *A Grammar of Contemporary English.* London: Longman.

Schibsbye, K. (1956). *Engelsk Grammatik.* Vol. 2. Copenhagen: Munksgaard.

Thrane, T. (1980). *Referential-Semantic Analysis. Aspects of a theory of linguistic reference.* Cambridge: CUP.

Thrane, T. (1983) The Universality of AUX. *AL(H)*, 18.2, 154-200.

Thrane, T. (1992a) The fallacy of descriptivism. In S. L. Hansen & F. Sørensen (eds) *Issues in Semantic Representation.* Copenhagen: Samfundslitteratur 105-125.

Thrane, T. (1992b) Dynamic Text Comprehension. In S. Jansen et al. (eds) *Computational Approaches to Text Understanding.* Copenhagen: Museum Tusculanum, 173-90.

Thrane, T. (1993) The Computations of Text Comprehension. In L. Ahrenberg (ed) *Papers from the 3rd NoTex, Linköping 1992.*

Thrane, T. (1994a) NP-structure and computation. In M. Herslund (ed) *Noun Phrase Structures.* Copenhagen Studies in Language, vol. 17, 13-43.

Thrane, T. (1994b) Constituency and semantic interpretation. In R. Eklund (ed) *NoLiDa '93: Proceedings of '9: e Nordiska Datalingvistikdagarna' Stockholm 3-5 June 1993*. Stockholm 1994, 277-289.

'Free Adjuncts' in English

Torben Vestergaard

1. Introduction

In this paper we shall be concerned with constructions such as the italicized parts of the following examples:

(1)   Black Bush comes from the oldest licenced whiskey distillery in the world, 'Old Bushmill's Distillery'. *Situated in the county of Antrim in Northern Ireland* it received its first official licence to distil in 1608. (back label)

(2)   ... the cockroach, *albeit groggy*, crawled out. (GW 25)

(3)   Terrex is easy to use *requiring only a short period of practice*. (Wolf)

The sequences in question are the constituents termed 'free adjuncts' by Zandvoort (1961) and 'supplementive clauses' by Quirk et al. (1972, 1985). The construction has received scant attention in English linguistics, unlike the corresponding construction in French, which, under the name of *attribut indirect* has been the subject of some investigation, the main problem being how to delimitate it from appositional constituents, cf. Prebensen 1973 and references therein; more recently it has been studied from an argumentation theoretical angle by Nielsen (1996b) under the name of 'free predicate'. The present paper will first attempt to distinguish the construction from related constructions, and then give a preliminary characterization of the semantic relations between it and the main clause in which it occurs. In particular, I shall argue that a functional perspective will allow us to give a more precise characterization of many instances of the construction than that of 'accompanying circumstances', a term by which the free adjunct constructions have often been labelled.

For present purposes we will define the object of analysis as subjectless non-finite or verbless adverbial clauses; as one of their main characteristics, and their main fascination, lies in the fact that they are more loosely attached to the main clause in which they occur than many other constituents, I shall retain Zandvoort's term 'free adjuncts'.

1.2. Data

The present paper is based on data culled from two main sources: journalism and brochures, a genre on the border-line between journalism and advertising, known to be a particularly target-rich area. The brochures can further be broken down into three types: industrial, consumer durables and tourism (for further information, see appendix). I am thus in no way suggesting that my data are representative of the occurrence of free adjuncts in English texts; on the contrary, I have selected text types in which I expected to come across a particularly prolific growth of the phenomenon.

In addition, I cite a couple of examples from outside my corpus.

2. Delimitation

2.1. Free adjuncts and other adverbial clauses

Zandvoort (1961: 35) talks about a free adjunct when a present participle (plus accompanying constituents) a) is equivalent to an adverbial clause, and b) 'there is a clear break between the participle ... and the rest of the sentence ...'.[1] On p. 35, fn. 4 he includes infinitival and nominal constructions among free adjuncts, on p. 52 he further adds that past participles may occur as free adjuncts, and judging from his cross-references on p. 210, his definition covers not only infinitival constructions playing the role of Greenbaum's (1969) conjuncts and style disjuncts (*to begin with, to be frank*) but also clear cases of infinitival purpose constructions. Quirk et al. (1972: 760 and 1985: 1123ff) are more restrictive in their definition of the phenomenon, which they refer to as 'subjectless supplementive clauses', only admitting participial or verbless clauses. I shall follow Quirk et al. in excluding clauses, of whatever form, functioning as disjuncts and conjuncts.

I agree with Zandvoort (1961: 36), and Quirk et al. (1972: 760), that non-finite clauses with overt subject, so-called absolute clauses, such as (4) also exemplify the construction:

(4)   Daniel's view of the symphony was boldly drawn ..., *the bucolic rhythms of the scherzo lurching like a juggernaut ...*

I shall nevertheless exclude them from consideration here, mainly because their textual frequency is so low that, within the scope of the present study, it has proved impossible for me to collect a sample big enough to allow reasonably well-founded conclusions.

The decision by Quirk et al. not to include infinitival purpose clauses among their supplementive clauses seems to be based exclusively on semantic considerations, for whereas one of the intriguing characteristics of other supplementive clauses/free adjuncts is their semantic indeterminacy, their 'chameleon-like semantic quality of adapting to context' (Quirk et al. 1972: 760), purpose clauses are both semantically quite determinate and syntactically easy to isolate: they can be opened by the connector *in order to* (Thompson 1985: 57).

---

[1] In writing, as will appear from the examples in the present paper, the 'clear break' is generally, but not invariably, signalled by a comma, see e.g. examples (1) and (3) above.

2.2. Free adjuncts vs. postmodifying clauses

As examples (1) - (3) show, free adjuncts can occur in three positions: initial, medial (i.e. immediately following the subject of the main clause) and final. Clauses in medial and final position create problems of demarcation, however, as the structures in question may also function as postmodifying elements in the Noun Phrase ('reduced relative clauses'). Thus in the following example, either interpretation would make sense

(5)   Frannie, *intelligent, articulate*, is increasingly stressed. (GW 29)

(Cf.'Frannie, *who is* intelligent and articulate,...' or 'Frannie, *though* intelligent and articulate,...' or 'Frannie, intelligent and articulate *as she is*,...'). In such cases, the principle I have followed, inspired by Quirk et al. 1972, has been to exclude all cases where the sequence in question could follow its putative Head in a sentence where *only* the postmodifier interpretation would be possible. Thus, on the strength of (5'), (5) is considered adverbial rather than postmodifying:

(5')   *Yesterday Al had an argument with Frannie, *intelligent, articulate*.

The following example (6) on the other hand, must be considered structurally ambiguous, and it is only because the context shows that the 'logical subject' of *speaking* is *Ifshin* rather than *McCain*, that it can be classified as postmodifying and thus excluded:

(6)   It was in 1970 ... that the navy pilot John McCain first came across Ifshin, *speaking on Hanoi radio about American war crimes against North Vietnam.* (GW 6)

Note further that insertion of *who was* before *speaking* would result in a grammatical sentence.

3. Internal structure of free adjuncts

3.1. Realizations

As is well known, Free Adjuncts can be realized by Present Participle clauses and Past Participle clauses:

(7)   The Opera Theatre, *seating 1,547,* is mainly used for performances of opera, ballet and dance. (Opera House)

(8)   *Originally designed for chamber music as well,* the Playhouse is panelled with the white birch plywood [of the concert hall]. (Opera House)

In addition, verbless clauses with an Adjective (Phrase) as their main lexical element are possible:

(9) If royal divorces were staged ... Hensher would be their perfect commentator: *sharp to field-pattern, not a little sententious, acidly voluptuous on dress-sense and dress-nonsense.* (GW 28)

Perhaps less well known are realizations by a Noun Phrase or a Prepositional Phrase:

(10) *Apparently an ordinary Essex town*, [Braintree] is thought to lie in a pocket of the paranormal. (GW 29)

(11) [The stage curtain is woven from Australian wool] *Of abstract patterns in bright warm colours* it is known as the curtain of the sun. (Opera House)

Finally there is the question of infinitival clauses. The motivation behind my decision to exclude infinitival purpose clauses from consideration, cf. above 2.1, was first and foremost that unlike the various other types, they form a syntactically and semantically homogeneous group, which is easily distinguishable from the other realizations of the construction. Second, infinitival purpose clauses are by far the most extensively studied, from syntactic, semantic, as well as pragmatic points of view (cf. Thompson 1985; Golkova 1968). But in principle, it might be possible to come across adverbial infinitival clauses which are neither purpose clauses, on the one hand, nor conjuncts or disjuncts, on the other. Though I will not exclude the possibility of such infinitival clauses *a priori*, the only one I have come across is the following, perhaps significantly (cf. below section 4) occurring in a translation from French:[2]

(12) This fresh, fruity red wine is made from the Gamay grape grown in the best area of the Beaujolais region. *To be served at a rather cool temperature (53° F to 61°F)*, it is a light and lively wine. It accompanies particularly well the [sic] roasted or grilled meat dishes ...

For the moment, I shall thus leave open the question of whether the construction can be realized by infinitival clauses.

The 'main clause' in which the Free Adjunct occurs may itself be a dependent, adverbial clause:

(13) Until Mr Yeltsin spoke out on Monday, *repudiating the remarks of his security chief General Alexander Korzhakov*, there was some doubts as to whether voting would take place at all on June 16. (GW 12)

(14) As she coaches a new generation of dancers, *passing on her knowledge of the role*, Seymour tends to sing the praises that the others so diligently count. (GW 27)

---

[2]The French original has
   Ce vin rouge, frais et fruité, provient du cépage Gamay cultivé dans les meilleurs terroirs du Beaujolais. *A servir plutôt frais (12° à 16° c)*, c'est un vin léger qui accompagne les plats de viande grillée ou rôtie, les pâtes, salades et fromages doux.

And one Free Adjunct may even be nested in another:

(15) Founded in 1789 and a world leader for 150 years, *having introduced the world's first lawn mower in 1832,* Ransomes went on to manufacture the very first commercially produced power-driven lawn mower in 1904. (Mountfield)

In terms of textual frequency, Present Participle clauses account for well over half of the examples, followed by Past Participle clauses, Adjectival, Nominal clauses, and finally verbless clauses with a Prepositional Phrase as their main constituent, cf. table 1.

	GW	Brochures	total
ing	37	29	66
ed	11	14	25
NP	5	11	16
AP	6	5	11
PP	2	1	3
total	61	60	121

Table 1. Frequency of realizations

3.2. Syntactic link with main clause

In the vast majority of cases the understood subject of the subjectless adverbial clause is felt to be identical with the subject of the main clause, as in all examples cited up until now. Where no such link exists, the non-finite clause is felt to be 'dangling':

(16) *Famed for their diuretic properties*, medieval apothecaries called them [:dandelions] *dens lionis* [ital.] (GW 24)

(17) *Based on our expert knowledge of specific hazards and risks in the food industry,* we often make recommendations for applications of our products which go well beyond current legal safety requirements. (Lever)

There is however, a series of borderline cases, where the adverbial clause is not felt to be 'dangling', although there is less than total identity between the subjects of the dependent and the main clause. In the first place, the implied subject of the dependent clause, though not identical with, may be at least somehow retrievable from the subject of the main clause:

(18) *A wizard of deadpan wit*, Lewis's celebrated books on Indochina and the Italian Mafia catalogue with anthropological exactitude the weirdest rites and rituals. (GW 29)

(19) *Forced to prowl round the outside of the garden squares where the very expensive cars were parked*, my mood darkened. (GW 24)

Second, cases in which the subject, if expressed, would have been generic *one*, also seem tolerable to most people:

(20) *Travelling west*, the city gives way to bushland as you cross the mighty Hawkesbury River and climb up the Blue Mountains. (Map)

Finally, the shared subject of the main clause and the dependent clause is normally the overt, grammatical subject, even when the main clause is in the passive; but in one or two cases, the implied subject of the adverbial clause would correspond more closely to the 'logical' active subject of the main clause (cf also Quirk et al. 1972: 757f):

(21) Larger machines have been developed *using either tough lightweight die-cast aluminium or superstrong steel.* (Mountfield)

'Dangling' clauses, as well as the more or less acceptable types exemplified in (18) - (21), are relatively rare. There is however a fairly frequent type of non-identity of subjects which seems to be absolutely normal and unremarkable. In this type, the link between main clause and dependent clause is provided, not by the implied subject of the dependent clause being more or less identical with that of the main clause, but by the subject of the dependent clause being the *entire main clause*, or at least a proposition contained therein. As Halliday (1994: 229) puts it, the 'domain' of the dependent clause may be 'some larger segment of the primary clause, up to the whole clause':

(22) Spain's new conservative prime minister, José María Aznar, was sworn in at the week-end, *bringing the first change in government in almost 14 years.* (GW 3)

In this example, it is not Mr Aznar who brought the first change in government in Spain, but his having been sworn in. As further examples of this type, consider the following:

(23) ... his refuelling stops on laps 30 and 50 of the 61-lap contest were relatively small, *giving his car maximum agility to lap the back-markers.* (GW 32)

(24) Ariens Rear Engine Riders are easy to maintain, *making the engine last longer and run cleaner – for a better environment.* (Ariens)

(25) After four years of research Utzon altered his design ... This enabled the roofs to be constructed in a pre-cast fashion, *greatly reducing both time and cost.* (Opera House)

In my data the 'Main-Clause-as-Subject' type accounts for 10 per cent of all instances (12 out of 121). It only occurs with present participle clauses, and the participial clause is invariably in final position (cf. further below section 3.2).

The adjunct clause may be headed by a conjunction indicating its exact semantic relation to the sentence as a whole:

(26) *By* fitting one of the XR accessory packs available, the XR converts to a lawn raker or powered edge trimmer. (Qualcast)

(27) *Though* odds-on favourite before the tournament began, he was dissatisfied with his form throughout ... (GW 32)

(28) *while* pretending to decentralise ..., Tory administrations have in fact presided over an extrordinary and unprecedented concentration of might ... (GW 29)

The existence of such cases would seem to contradict Thompson & Longacre's claim that free adjuncts, which they refer to as 'absolute clauses', carry 'no explicit signal of the relationship between the main and subordinate clause;' (1985: 201). Although clauses with conjunctions signalling the relationship account for 10 per cent of the cases in my data (12 instances), Thompson & Longacre would in general seem to be right when they state (1985: 203) that free adjuncts are used 'when there is no need to specify more than that the clauses are related.' Or as I hope to show in what follows: thanks to the position and form of the free adjunct it is very often possible to leave the nature of the semantic link between the main clause and the dependent clause unspecified.

3. Semantic relations

As indicated, previous research has been rather vague about the exact nature of the semantic link between free adjunct and main clause; or rather: it has been suggested that vagueness is a central property of the meaning of free adjuncts. Thus Zandvoort states (1962: 210) that the free adjunct 'usually expresses ATTENDANT CIRCUMSTANCES', and that these circumstances in many cases can be 'further specified as the expression of cause, reason, time, contrariety, etc.' And in the same vein Quirk et al. suggest that 'what they describe is a "contingency" or "accompanying circumstance" to what is described in the main clause.' And they further state that contingency may be interpreted

> as a causal or temporal connection, or perhaps most commonly of all, a circumstantial one ... (1972: 762)

And as mentioned above, Thompson & Longacre go even further, suggesting that the very vagueness of the relationship is the reason for using free adjuncts.

My main concern in this part of the paper will be to take a closer look at the somewhat vague terms 'attendant circumstances', 'accompanying circumstances', 'contingencies' in order to see if it might be possible to arrive at a more satisfactory, and more precise, specification of the meaning of the constructions given these labels. But before I go on to do so, let me note that there are in fact a considerable number of cases where the meaning of the adjunct is not vague, and which do not fall into the 'contingency' category. These fall in two clear groups: temporal and causal.

3.1. Temporal adjuncts

Temporal relations can be relations of anteriority, simultaneity or posteriority, or 'time before' – 'same time' – 'time after'. In my data, there are 18 instances of temporal free adjuncts, the majority of which (14 instances) comes from GW. Significantly (cf. below section 3.3), they denote time before (13 instances), or same time (5 instances), but not time after. Anteriority and simultaneity are illustrated in (29) - (30):

(29) Newcastle simply could not keep up the pace. *Having established their 12-point lead*, they then dropped 21 out of the next 45. (GW 30)

(30) *Speaking in Bonn*, Mr Zyuganov said: ... (GW 1)

Present participial clauses account for 14 of the temporal adjuncts; other realizations represented are past participle (2 instances), adjective phrase (1 instance), and noun phrase (1 instance).

3.2. Causal adjuncts

Under the term 'causal', I subsume various relations between two propositions which all share the property that the one, the Precedent (p), is a conceptual/logical pre-condition for the second, the Consequent (q). Pairs like cause-effect, reason-consequence, means-end are thus all considered causal. So, too, are cases where the cause-effect relationship is hypothetical, as in Conditional clauses, as well as cases where a 'cause', hypothetical or real, does not have the expected effect, as in Concessive and Adversative clauses. Below, I illustrate the main types where the relation between adjunct and main clause is considered 'causal', first, in (31) to (34), the adjunct is Antecedent and the main clause Consequent:

(31) *As the manufacturer of the largest range of garden power tools in the UK*, Black & Decker understand what you're looking for. (Black & Decker)

(32) The NLD won 32 per cent of the seats in the new parliament. *Stunned*, the junta responding by arresting 3,000 NLD workers and ... (GW 22)

(33) Larger machines have been developed *using either lightweight die-cast aluminium or superstrong steel*. (Mountfield)

(34) *Though odds-on favourite before the tournament began*, he was dissatisfied with his form throughout but mentally he remained unparalleled. (GW 32)

Causal and temporal relations share the feature of directionality (hence the '*post hoc ergo propter hoc*' fallacy), and in some cases it is hard to determine whether the adjunct is causal or temporal, or rather: it would be a mistake to insist on an either-or interpretation, as the construction is capable of expressing both relations at one and the same time:

(35)   Mr Yeltsin is still trailing by six points in the opinion polls, *having made up much lost ground*. (GW 1)

Is he trailing six points behind *after*, *because of* or *in spite of* having made up much lost ground?

As we saw above, temporal relations expressed by free adjuncts are overwhelmingly anterior and never, in my data, posterior. If the directionality feature were to surface in parallel fashion in causal relations, we would expect all, or at least most, causal adjuncts to express relations of the 'before'-type, i.e. to be Antecedents. This is certainly not always so; in both the examples below the adjunct clause is the Consequent and the main clause the Antecedent, (36) exemplifying the cause-effect relation, and (37) the reason-consequence relation:

(36)   ... all [the group's production plants] are strategically placed on the country's rail and motorway systems *offering the best possible communications throughout the UK and with the major European Ferry ports and the new Channel Tunnel terminal.* (Caradon)

(37)   The committee set up by the Government selected the site for the building. *Known as Bennelong Point*, it was named after the first Aborigine to speak English, who was born on the site. (Opera House)

On the face of it, this apparent lack of parallelism with time also shows up statistically: Although the majority of cause clauses are Antecedents and the minority Consequents (33 and 17 respectively), the difference is not great enough to be called overwhelming. It is worth noting, however, that the great majority of the Consequent clauses, 12 out of 17, are of the 'main clause as subject' type exemplified in (36) and in (22) - (25), above. As mentioned, this type invariably follows the main clause, and this lack of mobility throws some doubt on its adverbial status. If we disregard this type, then, we find the following realizations: present participle: 13, past participle: 11, noun phrase: 6, adjective phrase: 2, prepositional phrase: 1. It is perhaps worth mentioning that 'means' clauses (e.g. 33) account for 10 of the present participles. That is to say, in the other variants of the causal relation, the typical realization is past participle or noun phrase.

3.3. 'Accompanying circumstances'

As a first step towards an explicitation of the concept 'accompanying circumstances', I would like to ask what is achieved communicatively by using the free adjunct construction at all? For it will be apparent that in very many cases the information contained in the free adjunct might just as well have been given in a non-restrictive relative clause, or perhaps even in a co-ordinated main clause (cf. Quirk et al. 1972: 762):

(38) *Born 88 years ago in the terminal London suburb of Enfield*, Lewis himself now lives outside Braintree in a parsonage. (GW 29)

(38') Lewis himself, *who* was born 88 years ago ... now lives outside Braintree...

(39) *Powered by the Briggs & Stratton Quantum Precision XTE 55 engine with electronic ignition*, the Mountfield Multi-Mow 21 features a special 3 in 1 deck ... (Mountfield)

(39') The Mountfield Multi-Mow 21 is powered by the Briggs & Stratton ... engine ..., *and* it features ... a special 3 in 1 deck.[3]

There are two features that distinguish the original versions and the re-arranged versions of (38) and (39): first, in the originals the relevant sequences are non-finite, and second, they occur in thematic position (as 'marked theme', Halliday 1994: 44). The first question we need to ask, then, is this: what is achieved communicatively by presenting a given chunk of information in non-finite rather than finite form?

Halliday (1994: 75) in his discussion of the function of the finite element, says:

> The finite element ... brings the proposition down to earth, so that it is something that can be argued about. (Halliday 1994: 75)

'Something that can be argued about' is something that can be true or false, right or wrong. This is the feature Halliday calls polarity, and we can now say that when we present a proposition in non-finite form, we have taken it out of sentence polarity and presented it as something that is beyond dispute.

This status as something indisputable is further enhanced by placing the adjunct clause in thematic position, since the theme is the starting-point for the message (Halliday 1994: 39).[4] Moreover, if we consider the information structure of the sentence, there is, in unmarked cases, a tendency for Theme and Given information to coincide (Halliday 1994: 301). So the information presented in non-finite propositions in thematic position is both regarded as indisputably true and as information already known to the receiver. To see what this kind of information is good for, let us return to example (37) above, repeated here for convenience:

(37) The committee set up by the Government selected the site for the building. *Known as Bennelong Point*, it was named after the first Aborigine to speak English, who was born on the site. (Opera House)

---

[3] It is cases like these Steller & Sørensen (1976: 133) have in mind when they state that in some genres the construction is often used more extensively than is justfied. It is hard to disagree with them.

[4] In the first edition of the same work (1985), he also stated that the theme is 'what the clause is going to be about'(p. 39)

Conceptually, there is no doubt: the site is known as Bennelong Point (Consequent) *because* it is named after the first Aborigine to speak English (Antecedent), not the other way round. Nevertheless, this conceptual relation between the two propositions is almost suppressed by the sentence in its actual form, but it can be brought forward much more clearly if we re-arrange the propositions of the sentence so that 1) Antecedent and Consequent change places, and 2) the information of the Antecedent is represented as non-finite, and that of the Consequent as finite:

(37') *Named after the first Aborigine to speak English*, the site is known as Bennelong Point.

Both versions contain the same two propositions: 'the site is named after the first Aborigine to speak English' (p), and 'it is known as Bennelong Point' (q), and we are able to infer that q is because of p, but why is it that it is so much easier to make that inference on the basis of (37') than on the original (37)? The answer lies in the nature of the inherent relationship between Antecedent and Consequent: to say that 'q is because of p' is to provide a *reason* for q. And the explanation for why the original version of (37) tends to conceal the conceptual relation between the two propositions rather than reveal it is precisely that it does not really make sense to give reasons for believing in the truth of a proposition which, at the same time, by virtue of its non-finiteness and thematic position, is presented as being both beyond dispute and as known to both addresser and adressee beforehand.

When we adduce reasons for statements, opinions or beliefs, what we are trying to do is to back up statements about which there might be disagreement or doubt with other statements which, in the context at least, are regarded as beyond doubt (cf. Toulmin 1958; Perelman & Olbrechts-Tyteca 1969). Reasoning, in other words, is a process whereby we derive new knowledge from old knowledge. The new knowledge (the Claim in Toulmin's terminology) may not be quite certain, that is why we need to argue for it by backing it up with evidence (Toulmin's Data) consisting of old and certain knowledge. And as we have just seen, this is exactly how information encapsulated in a free adjunct in thematic position will be understood. Free adjuncts, then, particularly in thematic position, are eminently suitable for representing Data (cf. also Nielsen 1996b).

In a relatively large number of cases, 24 in all, the function of the free adjunct is in fact to back up claims made in the main clause, and interestingly, whereas the information given in the free adjunct is factual, i.e. information about which there can in principle be absolute certainty, the claims of the main clause are predictions, evaluations and the like, i.e. claims about which there can never be absolute certainty (for the distinction between factual and evaluative claims see Atelsek 1981). (40) and (41) are clear examples of this type:

(40) *At 38*, Hoddle will be the youngest England manager and the least experienced, having been a club manager only five years. (GW 30)

(41)   *Over 300 metres high,* it [Sydney Tower] is the highest public building in the southern hemisphere (map)[5]

Not surprisingly, the pattern recurs in cases where the relation between the fact (Datum) and the prediction/evaluation (Claim) is tenuous (example (42)), or where evaluative terms are smuggled into the supposedly factual Datum (example (43)):

(42)   *Cast in bronze or modelled in plaster or Sculpmetal (a clay-like medium with a metallic finish)* they [the sculptures] are made in such a way that they generate a deep ambiguity concerning their status. (GW 26)

(43)   *A significant and relevant museum for Sydney and Australia in the approach to 2000,* this place will join our city's major cultural institutions in showcasing our history, identity and contemporary culture to the world. (Museum)

In a variant, the adjunct containing the Datum occurs after the Claim, almost as an afterthought, but again providing evidence for the Claim of the main clause. The sentence final participial clause of (40), above, as well as the following are instances of this type:

(44)   The only discordant note was struck ... when Asako forgot her husband's name during her speech, *calling him Hiroshi instead of Satoshi.* (GW 25)

(45)   Both [lawn mowers] feature an advanced cylinder design which improves cutting and collection. And like all cylinder mowers they are energy efficient, *requiring smaller motors than other cutting systems.* (Qualcast)

This type, comprising a total of 12 examples, is the largest single subtype among 'accompanying circumstances'.

As we saw above in the discussion of (37), there are cases where, somewhat disturbingly, the adjunct is the vehicle of the Consequent rather than the Antecedent, and in like manner, there are a few cases where the adjunct clause carries the evaluative Claim rather than the (quasi-)factual Datum:

(46)   *Unique and highly recommended by Europe's consumer organisations,* this powerful machine really removes all 'thatch', undergrowth and moss from lawns and aerates down to grass root level. (Wolf)

Here, as in the case of (37), one might well speculate that the reason why Antecedent and Consequent have 'changed places', both in terms of finiteness and linear

---

[5]It might be objected that in these examples the adjunct simply expresses cause. This is not so, however; in (40) - (41) the adjunct provides the writer's justification or evidence for making the Claim of the main clause, whereas in a real causal relation, the cause in itself triggers off the effect, as in the following example:
   ... last autumn Barmby would have found the net with his eyes closed. But now, *off balance*, he put the ball well wide. (GW 30)

sequence, has to do with considerations of length, for as the bulk of the examples cited in this paper have shown, the normal pattern is for the initial adjunct clause to be shorter than the main clause, and this in turn would tally quite well with their functions, the adjunct clause providing the known facts upon which further evaluations are based. Such questions, however, are beyond the scope of this paper.

4. Conclusion

In this paper I have attempted to give an overview of the syntax and semantics of Free Adjuncts in English. The paper has of necessity been mainly exploratory, but I do hope that it has gone some way towards showing that the relation between the adjunct and the main clause is directional, as well as giving (some of ?) the reasons for this directionality. In saying that the relation is directional, I here mean that there is a conceptual sense in which the information expressed in the adjunct clause will most naturally precede, temporally or logically, that of the main clause. We have also seen, however, that there are reasons for this precedence relation to show up in actual linear sequence, as there are reasons to regard the marked theme position as particularly suitable for the role that free adjuncts normally play. If this is so, it is those cases where the adjuncts do not show up in thematic position that are the really interesting ones, and the ones that need explanation. It might well be that there are textual factors at work, as Thompson (1985) showed in the case of infinitive purpose clauses.

Another area awaiting further exploration is the discoursal function of the construction. It is such a favourite among brochure writers that there must be a reason for its popularity. And moreover, this popularity seems to be a cross-linguistic fact: in French as well as in English the brochure seems to be the home ground of the construction, cf. Nielsen 1996a.

A third area of future research would be its origin and spread: the construction seems to be widespread in all the Romance languages, whereas English is the only Germanic language where it is represented with anything like the same frequency and diversity of types as in French. Danish and Swedish accept it to a considerably lesser extent, and German even more reluctantly. There is thus every reason to believe that it has spread from French to English and from there into the other Germanic languages, but to my knowledge its route has never been charted.

Finally, let me note that although my main purpose in the second half of the paper has been to extend the scope of the concept of directionality by making inroads on the 'accompanying circumstances', there is still a large group of recalcitrant cases, illustrated in (38) and (39), above, which do not fit into any of the categories. Cases such as these are neither temporal, causal, nor directional in any other way. In fact I would claim that they do not denote accompanying circumstances at all, they simply present two disparate pieces of information, connected only by being information about the same entity, but they do so in such a way as to make it appear as if one is background, reason, etc. for the other. I do not think it would be unfair to say that such instances are parasitic upon a pattern that is otherwise both useful and convenient.

Added in Proof: When I wrote this piece, I was, regrettably and unforgivably, unaware of the existence of B. Kortmann, *Free Adjuncts and Absolutes in English* (London, 1991). This means that what I say in the first half of the paper is considerably less original than I first thought. As my main argument and general theoretical perspective in the second part of the paper are clearly different from Kortmann's, however, I nevertheless venture to publish it.

References

Atelsek, J. (1981). An anatomy of opinions. *Language in Society 10*, 217-225.

Golkova, E. (1968). On the English infinitive of purpose in functional sentence perspective. *Brno Studies in English* 7, 119-128.

Greenbaum, S. (1969). *Studies in English Adverbial Usage*. London: Longman.

Halliday, M. A. K. (1994). *An Introduction to Functional Grammar*. London: Edward Arnold (first edition 1985).

Nielsen, A. E. (1996a). *Argumentationsstrategier i franske præsentationsbrochurer. Fra det sproglige til det retoriske niveau*. Ph.D. thesis, The Aarhus School of Business.

Nielsen, A. E. (1996b). The argumentative impact of causal relations – An exemplary of the free predicate in the promotional discourse. *Argumentation* 10, 1-17.

Perelman, C. & L. Olbrechts-Tyteca (1969). *The New Rhetoric. A Treatise on Argumentation*. Notre Dame: University of NotreDame Press. (French original: *La nouvelle rhétorique: traité de l'argumentation*, 1958).

Prebensen, H. (1973). Apposition, attribut indirect et complement de circonstance en francais moderne. *Actes du 5ème congrès des romanistes scandinaves*. Turku: Turun Yliopisto.

Quirk, R. et al. (1972). *A Grammar of Contemporary English*. London: Longman.

Quirk, R. et al. (1985). *A Comprehensive Grammar of the English Language*. London: Longman.

Steller, P. & K. Sørensen (1976/1966). *Engelsk Grammatik*. Copenhagen: Munksgaard.

Thompson, S. A. (1985). Grammar and written discourse: Initial vs. final purpose clauses in English. *Text* 5, 55-84.

Thompson, S. A. & R. E. Longacre. (1985). Adverbial Clauses. In T. Shopen (ed) *Language Typology and Syntactic Description. Vol. II: Complex Constructions*, Cambridge: Cambridge University Press, 171-234.

Toulmin, S. (1958). *The Uses of Argument*. Cambridge: Cambridge University Press.

Zandvoort, R. W. (1961). *A Handbook of English Grammar*. London: Longman.

Appendix: Sources of Data.

Journalism
- the Guardian Weekly, 12 May 1996 (GW)

Brochures
- Industrial
  - Caradon Plastics (Caradon)
  - Chicago Bridge and Iron Company (CBI)
  - Lever Industrial (Lever)
- Consumer Durables
  - Ariens Rear Engine Riders (Ariens)
  - Black & Decker (Black & Decker)
  - Mountfield (Mountfield)
  - Qualcast (Qualcast)
  - Wolf Tools (Wolf)
- Tourism
  - The official map to Sydney (Map)
  - Museum of Sydney (Museum)
  - Sydney Opera House (Opera House)

The Aspectual Complexity of the Simple Past in English. A Comparison with French and Danish

Carl Vikner and Sten Vikner

Throughout his work, Niels Davidsen-Nielsen has consistently shown how fruitful and productive the comparative study of English and Danish can be, e.g. in his 1990 book *Tense and Mood in English. A Comparison with Danish*. In our contribution to this festschrift, we will take the same approach and discuss a topic from the comparative study of tense in English, French, and Danish.

We want to investigate some problems connected with the semantics of the English simple past, which sometimes is ambiguous and sometimes is not, as far as the distinction between telic and atelic interpretation is concerned.[1] In this connection we have found it useful to compare the English simple past with French passé simple and imparfait, which are consistently unambiguous in this respect, and the Danish simple past, which with most verbs[2] is consistently ambiguous in the same respect.

1. Making time go by

There is a clear distinction between the interpretations of English sentences with the simple past, e.g. *smiled*, and the past progressive, e.g. *was smiling*, cf. the following examples:[3]

(1)   Marianne looked at Niels. He smiled.
(2)   Marianne looked at Niels. He was smiling.

The two predicates *smiled* and *was smiling* are both instances of past tense, that is, they both describe an eventuality which precedes the point of utterance, but coincides with the point of reference in a Reichenbachian analysis (Reichenbach 1947: 290, S. Vikner 1985, Davidsen-Nielsen 1990: 59ff). Nevertheless, the two predicates have different interpretations. The most prominent interpretation of (1) is the one which sees it as describing an episode where Niels starts smiling when or

---

[1]We would like to thank Robin Cooper for bringing these problems to our attention, Roger Schwarzschild and Rex Sprouse for helpful comments and discussion, and Irène Baron and Anthony Hull for native speaker judgments.
[2]The qualification alludes to the verb pairs *være/blive* and *have/få* to which we return in section 3.2.1 below.
[3]These examples are adapted from Kamp & Reyle 1993: 547, cf. also Ogihara 1990: 11.

after Marianne starts looking at him. The description in (2), on the other hand, suggests that Niels is already smiling when Marianne starts looking at him. Thus, in (1) we get the impression that the *smiled*-sentence is moving the narrative time forward, whereas no such moving of the time takes place with the *was-smiling* sentence in (2). This effect comes about because *smiled* in (1) introduces a new reference point which follows the reference point of *looked at*, whereas in (2) *was smiling* takes over the reference point of *looked at* (see e.g. C. Vikner 1986: 82f).

In French a similar effect is obtained by means of the passé simple[4] and the imparfait respectively, so that (3) and (4) below are equivalent to (1) and (2) respectively:

(3)   Marianne regarda Niels. Il sourit.

    'Marianne looked at Niels. He smiled (passé simple).'

(4)   Marianne regarda Niels. Il souriait.

    'Marianne looked at Niels. He smiled (imparfait).'

In Danish, however, the situation is different. Danish, like German and most other Germanic languages, has only one past form corresponding to the two forms in English and in French. So if we try to reconstruct examples (1) - (4) in Danish we get the following example:

(5)   Marianne så på Niels. Han smilede.

    'Marianne looked at Niels. He smiled (simple past).'

In (5) the sentence *Han smilede* is ambiguous between the two readings in (1) and (2) (and (3) and (4)).[5]

Thus we are faced with the following problem: Why does the time move in (1) and (3), but not in (2) and (4), and why may (5) be interpreted either way? In other words, why does *smiled* (and *sourit*) introduce a new reference point, while *was smiling* (and *souriait*) does not?

In the following we will try to answer these questions. In section 2 we first give a short description of processes, states and events. Then, in section 3, we discuss the aspectual properties of the English simple past, and in section 4 the problem of whether a progressive sentence describes a process or a state. Finally, in section 5, we consider the use of the English simple present.

---

[4]The use of the passé simple in modern French is limited to literary style. In everyday language it has been replaced by the present perfect. This means that the French present perfect has become ambiguous between a perfect sense and a past sense, which is why we prefer to retain the unambiguous passé simple in our examples.

[5]An unambiguous rendering of *He was smiling* can be obtained in Danish with expressions like *Han sad og smilede* ('He sat and smiled'), *Han stod og smilede* ('He stood and smiled'), etc.

2. Processes, states and events

The notion of a process will be a major issue in our discussion. Therefore, we start with a brief sketch of our conception of processes.

We follow a view which has gained general recognition in the literature on tense and aspect and which has it that one can distinguish four main types of eventualities (or situations). The four types have been described by Vendler (1967), who calls them states, activities, accomplishments and achievements. Partly following Bach (1981: 61), we will use the following designations, which appear to us to be more intuitively transparent: states, processes, complex events and atomic events.

Here follow some sample sentences which in their most natural readings are interpreted as descriptions of different types of eventualities, i.e. as belonging to different aspectual classes. States: *She was intelligent, She had a bicycle*. Complex events: *She wrote a novel, She mowed the lawn*. Atomic events: *She began to sing, She found a ten-pound note*. It is much more difficult to give straightforward examples of sentences describing processes, because the very sample sentences in English constitute part of our problem. Vendler's exemplification of the notion of a process (activity) goes like this: "running, walking, swimming, pushing or pulling something, and the like are almost unambiguous cases of activity" (Vendler 1967: 107). That is, he presents no complete process-describing sentences. If we have recourse to other languages, the exemplification is somewhat easier. Thus, in their most prominent reading French *Elle nageait dans la piscine*, German *Sie schwamm im Schwimmbecken herum* and Danish *Hun svømmede rundt i bassinet* (which all translate as "She was swimming around in the pool"), are taken to be process descriptions.

Let us now have a closer look at processes.[6] Processes are like events in certain respects, and like states in others.

Processes and events are alike in that they are dynamic eventualities, i.e. in an event and in a process some kind of change necessarily occurs. An atomic event consists only of one such change from one state to another. Complex events and processes consist of series of subevents. States, on the other hand, are incompatible with any kind of change. Complex events and processes may contain gaps, at least if the gaps do not exceed some pragmatically determined maximum length. In the process of writing a novel, for instance, it is normal that from time to time the author is busy doing something else than tapping at a keyboard, and yet we would still say that he or she is engaged in the process of writing a novel. Such gaps are impossible with states. Cf. Dowty 1979: 139, Gabbay & Moravcsik 1980: 64f.

---

[6]The following short description is partly similar to points of view put forth, for instance, in Vendler 1967, Mourelatos 1978: 424ff, Platzack 1979: 67-121, Bach 1981: 67ff, Krifka 1989: 173ff, Smith 1991: 44f, Kamp & Reyle 1993: 563ff, but it also differs from these in some respects, most notably with regard to the issue of starting points (cf. also C. Vikner 1986: 70f; 1994: 144ff).

Processes and states, which we will comprise under the designation atelic eventualities, are alike in that they are homogeneous, i.e. any part of an atelic eventuality is of the same sort as the whole. Probably related to this, atelic eventualities do not include an initial or a final endpoint.[7] As a matter of fact, most eventualities must have started at some time and have stopped or will stop at some other time, but the beginning and the end of an atelic eventuality are in themselves atomic events and do not constitute parts of the atelic eventuality itself. When one describes an eventuality as atelic, e.g. with a process description like *Elle nageait dans la piscine*, this description abstracts away from the beginning and the end of the swimming process. This process is described as going on, the beginning and the end of it are, so to speak, invisible in the process description, i.e. for such a sentence to be a true description of the eventuality E going on or holding at a certain time t it must be the case that E started before t and will continue for some time after t.

Thus we can illustrate the internal structure of the four eventualities informally as shown in figure 1:

State: _____

Process: •••–•••–•–••••–•••–•–••••

Complex event: |••–•••–•••|

Atomic event: •

Figure 1: Eventuality structures.

In narrative texts event descriptions have the effect of making narrative time move forward by introducing a new reference point following the preceding one. Atelic descriptions, on the other hand, do not have this effect, they describe eventualities which hold at the time of the current reference point, i.e. the reference point of the preceding eventuality description (cf. for instance Kamp & Rohrer 1983, Cooper 1986: 32ff, Dowty 1986: 37f, Krifka 1989: 174, Parsons 1990: 214). That is why in a narrative discourse like the following, the second sentence (a state description) does not move narrative time forward:

(6)   Marianne looked at Niels. He was fast asleep.

Whereas time does move, when the second sentence is an event description:

(7)   Marianne looked at Niels. He stopped talking.

---

[7]For a somewhat different view of the endpoint property, see Smith 1986: 100f; 1991: 37 and 45.

It is well-known that expressions containing verbs that lexically denote a certain kind of eventuality for several reasons may be involved in aspectual shifts resulting in their denoting a different eventuality (cf. for instance Mourelatos 1978: 419 and Dowty 1979: 60ff). Most important for our purpose is the aspectual shift whereby a process description is changed into an event description. This may come about either by making visible and picking out the beginning of the process (the so-called inceptive use) or by including both the beginning and the end of the process into the description (cf. C. Vikner 1986: 92 and Smith 1991: 48f).

3. Simple past: states, events or processes

3.1. Compositionality of aspect

The aspect of a sentence is built up compositionally of contributions from various parts of the sentence. The lexical aspect of the verb is only one of these, along with e.g. the semantics of complements and adverbials. One of these contributors may be a morphological tense-aspect element in the verbal inflection. In French, for instance, the two past tenses, the passé simple and the imparfait, may be conceived of as aspectual functions which ascribe a certain aspect to a sentence such that a sentence in the passé simple always describes a telic (or perfective) eventuality, and a sentence in the imparfait an atelic (or imperfective) eventuality (C. Vikner 1986: 89ff, see also Kamp 1981: 45ff and Kamp & Rohrer 1983). This theory, together with the above mentioned principle of the movement of narrative time, gives an explanation of the two French examples (3) and (4). The possible interpretations of the Danish example (5) may be explained by assuming that the Danish simple past is aspectually neutral, i.e. it does not contribute to the aspectual composition. This would permit the second sentence in (5) to be interpreted either as an event description or as a process description.[8] Now, it is tempting to assume that English is like French here, i.e. that the English simple past behaves like the French passé simple, and the English past progressive like the French imparfait.[9] However, this assumption does not stand up to a closer scrutiny, as will be clear from the following.

We would like to propose the alternative hypothesis that the English progressive is an aspectual function which always gives process descriptions, whereas the English simple past is aspectually neutral apart from the fact that it cannot describe processes. This hypothesis, together with the principle of the movement of narrative time, accounts for the English examples (1) and (2).

---

[8]Actually, in (5) the first sentence too may be interpreted either as an event description or as a process description, so that (5) exhibits a fourway ambiguity much like the one discussed in connection with (8) below.
[9]As a matter of fact, Dowty (1986: 60) considers the possibility of ascribing identical semantics to the French imparfait and the English progressive.

Our view of aspect in English, French and Danish can thus be illustrated as follows:[10]

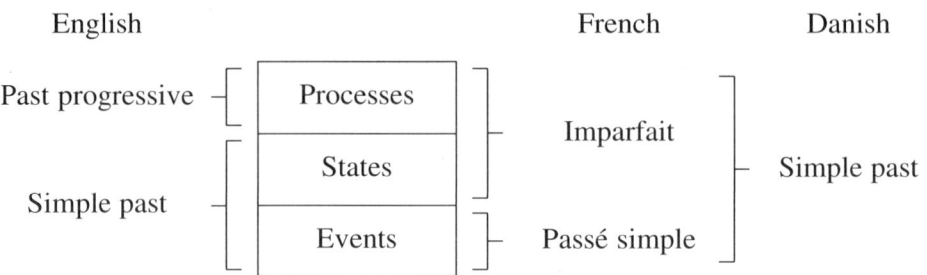

Figure 2: Aspects in the past tense in English, French and Danish.

There is no doubt that the progressive gives atelic descriptions. On the other hand, it is an open question whether these are state descriptions or process descriptions. There is no consensus in the literature on aspect on this point. We will return to the progressive problem below in section 4. In the remaining part of the present section we will have a closer look at the English simple past.

3.2. Simple past and states

If, contrary to our hypothesis, the English simple past were an aspectual function of the same kind as the French passé simple, all sentences in the simple past should describe events. This is not the case. Simple past sentences may very well describe states. This is seen both in connection with underlying (or lexical) state descriptions, and in connection with generic sentences.

3.2.1. Underlying state descriptions

If the underlying expression is a state description, the simple past sentence is ambiguous between a state description and an event description. This is clear in an example like (8):

(8)   They were married. They had a baby.

Here we have two sentences with underlying state predicates: *be married* and *have a baby*. In combination with the simple past, each of these predicates has two

---

[10]Here, as everywhere else in this paper, we have to omit any discussion of the use of the past and the present perfect.

readings, which give rise to four different interpretations of (8). In French, the aspectual difference between the passé simple and the imparfait has the effect that each of the four interpretations is expressed differently. The same is true in Danish, where the difference is marked lexically by means of the opposition between the state verb *være* ('be') and the event verb *blive* ('be, become'), on the one hand, and on the other hand between the state verb *have* ('have') and the event verb *få* ('have, get') (see e.g. S. Vikner 1988: 12f). The Danish and French data are shown in (9):[11]

(9a)   French: Ils étaient mariés. Ils avaient un bébé.

Danish: De var gift. De havde en baby.

'They were man and wife. They were parents.'

(9b)   French: Ils étaient mariés. Ils eurent un bébé.

Danish: De var gift. De fik en baby.

'They were man and wife. They became parents.'

(9c)   French: Ils furent mariés. Ils avaient un bébé.

Danish: De blev gift. De havde en baby.

'They became man and wife. They were parents.'

(9d)   French: Ils furent mariés. Ils eurent un bébé.

Danish: De blev gift. De fik en baby.

'They became man and wife. They became parents.'

Similarly, if we insert a simple past sentence with an underlying state description in (1), the result will also be ambiguous:

(10)   Marianne looked at Niels. He was confused.

This last sentence may mean either 'He was already in a state of confusion', and in this case time does not move, or 'He was thrown into a state of confusion', and then time does move with the occurrence of the new event.

3.2.2. Generic sentences

Another case where sentences in the simple past may describe states are generic sentences, which are discussed in detail in Krifka et al. 1995.

Generic or characterizing sentences are sentences which express generalizations,

---

[11]The sentence *Ils furent mariés* in the two last French examples can only be interpreted as an agentless passive, cf. e.g. *Ils furent mariés par un pasteur danois* ('They were married by a Danish priest'). The natural way of rendering the most salient event interpretation of *They were married* in French would be by means of the sentence *Ils se marièrent* ('They married (passé simple)'). This does not affect our main point here, however.

thereby abstracting away from particular events and facts. The generalization is often of a dispositional or habitual character, as in the example:

(11)   He smokes a cigar after dinner.

Adverbs like *usually, typically, always, often, every morning* etc. enforce a generic reading (cf. Krifka et al. 1995: 3, 7). It is generally agreed that generic sentences express a property and therefore are always aspectually stative (cf. Vendler 1967: 108f, Krifka et al. 1995: 17, Chierchia 1995: 207, Carlson 1995: 232).

It is interesting for our problem that the progressive is excluded in generic sentences (Krifka et al. 1995: 12), whereas the simple past has a "natural generic interpretation" (Chierchia 1995: 197). The following are examples of generic sentences in the simple past:

(12a)   He (usually) smoked a cigar after dinner.
(12b)   When Marianne looked at Niels, he was (always) confused.
(12c)   In 1989 he played tennis.

The last example is adapted from Krifka et al. 1995: 36. Because generic sentences are state descriptions, one would use the imparfait in French in examples like those in (12). Looked at in isolation, an English sentence in the simple past is often ambiguous between a generic and an episodic reading (i.e. a reading referring to a specific situation), whereas the use of the past tenses in French avoids this ambiguity, cf. (13):

(13a)   She got up at 6 o'clock.   Generic or episodic
(13b)   Elle se levait à six heures.   Generic
(13c)   Elle se leva à six heures.   Episodic

3.3. Simple past and events

What we tried to argue above, was that the simple past can describe states. According to our hypothesis, the only other possibility for the simple past is to describe an event (complex or atomic). That the simple past can describe events in sentences with verbs which are lexically stative was shown in (8) and (10) above.

With underlying event descriptions, there is no doubt that the event reading is preserved in simple past sentences, cf. the examples in (14):

(14a)   She wrote a novel.
(14b)   She mowed the lawn.
(14c)   She began to sing.
(14d)   She found a ten-pound note.

What happens then when an underlying process expression is combined with the simple past? In this case we think that a process interpretation is excluded and that the process expression is transformed into an event sentence. This may take place in one of two ways. Either the sentence is interpreted as describing the onset of the proces, this is the so-called inceptive or ingressive meaning, where the result is an atomic event description, or the process is seen as a completed whole with beginning and end, i.e. we get a complex event description.

An example of the first possibility is given in (15):

(15)   Mary ran at 2:30.

which normally will be interpreted as "Mary started to run at 2: 30" . This example along with its interpretation is taken from Vlach 1981: 276.

The second possibility, where the process description is tranformed into a complex event description with beginning and end may be illustrated as in:[12]

(16a) Mary slept badly last night.
(16b) Peter ate sweets all afternoon.

Thus we see that a situation may be described or viewed in two different ways, just as one and the same item may be described or viewed either as a mass (e.g. *some wood*) or as an individual (e.g. *a board*, *a piece of wood*).

Not all process expressions can be straightforwardly transformed into event descriptions. Often there are pragmatic/conceptual difficulties connected with imposing an event interpretation on a process expression. This is why sentences with process verbs in the simple past such as *She walked* often sound strange when seen in isolation, cf. Kamp and Reyle 1993: 563f and Sandström 1993: 188.

3.4. Simple past and processes

In our opinion, the process reading with simple past sentences is not available. Underlying state or event expressions cannot be transformed into process descriptions by combination with the simple past, and underlying process expressions when combined with the simple past are uniformly interpreted as event descriptions. Presumably the fact that the progressive unambiguously denotes a process, as argued in section 4 below, somehow blocks a process reading of simple past sentences.[13]

---

[12]See also Pustejovsky (1995: 65f), who characterizes *slept* as "an individuated event".
[13]This description is true only of colloquial English. In literary texts it is possible to describe processes by means of the simple past, cf. the following passage from Aldous Huxley: *Brave New World*, Penguin Books, 1955, p. 20f:
   "And in effect the sultry darkness into which the students now followed him was visible and crimson (...) among the rubies *moved* the dim red spectres of men and women with purple eyes and all the symptoms of lupus. The hum and rattle of machinery faintly *stirred* the air."
According to our informants, there is no semantic difference in such contexts between the simple past and the past progressive, and the use of the simple past has a distinctly literary flavour.

The unavailability of a process reading of the simple past with process verbs can be shown by contexts with *already*. The French equivalent of *already*, *déjà*, may normally only be combined with the imparfait, not with the passé simple (Togeby 1982: 347f). In other words, *déjà* forces the sentence to take on an atelic reading and only admits event readings under particular circumstances. In English, the event reading with *already* seems completely excluded, cf. the following examples where process verbs in the simple past are impossible:

(17a) When he came home, she was already sleeping.

(17b) *When he came home, she already slept.

The fact that sentences such as *He smiled – She ran – She swam – It rained* describe events and not processes has given rise to some curious effects in the literature on tense and aspect. This is most conspicuous in works by Anglophone linguists, and among them especially in the works of those who take the progressive to denote a state. This is not so surprising, because if *was smiling* is taken to describe a state, how do you describe the smile-process? A natural conclusion is that this is done by means of *smiled*. This results in many extraordinary statements about processes.

Often sentences in the simple past which in our view clearly must describe events are used as examples of process descriptions. In some cases with the inceptive reading:

(18) Max ran when I arrived. (Vlach 1981: 273)

In other cases denoting a complete delimited eventuality, i.e. a complex event, sometimes even combined with a delimiting adverbial or complement:

(19a) John pushed the cart for hours. (Mourelatos 1978: 426)

(19b) John ran (for an hour). (Bach 1981: 67)

(19c) Mary walked to her house yesterday. (Pustejovsky 1995: 13)

Note that the French equivalents of the examples in (18) and (19) would use the passé simple, as shown in (20):

(20a) Max courut quand j'arrivai.

(20b) John poussa le chariot pendant des heures.

(20c) John courut (pendant une heure).

(20d) Mary rentra à pied hier.

Most surprising, however, is the treatment of processes in Parsons (1990). Parsons uses the sentence *Mary ran* as a prototypical example (p. 21, cf. also p. 183). He furthermore admits to some uncertainty about the process notion: "I see a fairly clear distinction between events and states, and I see less clarity (along with less importance) about how processes fit in" (p. 34). In his definitive explanation of the difference between processes and events (p. 183f), he arrives at the conclusion that processes are a particular type of events, and he ascribes to them a culmination, which is in our opinion precisely a crucial defining property of events in contradistinction to processes. See also note 14 on p. 306, where he attributes to processes some properties that non-Anglophone linguists normally consider typical of events: "The past tense sentence must be made true by a process that has already culminated, and the usage principle that when we use a process sentence we implicitly limit our quantifiers to maximal processes yields the implication that no other process of the same kind is still going on." In other places he describes processes in a completely uncontroversial way, e.g. "Processes ... are like states in apparently having no natural finishing points" (note 26 p. 21), "a process is a spread-out homogeneous thing" (p. 317). It is our guess that these unusual suggestions have their roots in the interpretation of sentences like *Mary ran* as process descriptions.

To sum up: We think that with a process verb in the simple past, a process reading is excluded. This means that there are the possibilities generic state or event. The generic state reading is often impeded or ruled out for pragmatic reasons, so that only the event reading emerges, and this is exactly what happens in the example in (1).

4. Progressive: states or processes

The linguists who work on aspect are divided into two camps over the denotation of the English progressive. In one camp the progressive sentences are taken to describe processes, in the other to describe states. The process camp includes Vendler (1967), Mourelatos (1978), Dowty (1979: 163ff; 1986: 44) and Krifka (1989). In the state camp we find people like Vlach (1981), Bach (1981), Kamp & Reyle (1993: 508), Sandström (1993), Parsons (1990) and Cooper et al. (1996: 336ff). Even though it looks as if the state view is the more popular these days, we join the process camp, as will be apparent from the previous discussion.

The state view seems to be based on Vlach 1981. Vlach's argumentation builds on the observation that if we compare the three sentences in (21):

(21a)   Max was here when I arrived.
(21b)   Max was running when I arrived.
(21c)   Max ran when I arrived.

then (21a) and (21b) have an aspectual property in common, in that (21a) indicates that "Max must have been here for some period preceding and extending up to the time of my arrival", and similarly (21b) indicates that "Max was running for some period preceding and extending up to the time of my arrival" (Vlach 1981: 273f). As (21a) describes a state, Vlach concludes that this must be the case for (21b) too, and that is why he turns the property referred to into the defining property of statives in contradistinction to processes. In (21c), on the other hand, Vlach takes *Max ran* to describe a process which "took place at the time of or slightly after my arrival, not before" (Vlach 1981: 273). We believe that this reasoning is flawed. The aspectual property of an expression φ that when we have φ *when* ψ, the φ describes an eventuality that has started before the eventuality described by ψ occurs (cf. (21a) and (21b)), is common to atelic eventualities (i.e. states *and* processes). It is not a property that can be used for telling state descriptions apart from process descriptions. Therefore it cannot serve as an argument for including progressive sentences among state descriptions. In addition to this, the property which Vlach describes in connection with (21c) is a property that is typical of events, not of processes, cf. also Krifka (1989: 174f).

However, even if we give up Vlach's definition of states and let his defining property define processes too (which we think it should), this does not entail that a progressive sentence must denote a process, only that it may. We have three reasons for taking progressive sentences to describe processes and not states. First, we are impressed by the observation in Krifka (1989: 31f) that state predicates select a generic (kind-referring) interpretation of mass and plural terms, cf.:

(22a)   Dogs bark.

(22b)   Cats hate dogs.

By contrast, dynamic predicates select an object referring interpretation, as in (23), where the reference is necessarily to some specific dogs in a specific situation:

(23)   Dogs are barking.

Second, the eventualities described by progressive sentences admit of gaps. For instance, it is possible to say (24a) pointing to a chair which is empty because John for a moment has left his seat, but such a situation cannot be described by means of (24b), which conveys a state description. (24c) on the other hand gives a habitual reading, i.e. a generic state description.

(24a)   John is sitting there.

(24b)   John is in that chair.

(24c)   John sits there.

Now, as we showed in section 2, it is precisely a typical property of dynamic eventualities, as opposed to states, that they admit of gaps. Citing an example similar to (24a), Vlach (1981: 280) also notes this peculiarity of progressive sentences, though without drawing the conclusions drawn here.

Third, as Smith (1991: 37) points out: "In contrast with Activities, the event closest in temporal properties, states lack shifts or variation; this difference is reflected in the difference between *The child is asleep, The child is sleeping*." One might add that there is even a sharp contrast between progressive sentences and state sentences with respect to adverbial modification possibilities, as shown in (25a-b):

(25a) The child is sleeping fitfully.

(25b) *The child is asleep fitfully.

Sandström (1993: 83f) suggests that only state expressions can appear as complements to epistemic modals, observing that examples like (26a) and (26b) have an epistemic reading, whereas (26c) can express only obligation, not epistemic necessity:

(26a) He must have left.

(26b) He must be leaving.

(26c) He must leave.

If this reasoning is sound, it constitutes a serious argument in favour of the state reading of progressive sentences. However, we do not think that Sandström is right here. Epistemic modals are not restricted to taking state expressions as complements. Thus the following example with *must* plus the event verb *come* clearly has the epistemic reading 'it is necessarily the case that ...':

(27) He must come soon.

Admittedly, it is difficult not to connect an obligation reading with (26c). But imagine a diplomatic party with two spies waiting impatiently for the ambassador to leave the party. Knowing that the ambassador has an important appointment in a few minutes, one of the spies could utter (28) to the other, thus using *must leave* with an epistemic reading.

(28) He must leave soon.

Similarly, the following examples with *may* and an event expression, (29a), and a process verb, (29b), both can express epistemic possibility (as well as deontic permission):

(29a) He may come at any moment.

(29b) He may work.

Thus we do not agree with Sandström when she says that only state expressions may occur as complements of epistemic modals, and therefore the wellformedness of (26b) does not present a problem for our analysis of progressive sentences as denoting processes.

By analysing progressive sentences as denoting processes rather than states, we also avoid postulating the existence of a particular kind of state with a surprising amount of properties in common with processes, cf. e.g. Parsons 1990: 171, 234: "the "In-Progress" state", or Cooper et al. 1996: 338: "a state which temporally includes (or is equivalent to) some process of the appropriate type".

We would like to end this discussion of the progressive by addressing the difficulty of combining state expressions with the progressive. Vlach claims that his hypothesis gives an explanation for this difficulty:

(30)   *He is knowing the answer.

Vlach's position is that the progressive is an aspectual function taking a process expression as input and yielding a state description as output. This may be illustrated by the following formula:

(31) $\text{Progr}(E_{\text{Proc}}) = E_{\text{State}}$

In Vlach's (1981: 274) words: "The function of the progressive operator is to make stative sentences, and, therefore, there is no reason for the progressive to apply to sentences that are already stative". We do not find this particularly convincing. In French, nothing prevents the use of the imparfait in sentences that "are already" atelic.

We think, on the other hand, that the progressive is an aspectual function taking an expression of any aspectual type as input and yielding a process description as output:

(32) $\text{Progr}(E_x) = E_{\text{Proc}}$

Our hypothesis says that the progressive imposes a process reading on an underlying expression of whatever aspectual type. If this hypothesis is correct, then the explanation of the unacceptability of examples like (30) is that it is not all kind of state descriptions which may be transformed into process descriptions, and that in a case like (30) it is difficult to imagine a process interpretation of *know the answer*. In certain cases, however, it *is* possible to change a state expression into a process sentence in the progressive, cf. for instance (33):

(33a)   He is silly.
(33b)   He is being silly.

(33b) means something like "he is acting in a silly way". Here it is not difficult to imagine a dynamic sequence (i.e. a process) corresponding to such a description.

5. The simple present

Above, we have argued that, irrespective of the underlying aspect, simple past sentences in English always describe either a state or an event.

If we now take a look at sentences in the simple present[14], it turns out that the

---

[14] For relevant discussion of the English simple present, see for instance Dowty 1979: 135, 167, 189f, Bach 1981: 68f, 75ff, Davidsen-Nielsen 1990: 113ff, 126, Kamp & Reyle 1993: 538.

picture is very much the same here. However, there is one fundamental difference to be noted between past and present tense sentences. It stems from the conceptual impossibility of describing an event as occurring at the present moment (cf. Kamp & Reyle 1993: 536f). This impossibility is found not only in English, but in other languages as well.

Thus for instance, consider the two Danish sentences in (34), which differ only in that (34a) is in the simple past (*vaskede* 'washed'), and (34b) in the simple present (*vasker* 'washes').

(34a)   Hun vaskede bilen.
        'She washed/was washing the car'
(34b)   Hun vasker bilen.
        'She washes/is washing the car'

It is striking that whereas the simple past sentence in (34a) has three interpretations, as an event, as a process, and as a (generic) state, the simple present sentence in (34b) lacks the event interpretation and has only the two last interpretations.

Bearing this general constraint in mind, it is to be expected that if the characteristics of the English simple past carry over to the simple present, this last tense should be restricted to describing states to the exclusion of events, and as a matter of fact that is exactly the case. Thus the sentences in (35) have only a habitual or dispositional reading (see e.g. Davidsen-Nielsen 1990: 114f), i.e. they describe generic states: As with the English simple past a process reading is excluded, and as in other languages an event reading is impossible because an event cannot be co-temporal with the time of utterance.

(35a)   She washes the car.
(35b)   She walks.

It is also remarkable that (36) has only a state reading and does not present the four-way ambiguity seen with the corresponding simple past example, cf. (8) and (9) above.

(36)   They are married. They have a baby.

This is not the whole truth about the English simple present however. We have had to leave out any discussion of other uses, e.g. the performative use or the particular narrative use of the simple present, the so-called historical present (and its derivative, the so-called reportive use[15]), where the simple present functions as a stilistic substitute for the simple past. In this use, the simple present takes over the characteristics of the simple past, most notably the ability to describe events (but

---

[15]Cooper (1986: 26ff) gives a different account of the reportive reading.

still excluding processes). In this connection it is interesting that Cooper (1986: 29) notes that *John runs* with a reportive reading tends to mean *John begins to run*. This is completely parallel to the cases with the inceptive use of the simple past discussed in connection with (15) above.

In French, the aspectual difference between the passé simple and the imparfait is not found in the present tense, which has only one form, as in Danish. In these two languages, the sole present tense form therefore is aspectually neutral.

Marking the events as somewhat marginal in this connection, the aspects in the present tense in the three languages can be illustrated as follows:

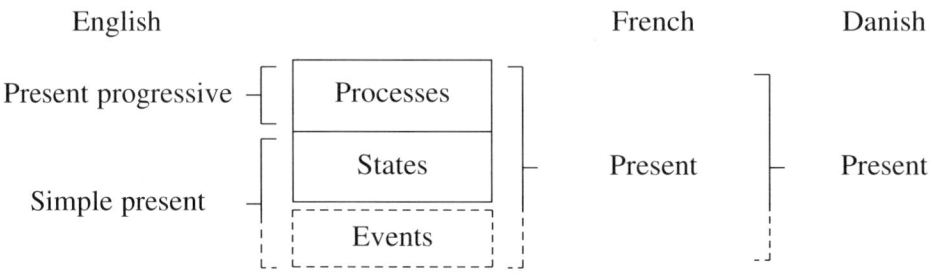

Figure 3: Aspects in the present tense in English, French and Danish.

6. Conclusion

In this paper we have presented arguments in favour of two hypotheses. First that in colloquial English the simple tenses cannot denote processes, but are neutral with respect to states and events. Second that the English progressive denotes processes. The two hypotheses are closely interconnected, because we suspect that it is due to the monopolization of the processes by the progressive that the simple tenses have been ousted from this domain.

The tense forms in French and Danish behave differently from the English ones (as summarized in figures 2 and 3). This means that when translating between the three languages, especially when translating from Danish into English or French, it is necessary to determine the kind of eventuality described by a given sentence (i.e. the aspect of the sentence) in order to choose the correct verb form in the target language. This aspectual determination may involve a number of different factors, such as lexical information and morphological and syntactic form not only of the verb but also of quantifiers, of complements, of modifying adverbials, etc.

References

Bach, E. (1981). On Time, Tense, and Aspect: An Essay in English Metaphysics. In P. Cole (ed) *Radical Pragmatics*, New York: Academic Press, 63-81.

Bach, E. (1986). The Algebra of Events. *Linguistics and Philosophy* 9, 5-16.

Carlson, G. N. (1995). Truth Conditions of Generic Sentences: Two Contrasting Views. In Carlson & Pelletier 1995, 224-237.

Carlson, G. N. & F. J. Pelletier (eds) (1995). *The Generic Book*. Chicago: The University of Chicago Press.

Chierchia, G. (1995). Individual-Level Predicates as Inherent Generics. In Carlson & Pelletier 1995, 176-223.

Cooper, R. (1986). Tense and Discourse Location in Situation Semantics. *Linguistics and Philosophy* 9, 17-36.

Cooper, R., R. Crouch, J. van Eijck, C. Fox, J. van Genabith, J. Jaspars, H. Kamp, D. Milward, M. Pinkal, M. Poesio & S. Pulman (1996). *Building the Framework*. FraCaS, Deliverable D15, University of Edinburgh, Centre for Cognitive Science.

Davidsen-Nielsen, N. (1990). *Tense and Mood in English. A Comparison with Danish*. Berlin: Mouton de Gruyter.

Dowty, D. R. (1979). *Word Meaning and Montague Grammar*. Dordrecht: Kluwer.

Dowty, D. R. (1986). The Effects of Aspectual Class on the Temporal Structure of Discourse: Semantics or Pragmatics? *Linguistics and Philosophy* 9, 37-61.

Gabbay, D. & J. Moravcsik (1980). Verbs, events, and the flow of time. In C. Rohrer (ed) *Time, Tense, and Quantifiers*. Tübingen: Niemeyer, 59-83.

Kamp, H. (1981). Evénements, représentations discursives et référence temporelle. *Langages* 64, 39-64.

Kamp, H. & U. Reyle (1993). *From Discourse to Logic. Introduction to Modeltheoretic Semantics of Natural Language, Formal Logic and Discourse Representation Theory*. Dordrecht: Kluwer.

Kamp, H. & C. Rohrer (1983). Tense in Texts. In *Proceedings of the 1981 Linguistics Conference in Konstanz, Germany*, 250-269.

Krifka, M. (1989). *Nominalreferenz und Zeitkonstitution. Zur Semantik von Massentermen, Pluraltermen und Aspektklassen*. München: Wilhelm Fink Verlag.

Krifka, M., F. J. Pelletier, G. N. Carlson, A. ter Meulen, G. Chierchia & G. Link (1995). Genericity: An Introduction. In Carlson & Pelletier 1995, 1-124.

Mourelatos, A. P. D. (1978). Events, processes and states. *Linguistics and Philosophy* 2, 415-434.

Ogihara, T. (1990). The Semantics of the Progressive and the Perfect in English. In H. Kamp (ed) *Tense and Aspect in English*, DYANA, Deliverable R2.3.A, Centre for Cognitive Science, University of Edinburgh, 3-38.

Parsons, T. (1990). *Events in the Semantics of English: A Study in Subatomic Semantics*. Cambridge, Massachusetts: MIT Press.

Platzack, C. (1979). *The Semantic Interpretation of Aspect and Aktionsarten. A Study of Internal Time Reference in Swedish*. Dordrecht: Foris.

Pustejovsky, J. (1995). *The Generative Lexicon*. Cambridge, Massachusetts: MIT Press.

Reichenbach, H. (1947). *Elements of Symbolic Logic*. New York: The Free Press. Paperback issue 1966, same publisher.

Sandström, G. (1993). *When-clauses and the temporal interpretation of narrative discourse*, University of Umeå, Sweden, Report 34.

Smith, C. S. (1986). A Speaker-Based Approach to Aspect. *Linguistics and Philosophy* 9, 97-115.

Smith, C. S. (1991). *The Parameter of Aspect*. Dordrecht: Kluwer.

Togeby, K. (1982). *Grammaire française* II. Copenhagen: Akademisk Forlag.

Vendler, Z. (1967). *Linguistics in Philosophy*. Ithaca: Cornell University Press.

Vikner, C. (1986). Aspect in French: The Modification of Aktionsart. CEBAL Series No 9, Copenhagen, Nyt Nordisk Forlag Arnold Busck, 58-101.

Vikner, C. (1994). Change in homogeneity in verbal and nominal reference. In C. Bache, H. Basbøll & C.-E. Lindberg (eds) *Tense, Aspect and Action. Empirical and Theoretical Contributions to Language Typology*. Berlin: Mouton de Gruyter, 139-164.

Vikner, S. (1985). Reichenbach Revisited: One, Two, or Three Temporal Relations. *Acta Linguistica Hafniensia* 19, 81-98.

Vikner, S. (1988). Modals in Danish and Event Expressions. *Working Papers in Scandinavian Syntax* 39, 1-33.

Vlach, F. (1981). The Semantics of the Progressive. In P. Tedeschi & A. Zaenen (eds) *Syntax and Semantics. Vol. 14, Tense and Aspect*. New York: Academic Press, 271-292.

List of contributors with their affiliation

CARL BACHE
Institute of Language and
Communication
Odense University
Campusvej 55
DK-5230 Odense M

JOHN M. DIENHART
Institute of Language and
Communication
Odense University
Campusvej 55
DK-5230 Odense M

PER DURST-ANDERSEN
Department of French
Russian Section
Copenhagen Business School
Dalgas Have 15
DK-2000 Frederiksberg

DORRIT FABER
Department of English
Copenhagen Business School
Dalgas Have 15
DK-2000 Frederiksberg

PETER HARDER
Department of English
Copenhagen University
Njalsgade 80
DK-2300 Copenhagen S

MICHAEL HERSLUND
Department of French
Copenhagen Business School
Dalgas Have 15
DK-2000 Frederiksberg

BENTE LIHN JENSEN
Department of Italian
Copenhagen Business School
Dalgas Have 15
DK-2000 Frederiksberg

PER ANKER JENSEN
Department of Modern Languages and
Language Technology
Southern Denmark
School of Business
Engstien 1
DK-6000 Kolding

STIG JOHANSSON
Department of British and American
Studies
University of Oslo
P.O. Box 1003, Blindern
N-0315 Oslo

ALEX KLINGE
Department of English
Copenhagen Business School
Dalgas Have 15
DK-2000 Frederiksberg

FRITZ LARSEN
Institute of Language and
Communication
Odense University
Campusvej 55
DK-5230 Odense M

BERIT LØKEN
Department of British and
American Studies
University of Oslo
P.O. Box 1003, Blindern
N-0315 Oslo

HANS F. NIELSEN
Institute of Language and
Communication
Odense University
Campusvej 55
DK-5230 Odense M

BENT PREISLER
Department of Languages and Culture
University of Roskilde
P.O. BOX 260
DK-4000 Roskilde

FINN SØRENSEN
Department of Computational
Linguistics
Copenhagen Business School
Dalgas Have 15
DK-2000 Frederiksberg

TORBEN THRANE
Department of English
The Aarhus School of Business
Fuglesangs Alle 4
DK-8210 Aarhus V

TORBEN VESTERGAARD
Department of Languages and
Intercultural Communication
Aalborg University
Kroghstræde 3
DK-9220 Aalborg

CARL VIKNER
Department of Computational
Linguistics
Copenhagen Business School
Dalgas Have 15
DK-2000 Frederiksberg

STEN VIKNER
Department of General and Germanic
Linguistics
University of Stuttgart
Postfach 106037
D-70049 Stuttgart